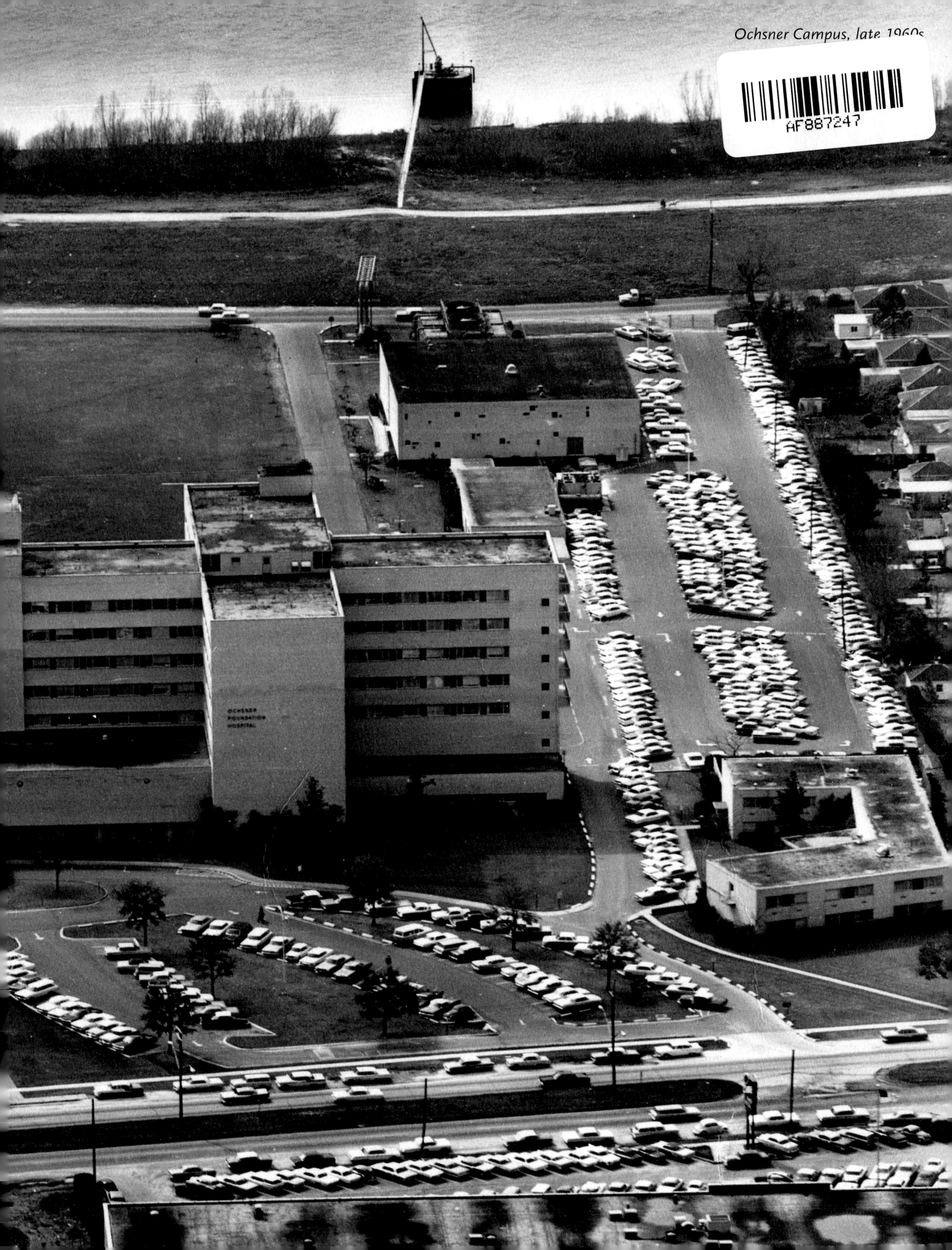

Ochsner Campus, late 1960s

OCHSNER

THE
DONNING COMPANY
PUBLISHERS

The Donning Company Publishers

184 Business Park Drive, Suite 206

Virginia Beach, VA 23462

Steve Mull, General Manager and Project Director

Barbara Buchanan, Office Manager

Anne Burns, Editor

Amanda D. Guilmain, Graphic Designer

Priscilla Odango, Imaging Artist

Tonya Washam, Marketing Specialist

Pamela Engelhard, Marketing Advisor

Cataloging-in-Publication Data

Beck, Bill.

Ochsner / by Bill Beck.

p. cm.

Includes bibliographical references and index.

ISBN 978-1-57864-597-8

1. Ochsner Health System--History. 2. Public health--Louisiana--New Orleans--History. 3. Medical care--Louisiana--New Orleans--History. 4. New Orleans (La.)--Social conditions. I. Title.

RA982.N452O253 2011

362.10976335--dc23

2011038201

Printed in the United States of America at Walsworth Publishing Company

DEDICATION

THIS BOOK IS DEDICATED TO THE GENERATIONS OF PATIENTS AND FAMILIES who have entrusted their healthcare to the professionals at Ochsner and to the tens of thousands of employees who have provided wonderful, personalized and loving care for our patients for 70 years.

DR. ALTON OCHSNER'S CREED

Develop to the utmost one's God-given talents.

Utilize every waking moment to improve one's self, spiritually, educationally, or physically.

Be honest with others and with yourself.

Be loyal. Loyalty is one of the finest of all attributes and it is found so infrequently.

Leisure, although beneficial, is too frequently abused because of the inability to utilize it in a beneficial manner. Such instances cause waste and may result in detrimental excesses, such as alcoholism and boredom. Mental activity delays deterioration of the mind as physical activity prevents muscular atrophy.

Develop and maintain a positive attitude.

Determination and industriousness result in unexpected positive results. Live every moment, minute, hour, and day to the fullest. Strive to make each day better than the previous one. Life is not eternal and every moment is so precious; none should be wasted.

CONTENTS

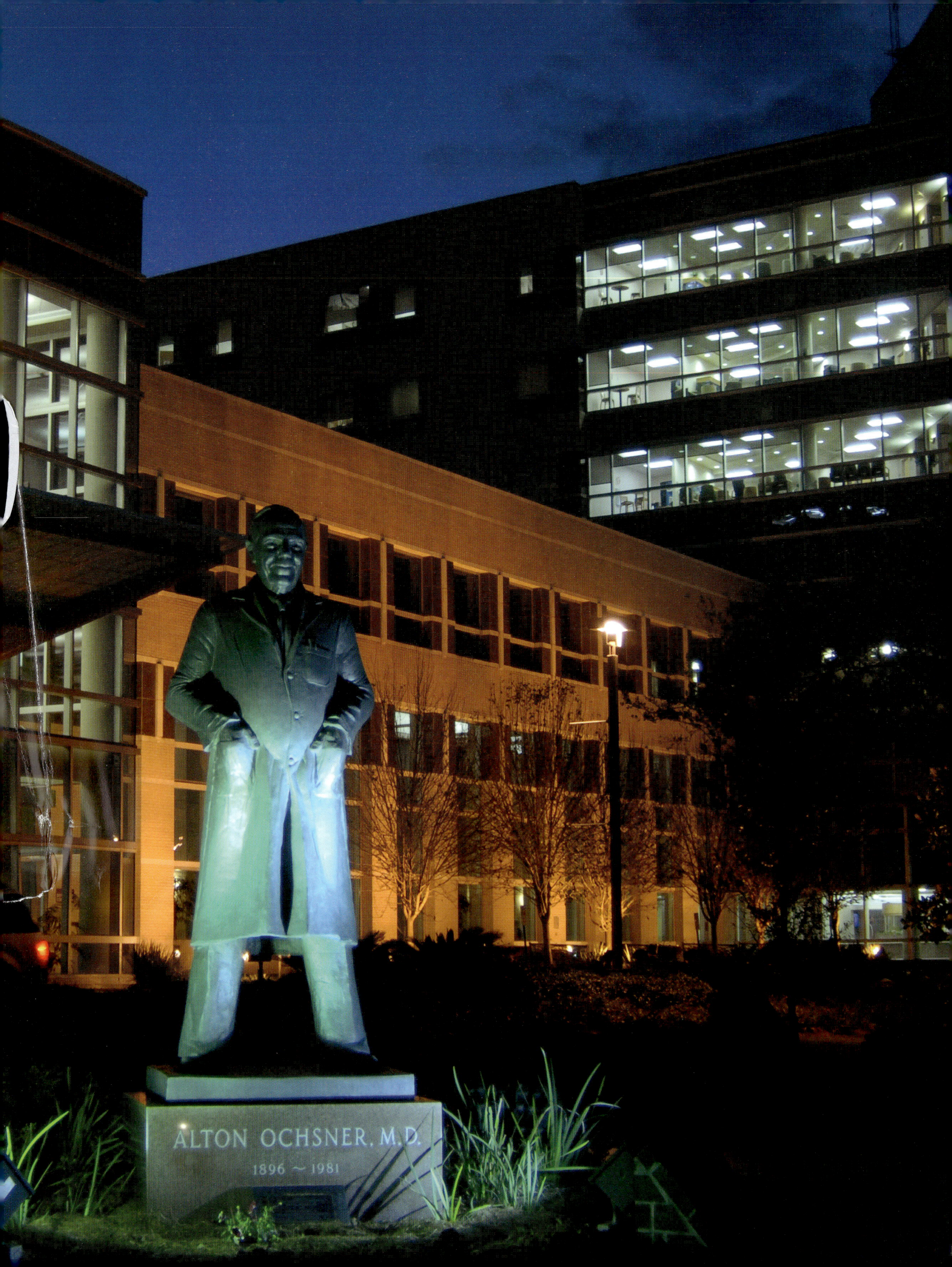
ALTON OCHSNER, M.D.
1896 ~ 1981

FOREWORD

BY FRANK A. RIDDICK JR., M.D., CEO EMERITUS

THIS VOLUME SPANS 70 YEARS OF OCHSNER HEALTH SYSTEM'S HISTORY. It reflects the vision of Alton Ochsner and his fellow founders in creating a center of excellence based on the group practice model where patients would benefit from the coordinated services of superlative physicians. Working together, those physicians could achieve the correct diagnosis and the most appropriate plan to solve the patient's overall health problems applied skillfully in an atmosphere of education and research.

From the beginning, the founders and their successors were challenged and opposed by supporters of the status quo and entrenched interests. The founders' vision led Ochsner's leaders to create a not-for-profit foundation to nurture education and research, to call on advice from community businessmen and to share decision-making with the growing professional staff to create a physician-driven organization, which reflects high ethical standards. Advances in medical science and technology spurred the organization to expand and mature to assure the best and latest care available to its patients and to the developing healthcare delivery system.

The changes in the environment of care and in the expectation of patients saw an evolution of Ochsner from a single site, highly specialized referral tertiary care center to one characterized by the addition of primary care services, community-based population care, decentralization into neighborhoods and later into the region, and the creation of an insurance mechanism, the Ochsner Health Plan, to help with the increasing burden of healthcare costs. The challenges of funding and supporting the satellite system created stresses not easily solved under the structural configuration of separate but allied organizations, Ochsner Clinic and Alton Ochsner Medical Foundation.

The difficulties of having two organizations, the Clinic and the Foundation, with duplication of management and support systems and the pressing need to assure congruence in vision, planning and initiatives to achieve the best outcomes were compounded by the fact that regulations and tax handling of the two often created barriers to an effective conjoined approach. These factors led leadership to the realization that unification into a single organization was essential. After three false starts, this was achieved in 2001.

Over the years, in varied configurations, under different payment mechanisms and in increasingly diverse locales, the nature of care at Ochsner has remained constant—focused on meeting the individualized needs of patients, their families and the community. Healthcare at Ochsner remains physician-directed, based on professional excellence and the latest medical information, in an environment of group practice. The lessons of Katrina show that Ochsner is positioned to continue addressing and meeting the needs of the community, the region and the nation effectively.

ACKNOWLEDGMENTS

BY BILL BECK

TO THOSE WHO HAVE NEVER DONE IT, WRITING A BOOK seems an eminently solitary task. The author wiles away the hours doing research, interviewing people and polishing drafts of the manuscript. His or her efforts are finally rewarded with a picture and short biography on the back end flap of the dust jacket.

Nothing could be further from the truth. Writing books is and always will be a team effort. The writer needs copious amounts of help finding all those research files and scheduling interviews. Someone on the home front provides the peace and quiet necessary to physically spend time at the computer writing. Legions of editors take what is frequently a disjointed jumble of words and turn them into a manuscript suitable for publishing.

Writing is only the first step in the book process. A competent staff in the publishing house keylines the manuscript, combines words and pictures in an attractive layout, proofs the final pages, prints and binds the book and delivers it where it needs to be when it needs to be there.

My list of thanks for all who helped with shepherding this book project from idea to printed page is long and, I hope, complete.

Dr. Patrick Quinlan and Warner Thomas wanted this story told. They graciously gave of their always-limited amount of time to walk me through the last 10 years of Ochsner history and to review the manuscript for errors and omissions.

Dr. Frank Riddick is the living memory of Ochsner and passionate about the institution he has served for nearly a half-century. Someone said that if Ochsner ever erects another statue out front, it will be of Frank Riddick.

Dr. Michael A. Sullivan was equally helpful, sharing his personal knowledge of more than 40 years of Ochsner history. The incomparable Ochsner Medical Library and Archives staff was able to track down every document and file requested, no matter how obscure. The Ochsner Medical Editing staff took a sow's ear of a manuscript and made a silk purse out of it. Along the way, the folks from Ochsner introduced this Hoosier to such New Orleans delicacies as muffalettas, king cake and olive salad.

Ochsner's Marketing staff was a catalyst for this project, coordinating interviews, archival research, in-house revisions and photo selection. The Marketing staff facilitated every part of this project and served as the liaison between Ochsner and The H Agency.

The H Agency was a driving force behind the project, serving as a buffer between the writer and Ochsner. They read every word of the manuscript and moved copy back and forth with aplomb, never losing sight of the end product. The H Agency also designed the layout of the book.

My assistant, Nicole Clegg, learned how to decipher my atrocious handwriting in the process of transcribing hundreds of pages of notes. Steve Mull of the Donning Company makes the publishing part of the book a snap. Steve and I have collaborated on close to a dozen books now, and I thoroughly value his professional approach.

My wife Elizabeth has been part of this book writing process for more than 20 years now. She continues to be my inspiration, and grandbabies Avery and Taggart think she's great, too.

And none of the above should feel the least bit responsible for any of the errors or omissions that have crept into the text. That's where the solitary part comes in. They were all on my watch.

INTRODUCTION

BY PATRICK QUINLAN, M.D., CEO
OCHSNER HEALTH SYSTEM

LATE IN HIS LIFE, DR. ALTON OCHSNER MADE AN OBSERVATION that strikes me as a fitting description for what Ochsner has stood for during the past two-thirds of a century.

Ochsner said doctors frequently concentrate on treating the disease and not the patient. The important thing is to treat the patient. Treating the disease will inevitably follow. It is a simple concept, really, but elegant in its grasp of the end goal modern healthcare should pursue.

Alton Ochsner and the other four founders of Ochsner Clinic set a course in 1942 to establish a multi-specialty private group practice in New Orleans. They faced opposition from the city's medical community and began their venture as the United States embarked upon a great war that would transform American society. Key principles and attributes never changed—they demonstrated courage, conviction and devotion to higher purpose.

The vision of the founders encompassed clinical practice, innovative research, and the education of further generations of physicians and other healthcare professionals. They never lost their focus on the patients and their families. Then, as now, our value is derived from our service to them, as defined by them.

Along the way, the founders and those who followed them wed Ochsner Clinic to the Foundation Hospital and emerged as the largest private not-for-profit healthcare system in the region, with eight hospitals and more than 38 neighborhood health centers. Ochsner stepped up when the community was reeling from the devastation wrought by Hurricane Katrina and invested in New Orleans when few else would; the legacy of courage, conviction and innovation lives on.

This book tells the story of how the legacy of Alton Ochsner and his colleagues continues on in the commitment of Ochsner and its more than 12,000 employees. It is a story that defines the Ochsner vision for the future and pays tribute to those who have laid the groundwork for this generation to carry that vision forward. The best is yet to come. To continue the story, visit ochsner.org/history.

This book has been made possible by generous support from the Othon Henry Ochsner I and Louise Catherine Schlichenmaier Ochsner family.

THE BIOGRAPHIES
OF OTHON HENRY OCHSNER I AND LOUISE CATHERINE SCHLICHENMAIER OCHSNER

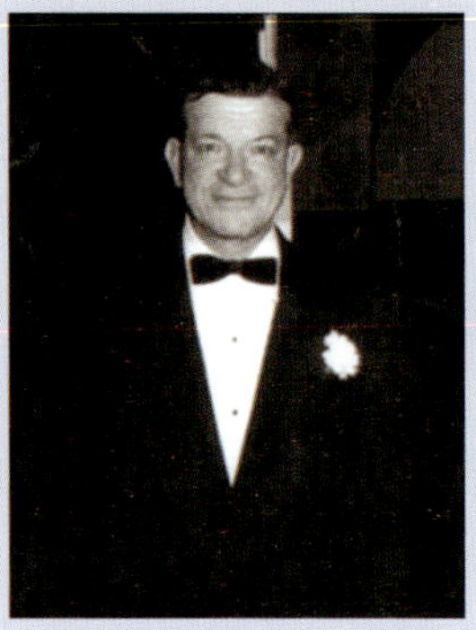

Othon
Chicago, 1950

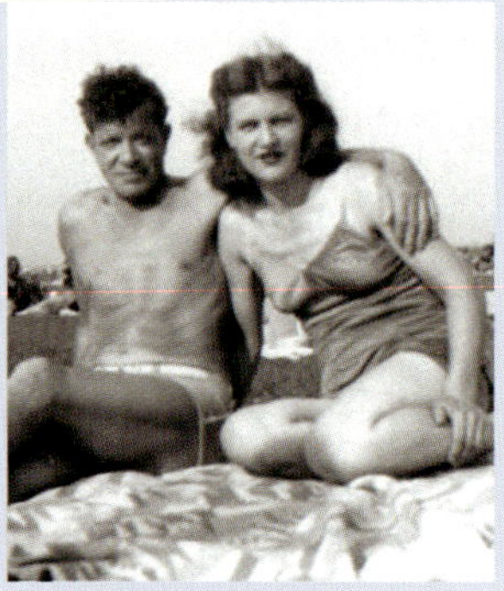

Othon and Louise
Foster Avenue Beach, Chicago, 1947

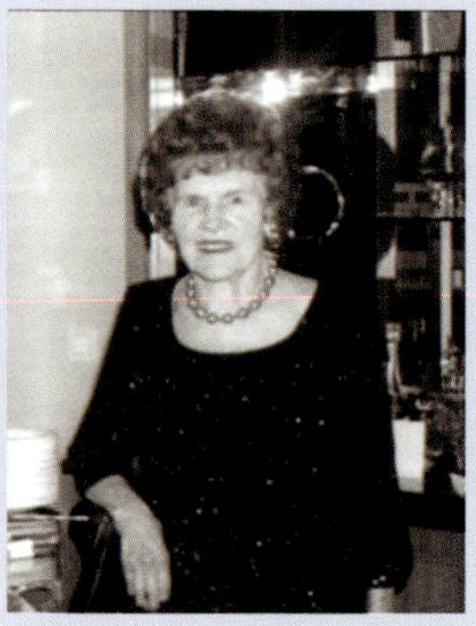

Louise on her 99th Birthday
Peninsula Hotel, Chicago, 2002

OTHON HENRY OCHSNER was born in 1895, the eighth of nine children of Anna and Henry Ochsner. He was born and educated in Oberhallau, Switzerland. In 1912, he moved to Zurich and began racing bicycles. In 1919, he became the Swiss Pursuit Champion. Othon also served his country as a Swiss Cavalry Officer.

In 1922, he emigrated from Switzerland to the United States. He spoke German, French, Italian and English. He worked at the Broadmoor Hotel in Colorado Springs as a Swiss gourmet chef. It was there that he met his future wife, Louise Catherine. During the courtship years, he wrote her beautiful poems. They were married in 1927.

Othon and Louise moved to Chicago and reared four children. He continued his cooking career at the Skyline Club and Biggs Catering Company before retiring from the Saddle and Cycle Club in 1960. He was a very creative and artistic individual who brought his talent to the culinary world, gracing serving tables with beautiful ice carvings and spectacular platings.

As an avid cyclist, he encouraged young cyclists by creating personal training programs and special diets for them to follow. He purchased Swiss racing equipment for his young charges on his numerous trips to Europe. He enjoyed riding his bicycle great distances well into his eighties when failing eyesight and prompting from Louise caused him to reluctantly stop.

In 1969, Othon and Louise co-founded Ochsner & Ochsner Importers and worked from the basement in their home. Their company grew rapidly and more space was required. They imported racing bicycle framesets, components, tires and clothing. Their partnership was incorporated in 1981 as Ochsner International, Inc. and Othon served as President and CEO until the Lord called him home on June 21, 1981.

LOUISE CATHERINE (SCHLICHENMAIER) OCHSNER was born in 1903, the third of eight children of German born Bertha Anna and Jacob Schlichenmaier. She was born and educated in Kansas City, Missouri and moved to Chicago in 1927 after her marriage to Othon Henry Ochsner.

Louise was a full-time wife and mother of four children until 1941 when she felt the call to support her country and worked in a military defense plant. After the war, Louise continued to work until retirement age. In her last position, she worked for thirteen years at the Walgreen corporate offices in the financial department.

Louise traveled the world with her husband and after his death, her travels continued well into her nineties. She traveled extensively within the United States, Mexico, Canada, the Caribbean, Europe, Africa, the Middle East and the Far East. She flew on the Concorde, sailed on the QE2, dined on the SS France and sipped tea on the Orient Express. She was a superb traveling companion through rough seas, tropical storms and a frightening cable car experience near Mt. Fuji. She always remained calm. Louise saw the pyramids along the Nile, visited Macau by rickshaw, viewed the Swiss Alps from a cog-train, observed the French countryside from the TGV, enjoyed Venice from a gondola, was awed by the stained glass windows in the Cologne Cathedral, gazed at the China Sea from a hydrofoil, rode a camel in Egypt, toured the Osaka Castle and saw the Tian Tan Buddha in Hong Kong.

Louise was a kind, deeply religious and inspiring person who taught her children strong moral, ethical and work principles by the way she lived rather than by words and rules. Louise and Othon were members of the Ravenswood Baptist Church and the Forest Glen Baptist Church both in Chicago. The Lord called Louise home on August 26, 2002.

THE
OCHSNER FAMILY
CORPORATE STRUCTURE

OCHSNER INTERNATIONAL, INC.

AUTOMOBILE DIVISION
Licensed Illinois automobile dealer specializing in buying and selling classic and collector motorcars.

BICYCLE DIVISION
We are the exclusive USA importers for the Alfa Romeo bicycles, and the distributor for the Ferrari city, mountain, and children's bicycles. We sell the complete collection of Ochsner bicycles and clothing.

OBERHALLAU WAREHOUSE
The warehouse is available to European, Southeast Asian and South American companies for all their warehousing needs—receiving, storing and shipping.

WINE DIVISION
Specializing in the buying and the selling of Chateau Mouton Rothschild wine. Wine is available for purchase by the bottle, the case or any vertical collection.

OCHSNER COOKBOOK AND MENU DIVISION
We have one of the largest collections of cookbooks and menus written by world class chefs and from famous restaurants.
A limited selection is available for purchase.

CORPORATE OFFICES
246 East Marquardt Drive, Wheeling, Illinois 60090 / 847-465-8200 phone / 847-465-8282 fax / www.ochsnerusa.com / www.ochsnerautos.com

OTHON H. OCHSNER II / oochsner@ochsnerusa.com / Son of Founders / President and CEO

DR. CATHERINE A. OCHSNER JOHNSON / Granddaughter of Founders / Treasurer and Corporate Physician

THE OCHSNER FOUNDATION AND MUSEUM
86 Albrecht Drive, Lake Bluff, Illinois 60044 / 847-615-0466 phone / 847-615-0886 fax

OTHON H. OCHSNER II / Son of Founders / Managing Director of Foundation and Museum

JEFFREY A. PELTZ, JR. / Great-grandson of Founders / Museum Curator

THE OCHSNER FAMILY NON-PROFIT ENTITIES

LOUISE CATHERINE SCHLICHENMAIER AND OTHON HENRY OCHSNER I FAMILY CHARITABLE FOUNDATION
Our mission is to perpetuate the values, interest and kindness of Louise Catherine Schlichenmaier and Othon Henry Ochsner I.

THE OCHSNER ART, AUTOMOBILE AND BICYCLE MUSEUM
Our museum features the works of Salvatore Dali, the celebrity cars of Queen Elizabeth, Howard Hughes, Steve McQueen, President Ronald Reagan, the President of Saudi Arabia and the 19th century Pierce-Arrow racing bicycle and racing tandem and an original Swiss Army bicycle. The museum is available for fundraising events.

THE OCHSNER LIBRARY
Our library was created to preserve world-renowned cookbooks and menus from around the world dating back to the 1800s. A collection of the Ochsner Guide to the Finest Restaurants in the World from 1984 to 1995 is on display in the library. Beginning in 1996, the Ochsner Guide became available online and today it includes hotels. We continually purchase items to add to our collection. The library is open for research by appointment only.

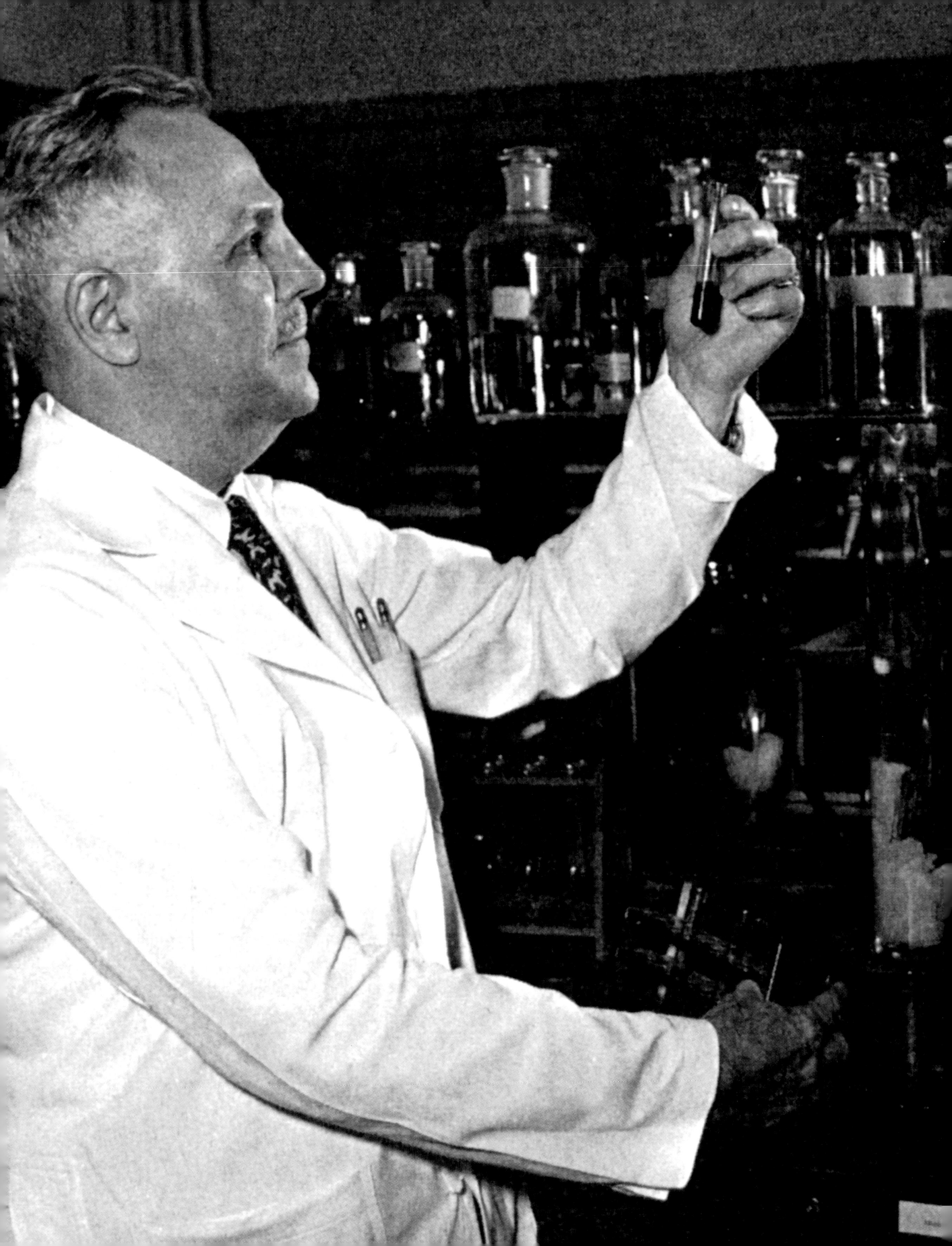

CHAPTER 1:

IN THE BEGINNING

THE DOORS OF OCHSNER CLINIC OPENED in the city's Physicians and Surgeons Building at the corner of Prytania and Aline streets during the first week of January 1942. It was in many ways an inauspicious start. New Orleans, Louisiana, and the nation were gripped with war fever. Elements of the Japanese Navy and Air Force had attacked the U.S. Navy's Pacific Fleet at Pearl Harbor just three weeks before, dragging the United States into a world war that had been raging in Asia and Europe.

The concept of a group practice was new to the Gulf South region and viewed as a threat by many in the medical community. Indeed, the five founders of Ochsner Clinic had been castigated by a number of their peers in New Orleans as Judases. The opposition to the formation of the Clinic went public on Good Friday in 1941 when anonymous detractors left chamois bags with thirty pieces of silver on the porches of each of the five founders.

Despite the opposition, the Clinic's rapid acceptance by residents of New Orleans and the Gulf South region was rooted in the city's proud tradition of medical accomplishments. From the mid-nineteenth century on, New Orleans was a medical center for the entire region, as well as for patients from Central and South America. The city's hospitals and infirmaries were known throughout the South, and Tulane Medical School was renowned for its curriculum and graduates.

Ochsner Clinic's rise to preeminence traced its start to the arrival at Tulane of a young doctor from the North during the waterlogged summer of 1927.

Alton Ochsner would put an indelible stamp on the practice of medicine in New Orleans.

Alton Ochsner was as comfortable in the laboratory as he was in the surgical suite.

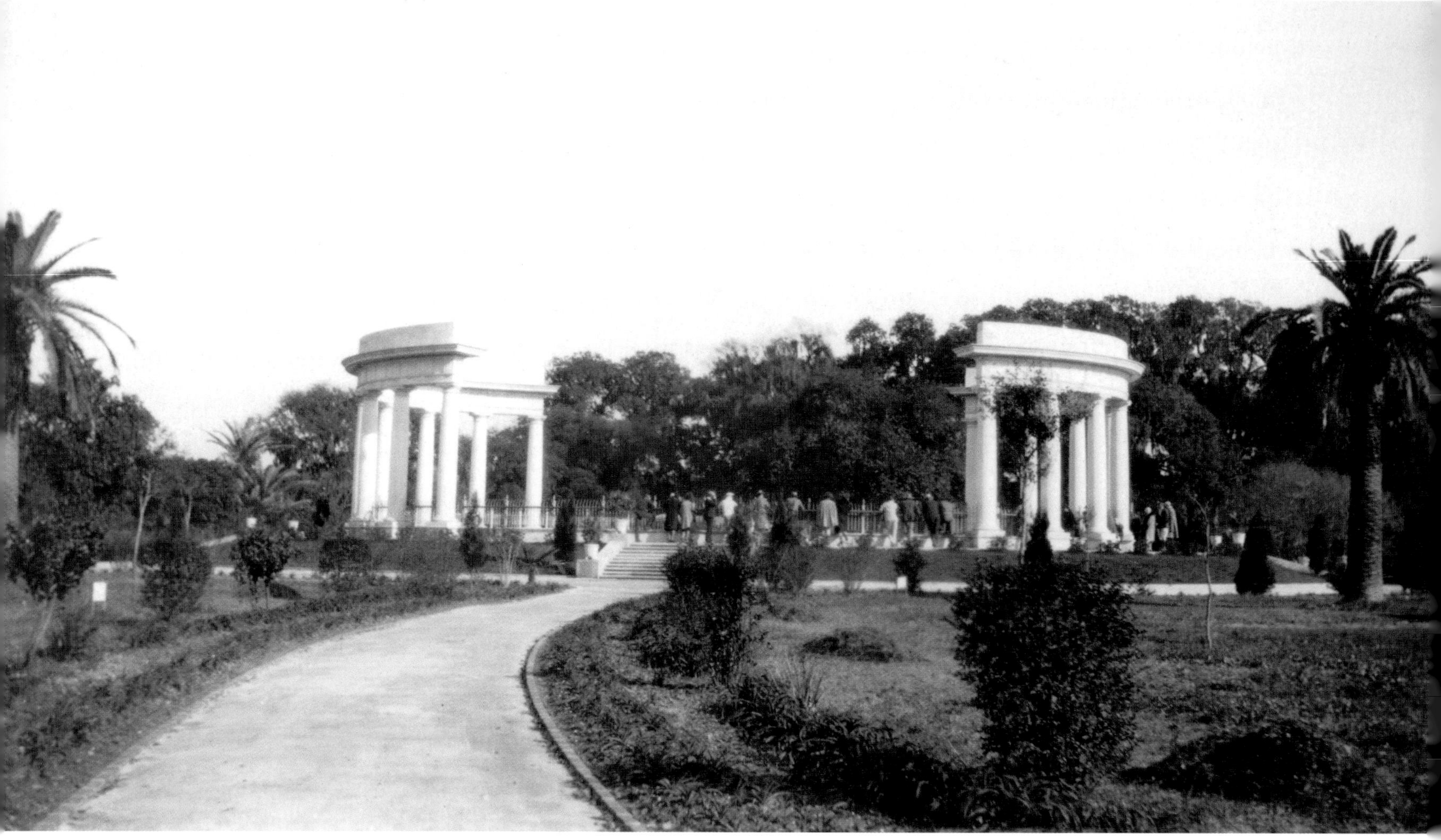

TULANE

Since the end of the Civil War, visitors from as far away as Natchez, Mississippi, and Memphis, Tennessee, had been coming to New Orleans seeking medical care. By the 1920s, the city hosted some of the finest hospitals in the Gulf South. Charity Hospital of New Orleans, which had been serving Louisiana residents for nearly two centuries, was widely considered to be one of the finest hospitals in the nation.

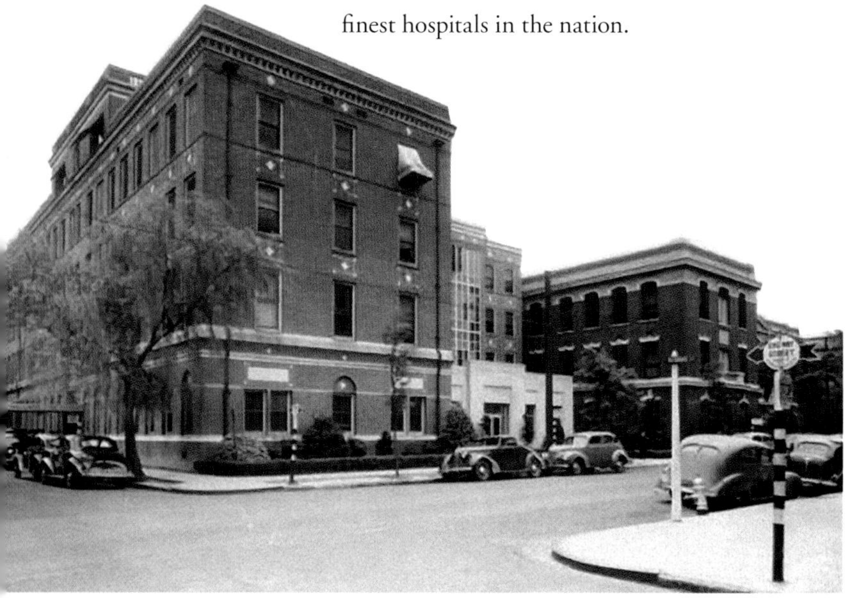

Alton Ochsner and the other Clinic founders practiced at Touro Infirmary during their years on the Tulane faculty. The Historic New Orleans Collection, accession no. 1979.89.7195.

The oldest of the city's colleges, founded in 1834, Tulane was the most influential institution of higher education in the South at the turn of the twentieth century. Both Tulane, which included the H. Sophie Newcomb Memorial College for Girls, and Loyola University were located along St. Charles Avenue, within walking distance of Audubon Park.

Part of Tulane's contribution to New Orleans' reputation as an early twentieth-century medical center was the Medical College of Louisiana (which became Tulane Medical School) and its most famous alumnus, Dr. Rudolph Matas.

Many of the founders lived in Uptown neighborhoods surrounding Audubon Park within walking distance of the Tulane campus. Louisiana Division/City Archives, New Orleans Public Library.

A SURGICAL PIONEER

Matas, a native of the Bonnet Carre area, was one of the most accomplished surgeons in North America. Dr. Will Mayo, one of the founders of the Mayo Clinic, called Matas "the most learned surgeon in the world."[1] The goateed Matas practiced surgery at New Orleans' Charity Hospital, Touro Infirmary and Eye, Ear, Nose and Throat Hospital.[2] For nearly a third of a century, from 1895 until 1926, Matas served as Distinguished Professor of Surgery at Tulane.[3]

His elevation to Emeritus Professor of Surgery at Tulane Medical School occasioned a nationwide search for Matas' successor as full professor. That search ended in Madison, Wisconsin, by way of small-town South Dakota, Chicago and Europe.

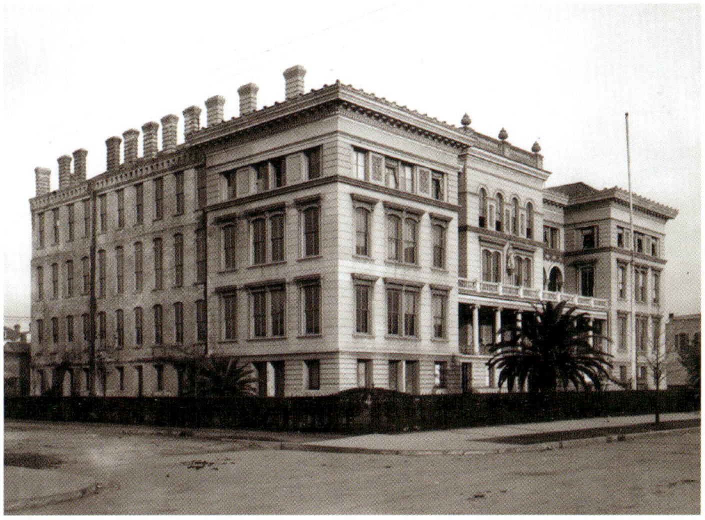

The founders of Ochsner Clinic developed collegial relationships when they taught at Tulane Medical School during the 1920s and 1930s. Louisiana Division/City Archives, New Orleans Public Library.

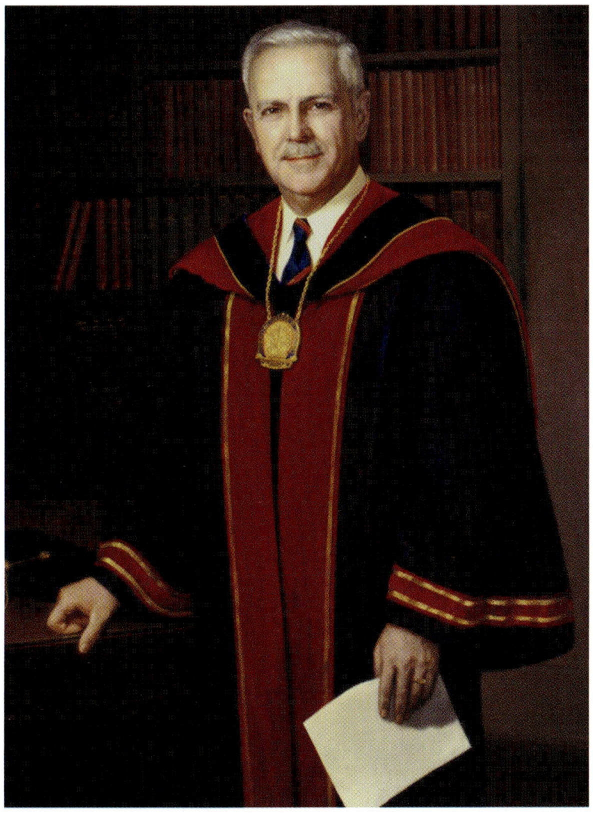

Alton Ochsner in his founder's portrait

A CONTROVERSIAL APPOINTMENT

The selection of Dr. Alton Ochsner to succeed Rudolph Matas at Tulane was initially somewhat of a surprise to the New Orleans medical community. Then 31 years old, Ochsner came to the prestigious professorship at Tulane from the staff of the medical school at the University of Wisconsin in Madison, where he was a junior member of the faculty.[4]

But Ochsner had impressive credentials—and connections—including training in Europe and experience with Dr. A. J. Ochsner, his father's cousin, a renowned Chicago surgeon.

Ochsner interviewed with a panel from the medical school and was convinced that the interview had not gone well,[5] but the young doctor had impressed the interviewers, and during the summer of 1927, Tulane asked him to take the position at a salary of $10,000 a year.

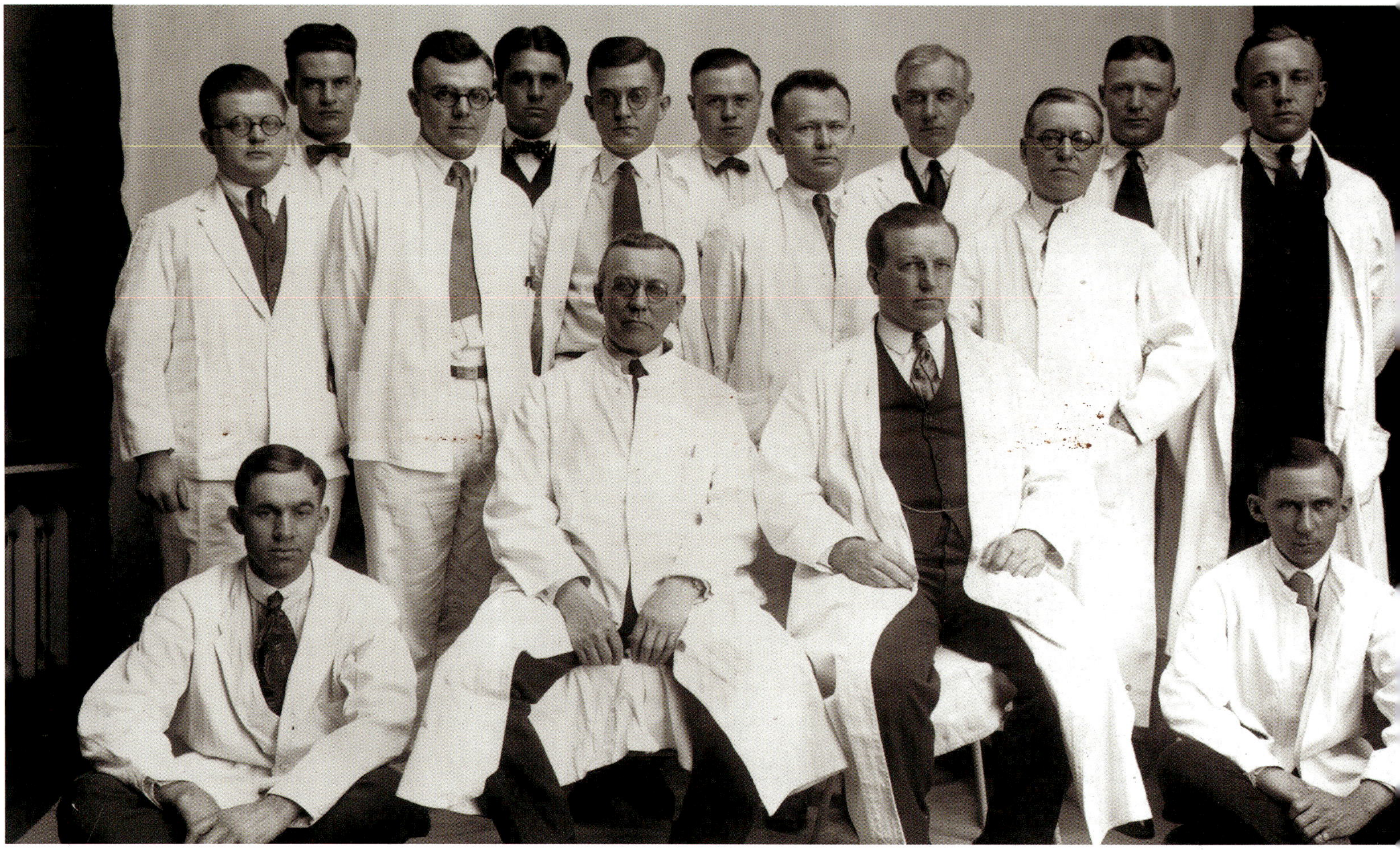

PIONEER YEARS

Born in 1896 in frontier South Dakota, Edward William Alton Ochsner, better known as Alton Ochsner, grew up in the railroad town of Kimball. Ochsner's parents, Edward Phillip and Clara Shontz Ochsner, left Bear Valley, Wisconsin, southwest of the Dells, to homestead in South Dakota in 1881.

Edward Phillip Ochsner, his wife and brother, Benjamin, quickly put down roots in the community. When South Dakota became a state, Edward Phillip Ochsner was elected the first sheriff of Brule County, South Dakota.

Edward Phillip and Clara Ochsner lived in a sod hut on the South Dakota prairie for several years before moving into the nearby town of Kimball, where Edward Phillip and Benjamin Ochsner started a hardware store. After five years, the brothers bought the Kimball Opera House and added a drugstore, grocery and dry goods emporium.[6]

• WHAT OCHSNER MEANS TO ME •

"Ochsner means a lot to me... it's a great place to work, the doctors, the nurses, the community... when you come to Ochsner they take care of you like a FAMILY."

Bobby Brown, Team Leader, Food/Nutrition Catering, Ochsner Medical Center

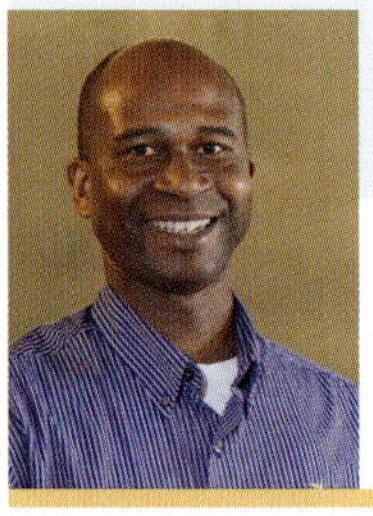

To watch the full interview with Bobby Brown, visit **ochsner.org/history**.

The faculty and staff at Barnes Hospital, the teaching hospital of the School of Medicine of Washington University in St. Louis, during the internship and assistant residency in medicine of Alton Ochsner, pictured standing third from left.

THE FOUNDERS: GUY CALDWELL

The first member of the Tulane faculty that Alton Ochsner confided in regarding a clinical group practice was Dr. Guy Alvin Caldwell. An orthopedic surgeon who had practiced at Shriners Hospital for Crippled Children in Shreveport and Shreveport's Charity Hospital in the 1920s and 1930s, Caldwell came to Tulane as Chairman of the Division of Orthopedics in 1938.

A courtly Mississippian, Caldwell did his undergraduate work and first two years of medical school at the University of Mississippi and then headed east to Columbia University College of Physicians and Surgeons in New York. He did his internship and residency at Presbyterian Hospital in New York.[7] Following this, he booked passage to France where he joined Presbyterian's former Chief of Surgery at the American Red Cross Hospital No. 2 in Paris. Caldwell helped treat French war wounded from 1915 to 1917. When the United States entered the war in the spring of 1917, the medical staff of the Paris hospital was commissioned in the U.S. Army Reserve. Caldwell was named Adjutant of the Hospital.[8]

Following the war, Caldwell mustered out at Fort McPherson, Georgia. While practicing in Atlanta, he made the acquaintance of Dr. Michael Hoke, who had conceived the idea of Shriners Crippled Children's Hospitals. Caldwell moved to Shreveport to become Chief Surgeon at the new Shriners Hospital. He would remain in Shreveport for the next 16 years.

Alton Ochsner hired Caldwell for the vacant chair in Orthopedics in 1938, partly because the mustachioed surgeon shared his enthusiasm for establishing a group practice. Caldwell also had the best head for business management. His essential grasp of medical administration put the Clinic on sound footing in the early years. In the 1940s and 1950s, Caldwell was always heavily involved in the Clinic's fiscal affairs, staff activities and labor relations.[9]

Caldwell was nationally known for his work in Orthopedic organizations. During World War II, he served as a consultant to the Surgeon General of the Army. From 1941 to 1950, Caldwell served multiple terms as Secretary, and later President of the American Board of Orthopedic Surgery. In 1951, he was elected President of the American Academy of Surgeons.[10]

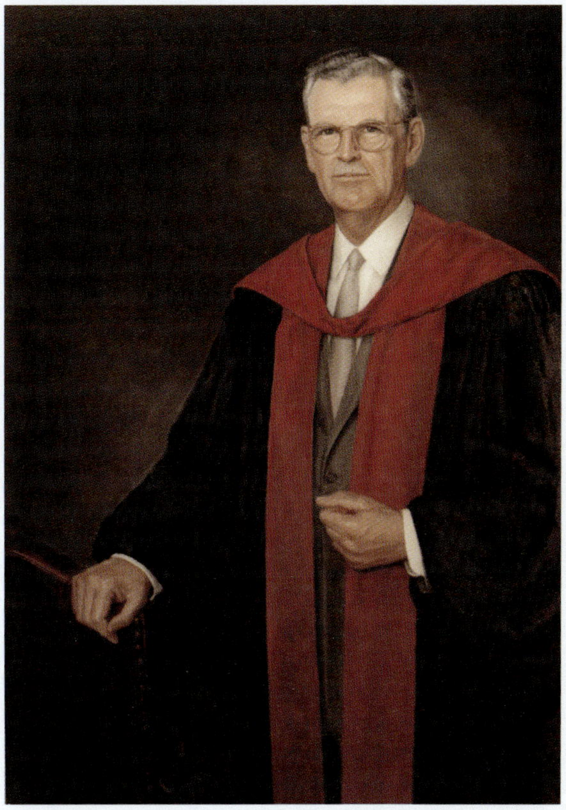

Founder Guy Caldwell, one of the finest Orthopedic Surgeons in the South, was an accomplished writer and authored the first history of the Clinic.

Caldwell served as a director and trustee of the Alton Ochsner Medical Foundation and found time to write a book on the early history of Ochsner Clinic. He was a member of the American Medical Association's Council on Medical Education and Hospitals, Chairman of the Advisory Council on Orthopedic Surgery of the American College of Surgeons, and a trustee of *The Journal of Bone and Joint Surgery*.[11]

Dr. Curtis Tyrone, one of the Clinic founders, paid special tribute to his colleague. Guy Caldwell, he said, "was the glue that held us together."[12]

Guy Caldwell died in New Orleans in November 1981, three months shy of his 91st birthday.

FAMILY LIFE

When Alton Ochsner was born in 1896, he had five older sisters. Two of the girls—Edna Pearl and Elizabeth—had been born in Wisconsin and made the journey as toddlers with their parents via oxcart to Dakota Territory. Four girls were born in South Dakota, Mabel Claire, Genevieve May, Ava Marie (called Mary) and Marguerite; Mabel Claire, born shortly after the family arrived in Dakota Territory, died of diphtheria at the age of four.[13]

Alton Ochsner grew up in rural, turn-of-the-century South Dakota. He had a scientific bent from an early age, inventing a battery-powered egg-candling machine to help with the onerous task of determining which eggs were for the store and which were for the incubator.[14]

By the time he entered school, several of Alton Ochsner's sisters were married. One of his fondest memories from high school was when brother-in-law Fred, Genevieve's husband, took young Ochsner on a deer-hunting trip to the nearby Black Hills.

In school, Ochsner excelled. The only boy in his class of 12 students, Ochsner graduated as valedictorian in 1914. That September, as British, French and German armies dug in along the Marne River, he boarded an eastbound train in Kimball and headed for college.

A. J.

Ochsner enrolled in the pre-medical program at the University of South Dakota at Vermillion, in the southeast corner of the state. A. J. Ochsner, his father's cousin, encouraged Alton Ochsner's interest in medicine. A. J. was the longtime Chief of Surgery at Augustana Hospital in Chicago. Over the years, he made periodic trips to South Dakota to hunt prairie chickens and visit his cousin.

Ochsner worked his way through school at the University of South Dakota. He was awarded a Bachelor of Arts degree in May 1918 and spent that summer as an extern at Augustana Hospital. A. J. insisted Ochsner complete his last two years of medical school at Washington University in St. Louis because he felt it was one of the finest medical schools in North America.

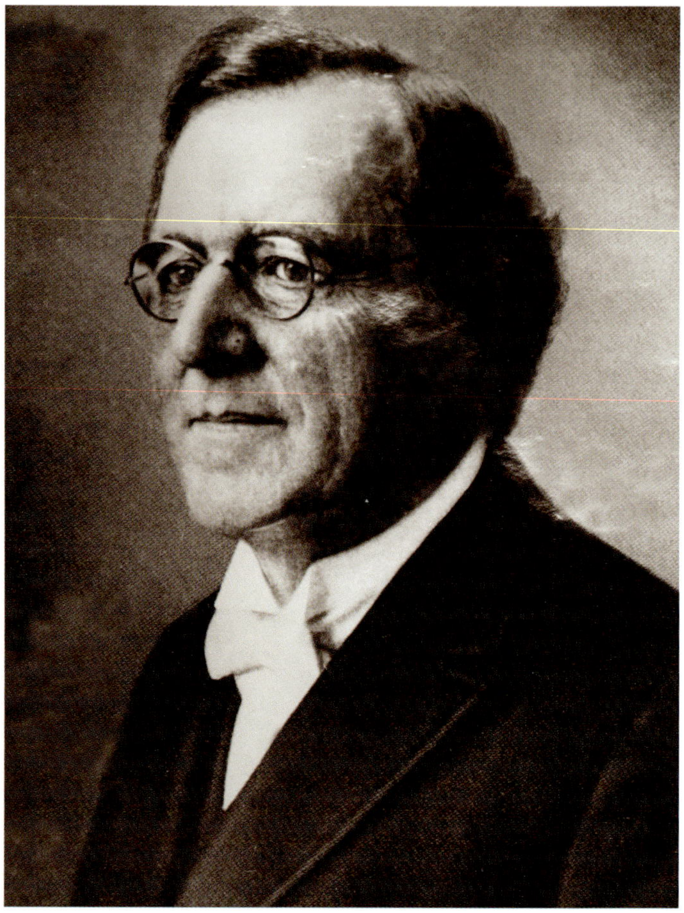

Albert John "A. J." Ochsner, Alton Ochsner's older cousin and mentor, was a renowned surgeon at Augustana Hospital in Chicago.

'HE IS GOING TO KILL ME'

Ochsner and Roy Rudolph, his lifelong friend, enrolled at Washington University during the fall of 1918. The war was still raging in Europe, so both joined the ROTC. The two earned their medical degrees in 1920 and spent the next year in post-graduate training at Barnes Hospital in St. Louis. In 1921, Ochsner moved to Chicago to do a surgical residency under the tutelage of his father's cousin.

A. J. was a hard taskmaster. He expected his cousin's son to get up and go horseback riding with him each morning, even if he had pulled a night shift at the hospital the evening before. When Ochsner protested he was tired, A. J. cut him off. "You are an Ochsner and you can take it," A. J. told him.[15] A. J. "is going to kill me," Ochsner wrote his sister, Mary.[16]

However, there was a purpose to A. J.'s rigorous training. Surgeons prided themselves on being the iron men of early twentieth-century

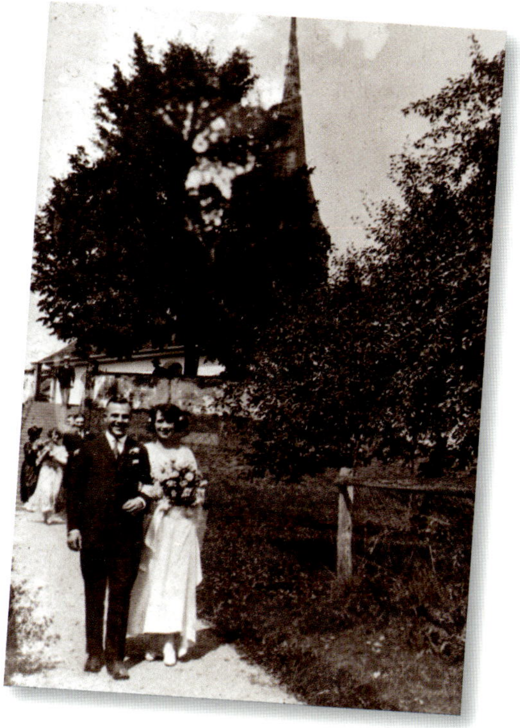

Alton Ochsner and Chicagoan Isabel Lockwood are wed in Zurich, Switzerland, in September 1923.

medicine. The stamina needed to spend hours in the surgical suite, often with little sleep, required physical strength along with intellectual capacity. In later life, younger colleagues often found it difficult to keep pace with Ochsner.

A. J. didn't fail to nurture Ochsner's intellectual advancement either. In 1921, he sent Ochsner to Europe to study under two of the preeminent surgeons in the world and to introduce American intra-operative blood transfusion techniques.

During those two years in Europe, Ochsner married Isabel Kathryn Lockwood. The young couple returned from the continent in 1923. Ochsner set up a surgical practice in Chicago, but his heart was in academia and not in the pure practice of surgery. When the University of Wisconsin in nearby Madison responded with an offer of a professorship in the medical school, Ochsner jumped at the chance.

Ochsner, Isabel and their firstborn, Alton Jr., "Akky," moved to Madison in 1925. "Practically all the faculty were young and enthusiastic," Ochsner recalled years later. "It was a delightful town in which to live, a university town which was beautiful, and we enjoyed it very much."[17] The chance to succeed the legendary Rudolph Matas at Tulane, however, was a once-in-a-lifetime opportunity.

THE FOUNDERS: EDGAR BURNS

By the 1930s, Dr. Edgar Burns was one of the best-known Urologists in the Gulf South region. A native of a small town in northern Alabama, Burns did his undergraduate work at the University of Mississippi and attended medical school at Northwestern University in Evanston, Illinois.

One of the founders of Ochsner Clinic, Burns came to New Orleans during the early 1920s to partner with Dr. Joseph Humes, an early pioneer in Urology in the city. By the late 1930s, Burns, like the other founders, was a department chair at Tulane Medical School. Alton Ochsner and Dr. Guy Caldwell had conceived the idea of a group practice, and the two immediately talked to Dr. Francis LeJeune Sr. and Burns about their interest in joining the practice. It was Burns who suggested bringing in Dr. Curtis Tyrone, the city's most accomplished OB/GYN specialist, as a fifth founding partner.

"Al Ochsner and Guy Caldwell have asked me to join in a group," Burns told Tyrone. "I told them I would consider it, but there is one condition. I won't come unless you also invite Curtis Tyrone."[18]

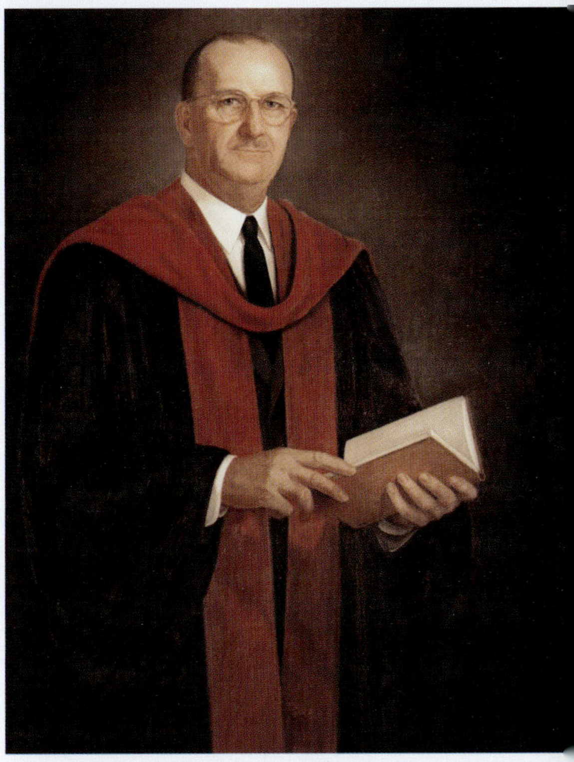

Edgar Burns, a pioneer New Orleans Urologist and a founder of Ochsner Clinic, had one of the strongest work ethics in the city.

Burns served as President of the American Board of Urology, the Clinical Society of Genitourinary Surgeons and the American Urological Society and was a member of the society's Board of Examiners for 15 years. In 1964, he was awarded the American Urological Association's Ramon Guiteras Award. Five years later, the American Association of Gastrourinary Surgeons honored him with the award of the Keyes Gold Medal.[19]

Six feet four inches tall and always impeccably dressed with his trademark bow tie, Burns was an excellent golfer. He was, his daughter recalled, "a wonderful, loving, concerned, all encompassing father."[20]

Burns chaired the committee that put a Clinic succession plan into place. When Dr. Merrill Hines, the Clinic's Medical Director, was injured in an automobile accident, Burns and his committee were responsible for selecting Dr. Frank Riddick as the Clinic's Associate Medical Director, a decision that would stand the Clinic in good stead for many years into the future.

Dr. William Brannan, former head of the Ochsner Urology Department and a Burns hire in 1957, recalled that Burns "was well organized and ran a tight ship. He was a man of great integrity and well respected throughout the United States."[21]

Edgar Burns died in New Orleans of coronary disease at the age of 79 in 1973, just months shy of his announced retirement from his beloved Ochsner Clinic.

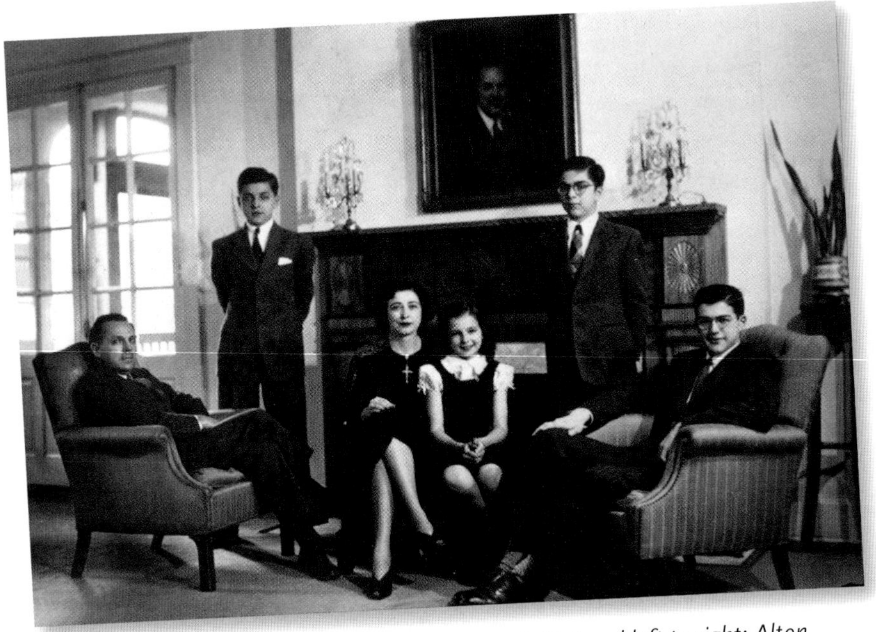

The Ochsner family sits for a portrait, 1940. Pictured left to right: Alton Ochsner, John, wife Isabel, daughter Isabel (Sis), Mims and Alton Jr. (Akky).

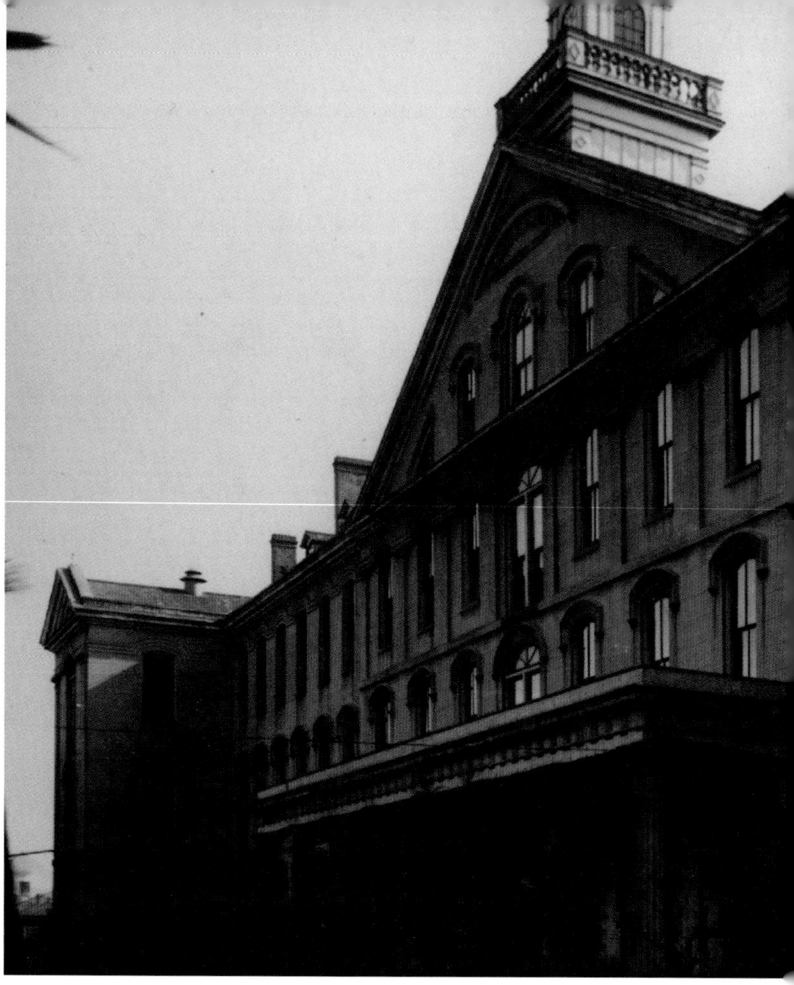

WATERMELON AND SALT

Alton Ochsner arrived at Tulane in the heat and humidity of a New Orleans June. Isabel, who had recently delivered their second son, John, stayed behind with the two boys at the Chicago home of her parents while Ochsner plunged into work at Tulane and found a place for the family to live.

One of his first tasks was appointing an associate professor of surgery. He selected Dr. Mims Gage, "who proved to be the finest friend I ever had, and because of his loyalty he made things very much easier for me."[22] Ochsner soon discovered the wisdom of A. J.'s rigorous training regimen. New Orleans was unbearably hot for someone who had spent recent summers in Wisconsin, and there was no air conditioning. The operating rooms in Charity Hospital had skylights and were almost like hothouses during the summer months.[23]

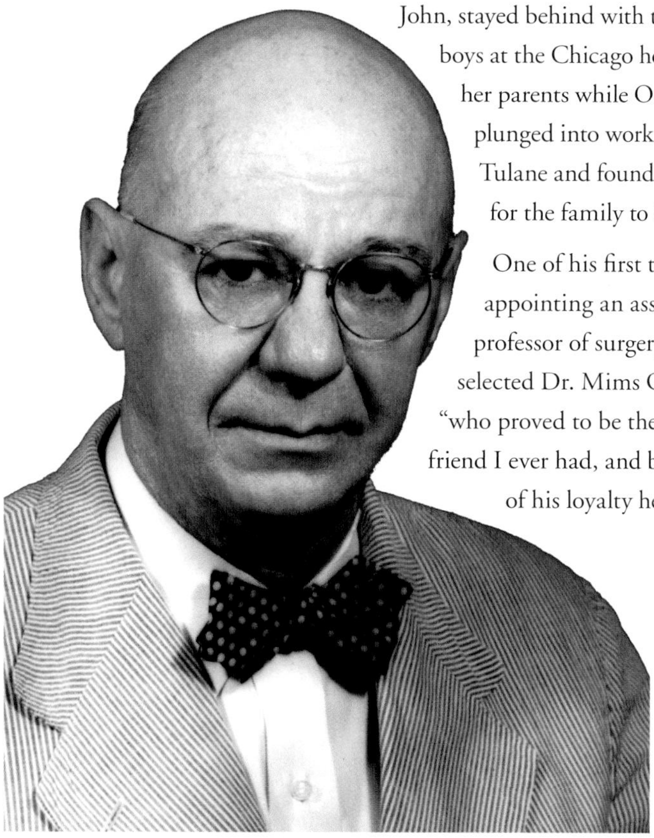

Mims Gage was Alton Ochsner's best friend and an accomplished surgeon in his own right. Ochsner thought so highly of Gage he named his youngest son Mims.

Five or six days after arriving, Ochsner was asked to perform a very rare brain tumor surgery at Charity. The operation lasted six-and-a-half hours, and Ochsner finished in a state of complete exhaustion. He had lost more than 10 pounds, was nauseated and wondered how he could make it through the rest of the day. He and Gage went down to Gluck's Restaurant to have lunch, "and the only thing that I wanted was watermelon with salt on it."[24]

THE BULL PEN

Alton Ochsner was an immediate hit with the Tulane medical students. Just 10 years older than most of them, he could understand their hopes and fears and aspirations. He was always interested in teaching and enjoyed every minute of it. He was convinced that learning medicine from textbooks was obsolete and introduced reading lists from medical periodicals to give students an appreciation of the latest medical advancements being discussed in current literature.

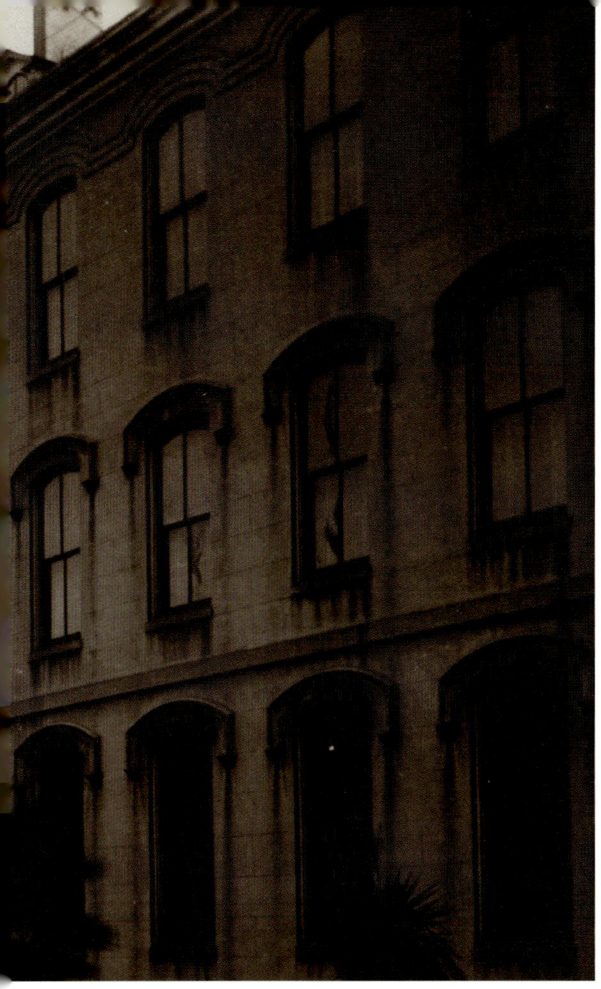

Charity Hospital, a healthcare system unique to New Orleans, was among the city's oldest and most respected healthcare facilities during the 1920s. Louisiana Division/City Archives, New Orleans Public Library.

His most lasting innovation was what he called the "bull pen." Ochsner explained later that the concept "consists of a senior student being given a patient he has not seen before and doesn't know anything about 20 to 30 minutes before the presentation."[25] During that short period of time the senior student took a history and did a physical examination.

"And then he is brought in before his class and the junior class," Ochsner continued, to present the case and make a diagnosis, following which he is quizzed by his classmates and professors. "This is quite a psychic ordeal, performing before all your schoolmates, but is an important part of training because it teaches one to think under stress."[26] The bull pen is still in use at Tulane, a legacy of the era of Alton Ochsner.

THE FOUNDERS: FRANCIS LEJEUNE

Dr. Francis E. "Duke" LeJeune Sr. was the only Louisiana native among the five founders of Ochsner Clinic. Born in Lafourche Parish, LeJeune grew up in Thibodaux, the son of a sugar mill engineer. When he was 11, LeJeune moved to Puerto Rico with his family where his father spent three years as the manager of a sugar property near San Juan.

"That's where Dad learned to speak Spanish," explained his son, Dr. Francis "Duke" LeJeune Jr. "Since the family spoke French at home, he really didn't learn English until he grew up."[27]

The family returned to Thibodaux in time for Francis LeJeune Sr. to attend school at Thibodaux College High School. He earned his Bachelor of Science Degree at Jefferson College in Convent, Louisiana, in 1914 and spent a year in the United States Army before enrolling in the College of Engineering at Tulane.[28] After two years, LeJeune discovered that "calculus was not to his liking," his son explained, and enrolled in Tulane Medical School. "His father told him that if he didn't make it, he'd be going into the sugar mill."[29]

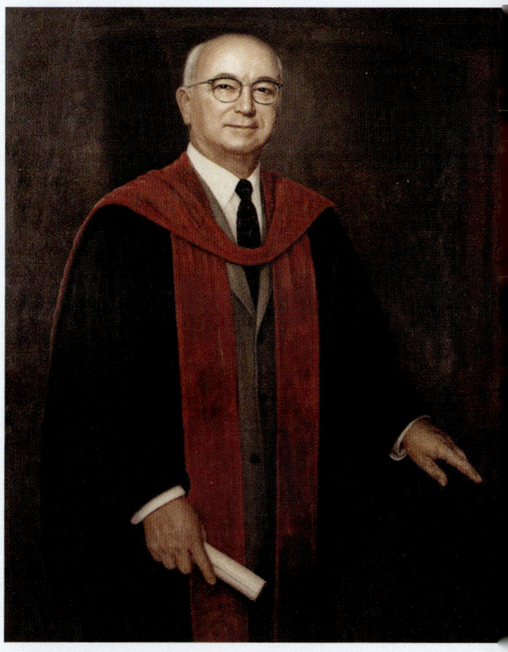

Founder and Otolaryngologist, Francis E. "Duke" LeJeune Sr., the only Louisiana native among the founders.

LeJeune earned his degree from Tulane in 1920, interned at Charity Hospital in 1920–1921 and did his residency the next year at the city's prestigious Eye, Ear, Nose and Throat Hospital. He joined the practice of Dr. Clyde Lynch in 1922 and was in private practice in New Orleans from 1922–1942.[30]

A pioneer in Otolaryngology, LeJeune was a respected professor of Otorhinolaryngology at Tulane in 1941 when Alton Ochsner approached him about joining a proposed group practice. Ochsner had met LeJeune more than a decade before when the ear, nose and throat specialist had performed mastoid surgery on two of Ochsner's sons. "If you don't come in," Ochsner told LeJeune in 1941, "I'll drop the matter."[31]

LeJeune did come in, and his expertise in Otolaryngology quickly gave the new Clinic a cachet of respectability in Louisiana medical circles. LeJeune and Alton Ochsner became the best of friends, as did their wives, Anna Lynne LeJeune and Isabel Ochsner. "Dad and Alton Ochsner loved to go fishing," said Duke LeJeune Jr. "They would go tarpon fishing at the mouth of the river every spring. It was always a treat for us kids to go fishing with Dr. Ochsner, Dad and Mims Gage."[32]

Francis LeJeune Sr. saw the first two patients in Ochsner Clinic in January 1942. His reputation and skill were critical to laying the medical foundations of the Clinic as one of the preeminent healthcare facilities in the Gulf South region. Like the other founders, LeJeune paid a price for his decision to be a part of the first multi-specialty group practice in the South. "Until I went into the Clinic," he once joked, "I didn't have an enemy. Now, I'm an SOB."[33]

The second doctor in history to win all three ENT prizes, including the Casselberry, Newcomb and deRoaldes Awards, LeJeune died in New Orleans in October 1977 at the age of 83.[34]

'IN POLITICS'

Alton Ochsner's appointment to the prestigious post at Tulane Medical School was not universally accepted in the New Orleans medical community. Matas' long tenure as Chair of the Department of Surgery meant that any number of prominent local physicians had waited a generation for the position to open. When Dr. Charles Bass, Dean of Tulane Medical School, replaced Matas with a 31-year-old from out of town, there were plenty of hurt feelings.

During the summer of 1930, the prestigious University of Virginia contacted Ochsner concerning his interest in appointment as Chair of Surgery in the school's medical college. Ochsner could not help but be interested. He wrote a letter to an old friend at Columbia University's College of Physicians and Surgeons informing him of the approach by the University of Virginia, adding that he was growing somewhat tired of New Orleans. Charity Hospital, he said, was embroiled "in politics."[35]

Since nothing came of the University of Virginia approach, the matter should have ended there. However, someone stole a copy of the letter and leaked it to Louisiana Governor Huey Pierce Long.

THE 'KINGFISH'

Huey P. Long, "the Kingfish," dominated Louisiana politics for a generation, first as the state's populist governor and later as a United States Senator. While in the Governor's Mansion in Baton Rouge, he proceeded to expand and nurture Louisiana State University (LSU). Long, who had been refused an honorary degree by Tulane, particularly wanted to establish an LSU Medical School in New Orleans to compete with Tulane.

Alton Ochsner, along with several faculty members at Tulane, felt that an LSU Medical School would be redundant, which earned them the ire of the Governor. Long viewed Ochsner's opposition to LSU Medical School as outright disloyalty. When the letter came into the Governor's possession in 1930, he unilaterally banned Ochsner from practicing at Charity Hospital. "As it turned out, it was the best thing that probably ever happened to me," Ochsner said years later, "because I then concentrated on doing research."[36] Ochsner also took time to develop a private practice, which took off during the years he was banned from Charity. The Tulane board subsidized 10 beds at Touro Infirmary so that Ochsner could continue doing surgery, and he also joined the consulting staff of Illinois Central Railroad Hospital.

The ban lasted two years. When the accreditation committee of the Association of Southern Universities refused to issue LSU the coveted "A" rating, Long personally recruited Dr. Urban Maes as the school's new Chair of Surgery to get the "A" rating for LSU. Maes said he would take the

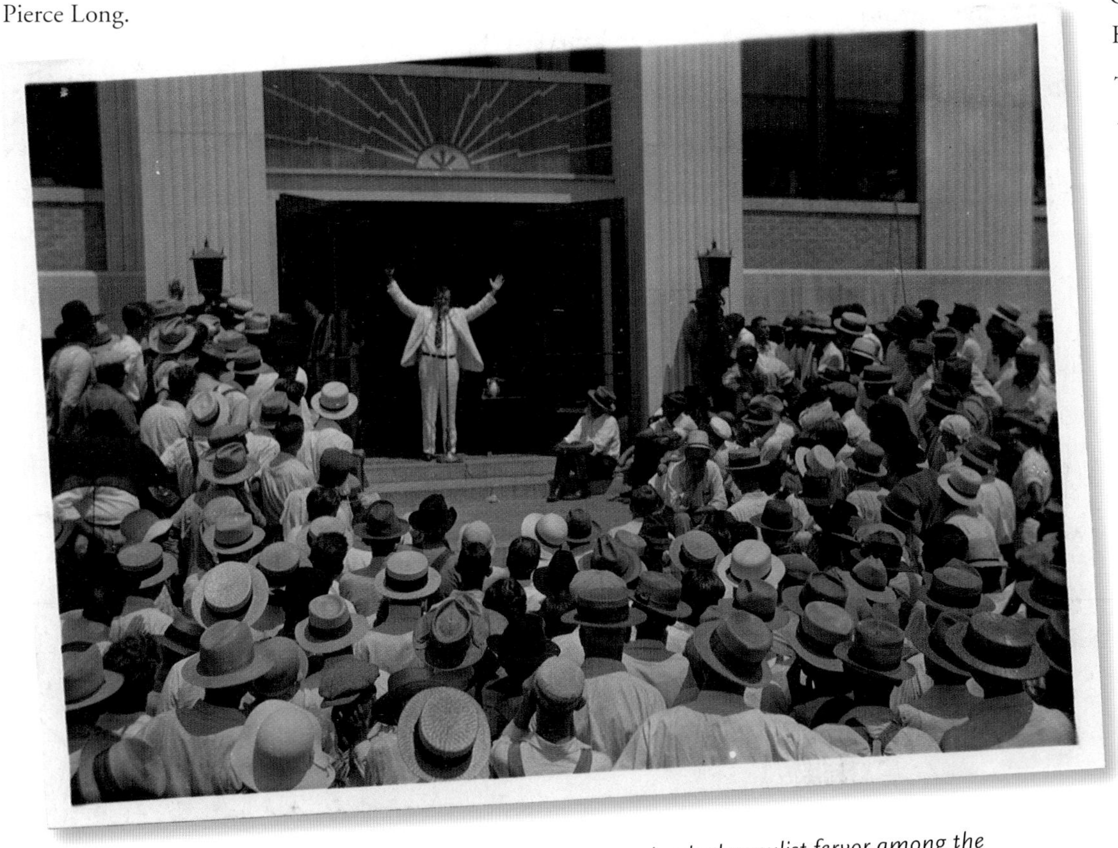

Governor Huey Pierce Long unleashed populist fervor among the Louisiana electorate and dominated state politics during the early 1930s.
Louisiana Division/City Archives, New Orleans Public Library.

job on two conditions: Alton Ochsner would be reinstated at Charity, and Long would pledge to keep politics out of the university and the hospital.[37]

When Long was shot at the state capitol in Baton Rouge in September 1935, the call went out to the best surgeons in the state to attend to the critically wounded Senator. The Long staff called Urban Maes, who was going to bring Dr. James "Jimmy" Rives, his second-in-command. The pair could not reach Baton Rouge in time because of construction on U.S. Highway 61. Ochsner was never called upon to attend the stricken Long. Senator Long died at Baton Rouge's Our Lady of the Lake Hospital in the early morning hours of September 10, 1935.[38]

The death of Huey Long laid to final rest the imbroglio between Tulane and LSU that involved Alton Ochsner. Tulane's Chair of Surgery went on to describe in the late 1930s the connection between cigarette smoking and lung cancer, a discovery that would establish Ochsner's reputation as a first-rate medical researcher.[39] By that time, Ochsner and a number of his Tulane colleagues were also discussing a radical new approach to the practice of medicine in New Orleans.

THE FOUNDERS: CURTIS TYRONE

Dr. Curtis Tyrone was the last of the founders of Ochsner Clinic to be brought aboard the fledgling organization. Edgar Burns told the other founders that he wouldn't join the Clinic unless they extended an invitation to Tyrone.

One of the best-known OB/GYN specialists in the Mid-South at the time, Tyrone was also the youngest of the five founders. At the age of 27, he had been hired as an instructor of Clinical Obstetrics at Tulane in 1925.[40]

A native of rural Mississippi, Tyrone grew up poor and intended to be a history professor when he got the chance to attend Mississippi College. Instead, he graduated from Tulane Medical School and interned at Touro Infirmary.[41] Following his internship, Tyrone joined the well-established practice of Dr. Charles Jefferson Miller. When Miller died suddenly in 1936, Tyrone inherited the practice.

Tyrone's charm and outgoing personality endeared him to his patients, who made him New Orleans' most popular Obstetrician and Gynecologist in a community where word of mouth was everything when it came to physicians' references. When Tyrone agreed to join the Clinic staff as a founder in 1941, he brought with him what was one of the city's most lucrative practices.

"Dr. Tyrone used to say that the best referrals did not come from other physicians but from happy, satisfied female patients who were members of the bridge clubs," explained Dr. George T. Schneider, whom Tyrone hired at Ochsner in 1949.[42] In the more than 40 years he practiced medicine in New Orleans, Tyrone delivered thousands of babies.

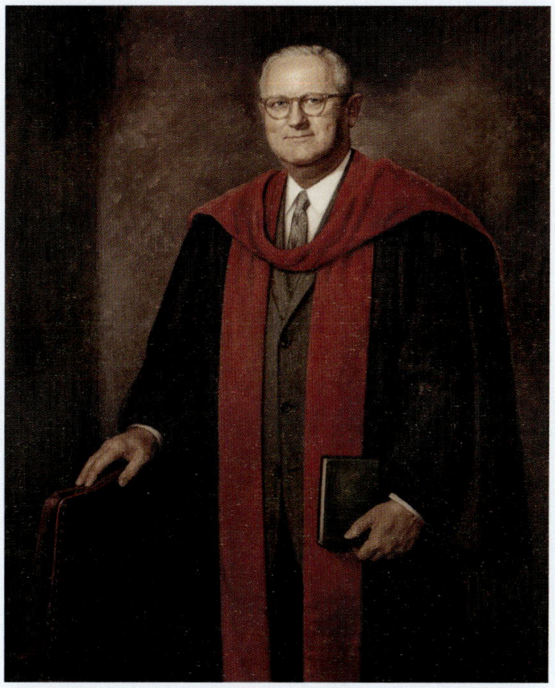

Curtis Tyrone, the energetic Gynecologist who became the fifth founder of Ochsner Clinic.

In later years, Tyrone took great pride in pointing out the young ladies he had delivered who served as that year's queen or maids at the many Mardi Gras balls.[43]

Tyrone was never as involved in medical societies as were his founder colleagues. "I'm no orator," he frequently told associates.[44] Instead, his passion was work. Tyrone frequently worked nights, and his work ethic more than once caused him to make threats to pull his practice out of the Clinic. He told colleagues before his death that he never regretted being a part of the growth of the Clinic and its reputation.

One surgeon who knew him described a Tyrone operation almost the way one would write a review of a play, calling the operation "a symphony, an artistic as well as an effective performance."[45]

Curtis Tyrone died in New Orleans in July 1982 at the age of 84.

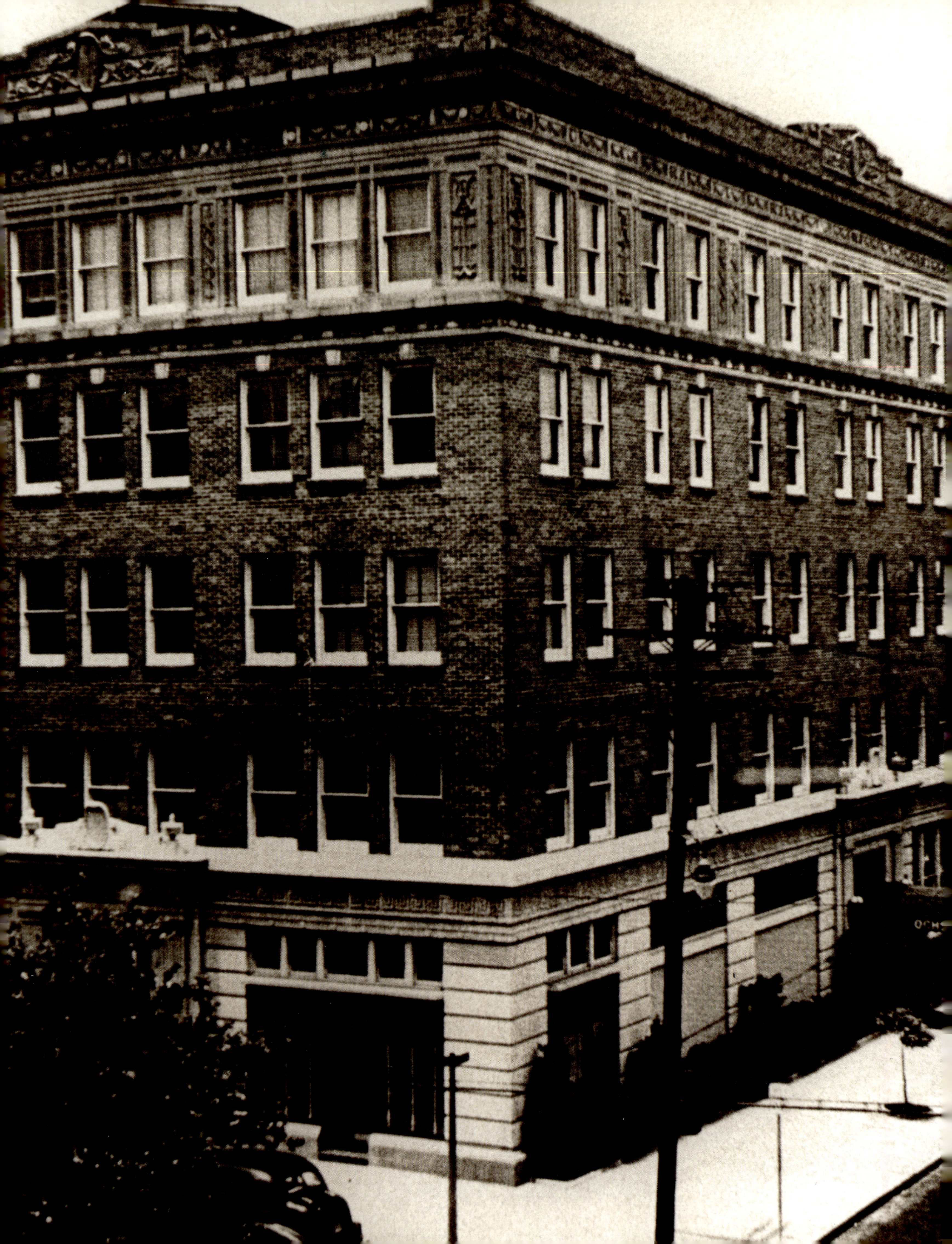

CHAPTER 2:

THE FOUNDING FATHERS

ALMOST FROM THE TIME HE ARRIVED IN NEW ORLEANS, Alton Ochsner dreamed of creating a new model for medical practice in the Gulf South region. Ochsner, who met Drs. Will and Charles Mayo through his father's cousin, A. J. Ochsner, admired the private, not-for-profit group practice that the Minnesota brothers established in the southern Minnesota community of Rochester. He would have been in total agreement with the Dutch surgeon who called the Mayo Clinic "a work of art, science and social service more complete than any other institution modern medical science has produced."[1]

Sometime during the late 1930s, Ochsner began talking with his colleagues about the possibility of establishing an integrated group practice in New Orleans. In January 1942, Ochsner Clinic opened in the Physicians and Surgeons Building at the corner of Prytania and Aline streets. Even though America had been thrust into World War II three weeks before, the Clinic was a success from the start. Ochsner Clinic was so successful, in fact, the partners inaugurated the postwar era in New Orleans by forming a not-for-profit foundation and establishing a hospital at an inactive U.S. Army post in Jefferson Parish.

LOSING ITS REPUTATION

Since arriving in New Orleans in 1927, Alton Ochsner recognized the fact that the city had long been a great medical center, drawing in talent and patients from across the area. By the late 1930s, however, Ochsner and some of his colleagues from Tulane Medical School felt that "New Orleans was beginning to lose this reputation, because good medicine was being practiced in other cities as well."[2]

The first Ochsner Clinic at the corner of Aline and Prytania streets in Uptown New Orleans was in the heart of the city's medical district.

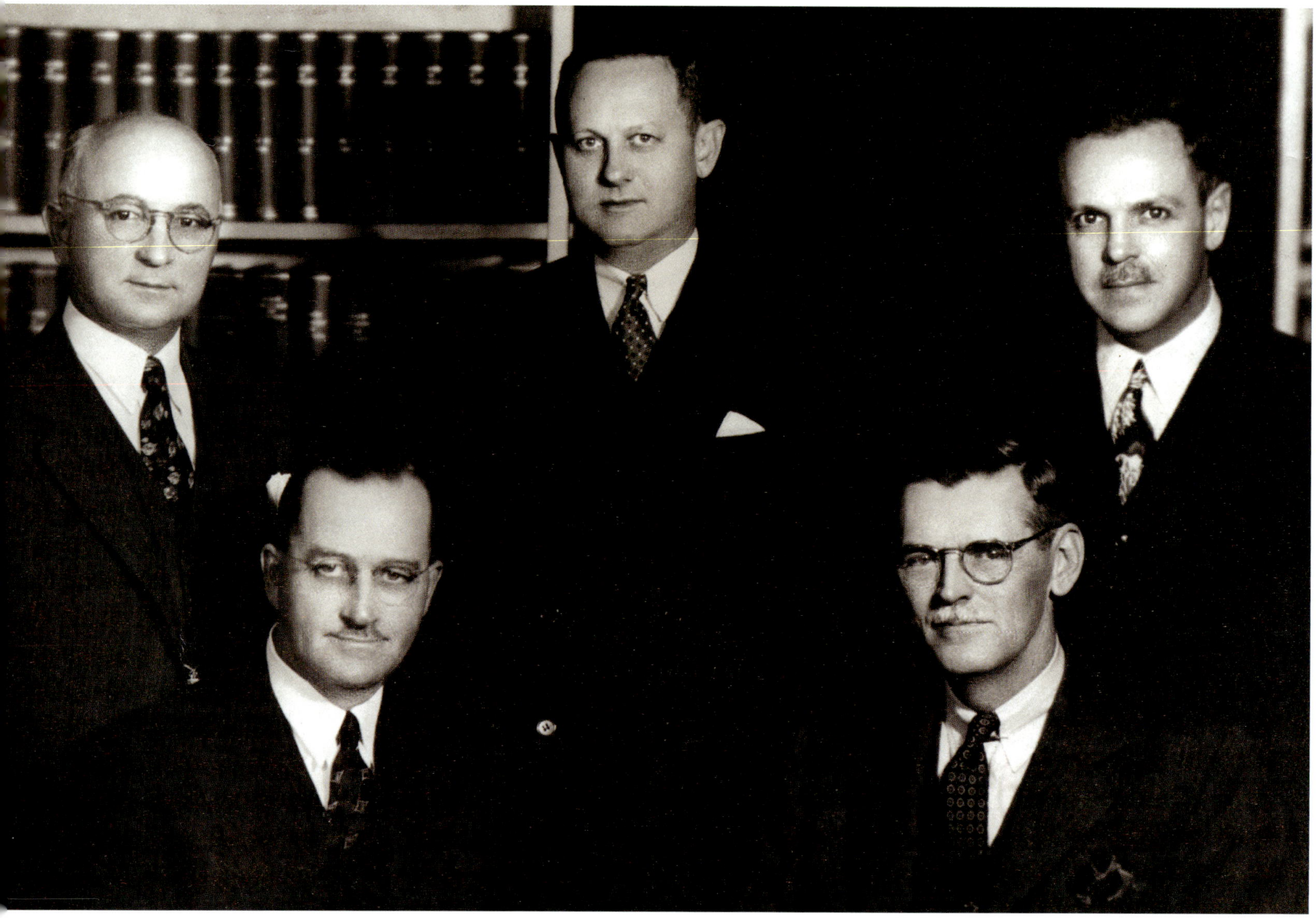

Ochsner did what he could to turn this perception around. As Chair of Tulane's Surgery Department, Ochsner recruited a number of top-flight doctors for the Green Wave faculty, including Guy Caldwell, who moved to New Orleans from Shreveport to take over the Division of Orthopedics at Tulane Medical School.[3]

Ochsner suspected the Tulane administration was responsible for the perceived malaise he saw in the local medical community. The university recoiled from the battles with Huey Long over establishment of LSU Medical School in New Orleans, and as a consequence, administrators were reluctant to take a strong leadership role in the community.

Ochsner felt the problem was most acute in the refusal of Charity Hospital, Tulane's teaching arm, to admit private patients. "I felt the private patients, at least those with difficult diagnostic problems, were not getting the proper care, such as was possible in university hospitals and in organized clinics," he said.[4]

A TULANE CLINIC

Ochsner wanted Tulane to sponsor a clinic, modeled on successful clinics already in existence, including the Mayo Clinic in Minnesota, the Cleveland Clinic and the Lahey Clinic in Boston. During the late 1930s, Ochsner approached the Board of Trustees at Tulane Medical School with his idea. The board considered it and reluctantly told the Chair of the Department of Surgery that the medical school wasn't ready to take such an ambitious step at the time.

Ochsner went back to Tulane's Board of Administration and received approval to start a clinic, provided Ochsner and any members of the medical school faculty agreed to remain at Tulane.[5] In short order, Ochsner and Guy Caldwell approached physicians Edgar Burns, Duke LeJeune Sr. and Curtis Tyrone about joining the proposed group practice. All agreed the idea was sound.

The five founders, seen here in the spring of 1941, felt so strongly about opening the first private group practice clinic in New Orleans that they each contributed $4,300 to the effort, a small fortune at the time. Seated left to right are Edgar Burns and Guy A. Caldwell. Standing left to right are Francis E. LeJeune Sr., Curtis Tyrone and Alton Ochsner.

Getting approval from the Tulane Board of Administration to start the Clinic was one thing. Finding the financing that would make the Clinic a reality was another.

In the tight money economy of 1940, Ochsner estimated that financing the new venture would require an investment upwards of $150,000. The partners made the rounds of New Orleans banks, and most, although not dismissing the idea out of hand, were unwilling at the time to advance the money needed to start the Clinic and see it through its first year of operations.[6]

Duke LeJeune Sr. discussed the project's financial needs with Hibernia National Bank President A. P. Imahorn, who expressed interest in helping the doctors get the Clinic off the ground. At about the same time, Caldwell was treating Mrs. Rudolph Hecht, the wife of Hibernia's chairman, and had the chance to discuss the project and its financing needs with the Hibernia executive.[7]

Caldwell arranged a luncheon meeting for Hecht and Ochsner, and the banker told Ochsner the only collateral he needed was his name. With Hecht and Imahorn backing the venture, Hibernia's Board of Directors approved a line of credit for the Clinic.

• WHAT OCHSNER MEANS TO ME •

"I'm proud to work at Ochsner. Even though we have several different community hospitals, everyone works together as one TEAM. We share the same commitment. We focus on the patient, on how to improve patient satisfaction and, most of all, on improving the quality of care."

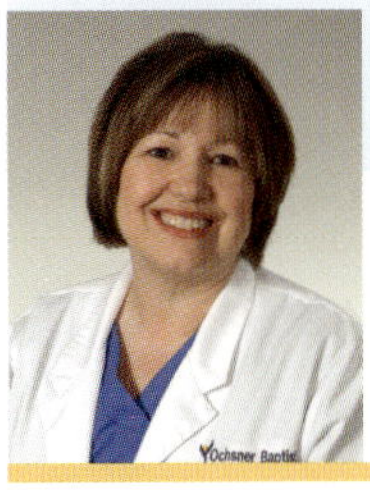

JoAnn Cardaro, Unit Director of the Med Surg Unit and ICU, Ochsner Baptist Medical Center

To watch the full interview with JoAnn Cardaro, visit **ochsner.org/history**.

THIRTY PIECES OF SILVER

Catherine Burns Tremaine recalled the April night in 1941 that her family arrived home from dinner at New Orleans Country Club. Then a teenager, she remembered that the family home in the Garden District was an old Greek Revival house with a wraparound front porch. A shelf and a mailbox hid behind the shutter to the right of the front door. Her father, Dr. Edgar Burns, noticed that the shutter was ajar and retrieved a chamois bag that contained thirty dimes.[8]

Inside the bag, a typewritten note said simply: "To help pay for your clinic. From the Physicians, Surgeons and Dentists of New Orleans."[9] Each of the five founders received a similar bag of dimes.

The reference to the thirty pieces of silver that the Roman authorities paid Judas Iscariot to betray Jesus Christ was hardly lost on Burns and the other four founders of the Clinic, given that predominantly Catholic New Orleans was getting ready to celebrate Easter in two days, after the bags were delivered on Good Friday.

"There was great polarization in the medical community" about the Clinic, explained Francis "Duke" LeJeune Jr.[10] The thirty dimes had arrived at the LeJeune home via Western Union courier fairly late that evening as the LeJeune family prepared for bed. At first, LeJeune recalled, his father thought the thirty dimes a touching gesture of support until he realized that it was anything but.[11]

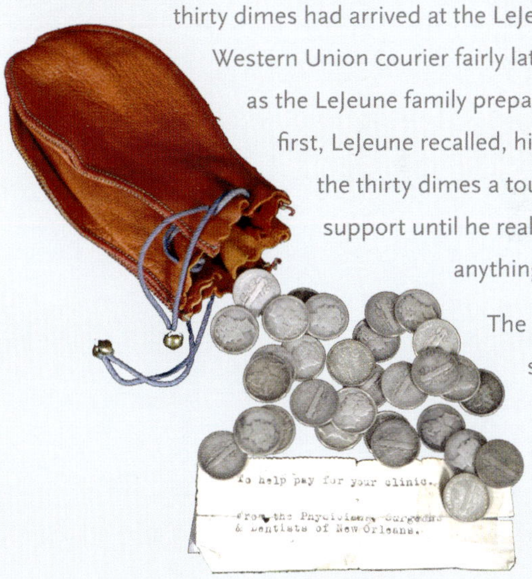

The 30 pieces of silver, a small leather bag with 30 dimes in it, that each founder received during Easter Week, 1941.

The thirty pieces of silver became part of Ochsner Clinic legend. The five founders had a pretty good idea of those behind the sophomoric prank, and LeJeune claims his father told him years later who the perpetrators were.[12]

The veiled threats never deterred Ochsner and the other founders from going ahead with establishing a group practice. "The joke in our house was that Alton Ochsner went out and spent the thirty dimes on lunch the next day," LeJeune said.[13]

THE PHYSICIANS AND SURGEONS BUILDING

With the loan in hand, Ochsner and his partners approached Stanley Lemarie of the New Orleans commercial real estate firm of Leo Fellman and Company to find property in the upscale residential neighborhood anchored by St. Charles Avenue. The partners hoped to build a two- or three-story building in the vicinity of Touro Infirmary with its 300 beds.

Lemarie quickly reported back that the partners could purchase the five-story Physicians and Surgeons Building at the corner of Aline and Prytania streets. The building's tenants included 25 physicians and a ground-floor drugstore. Immediately across Prytania Street was Touro Infirmary. The well-known New Orleans Medical Arts Building was just a half-block away.

The partners' bid to purchase the Prytania Street property brought the proposed Clinic into the public spotlight. City regulations required approval of 70 percent of the property owners in the area, and Ochsner and his partners had petitions signed by more than that number of local residents. A reporter from the *States-Item* dubbed the plan the "Little Mayo Clinic."[14] The New Orleans Clinic would do its best to live up to its initial reputation.

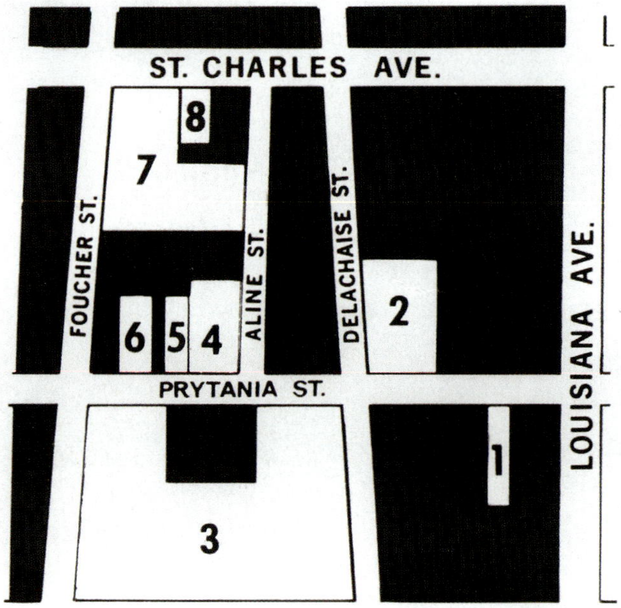

1. Caldwell Building. 2. Medical Arts Building. 3. Touro Infirmary. 4. Original Ochsner Clinic. 5. Research and Clinic Administration Building. 6. Matas Building. 7. Clinic Parking Lot. 8. Georgetown House (old Briede home).

A map of the Clinic area.

'NAMED FOR PAPA'

Approval of the plans from the Commission Council followed rapidly, and the partners spent much of the spring of 1941 working with attorney J. Blanc Monroe in drawing up articles of incorporation and a partnership agreement. The son of a former Louisiana Supreme Court Chief Justice, Monroe was a principal in the New Orleans firm of Monroe & Lemann and counsel for the banks, railroads and shipping companies that served as pillars of New Orleans commerce.[15]

Monroe immediately advised the partners that the first thing they needed to do was to come up with a name. Throughout 1940, the partners informally discussed a name but never came to a decision. Finally, in March 1941, Caldwell, Burns, LeJeune and Tyrone made a unilateral decision. They elected to call the new venture "Ochsner Clinic," in honor of the man who had recruited them.

Alton Ochsner was at a conference in Ogden, Utah, when he received a telegram from his partners on March 27. "Junior was born tonight and named for Papa," Duke LeJeune Sr. informed Alton Ochsner, the new President of Ochsner Clinic.[16]

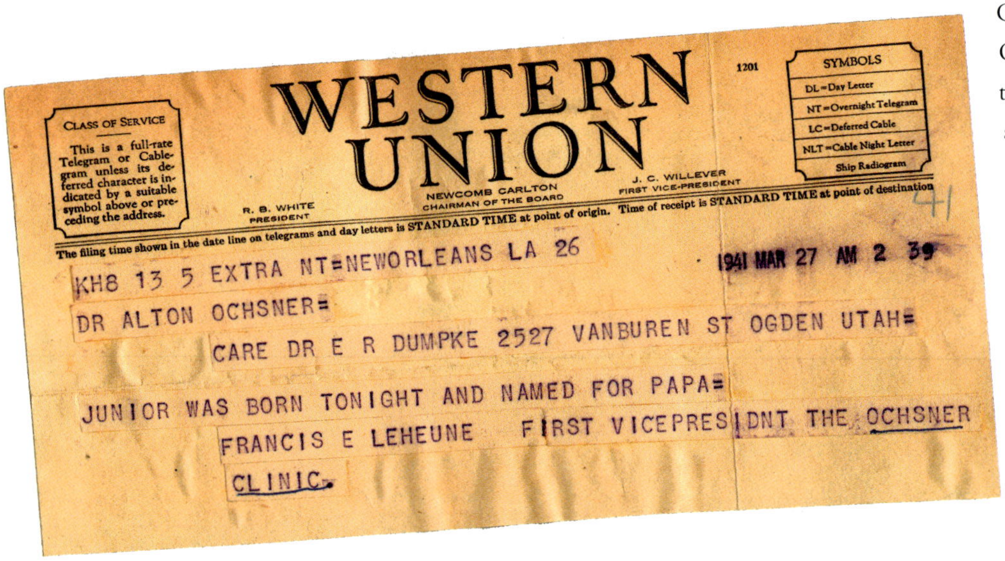
WESTERN UNION

CLASS OF SERVICE — This is a full-rate Telegram or Cablegram unless its deferred character is indicated by a suitable symbol above or preceding the address.

R. B. WHITE, PRESIDENT — NEWCOMB CARLTON, CHAIRMAN OF THE BOARD — J. C. WILLEVER, FIRST VICE-PRESIDENT

1201

SYMBOLS: DL=Day Letter; NT=Overnight Telegram; LC=Deferred Cable; NLT=Cable Night Letter; Ship Radiogram

The filing time shown in the date line on telegrams and day letters is STANDARD TIME at point of origin. Time of receipt is STANDARD TIME at point of destination

KH8 13 5 EXTRA NT=NEWORLEANS LA 26 1941 MAR 27 AM 2 39

DR ALTON OCHSNER=

CARE DR E R DUMPKE 2527 VANBUREN ST OGDEN UTAH=

JUNIOR WAS BORN TONIGHT AND NAMED FOR PAPA=

FRANCIS E LEHEUNE FIRST VICEPRESIDNT THE OCHSNER CLINIC.

The "named for papa" telegram informed Alton Ochsner that his partners had selected the name Ochsner Clinic for their new private group practice.

BUILDING A STAFF

With all of the incorporation papers filed, the five partners moved ahead to tap the bank line of credit. They each pledged $4,300 and borrowed more than $80,000 from Hibernia National Bank to meet the $101,000 purchase price for the property on Prytania Street.

Once that was accomplished, the partners proceeded to assemble a top notch staff. Junius Underwood was the first hire as the Clinic's office manager. Underwood, who worked for a local agency that collected debts for physicians, began outfitting the Clinic's offices and hiring office staff. Early employees included Enid Cary, Sidney Broussard and Josephine Thomann. Selma DeBakey, Dr. Michael DeBakey's sister, was the Clinic's first medical editor, and Julie Carnahan and Mary Heroy were the first two nurses hired.[17]

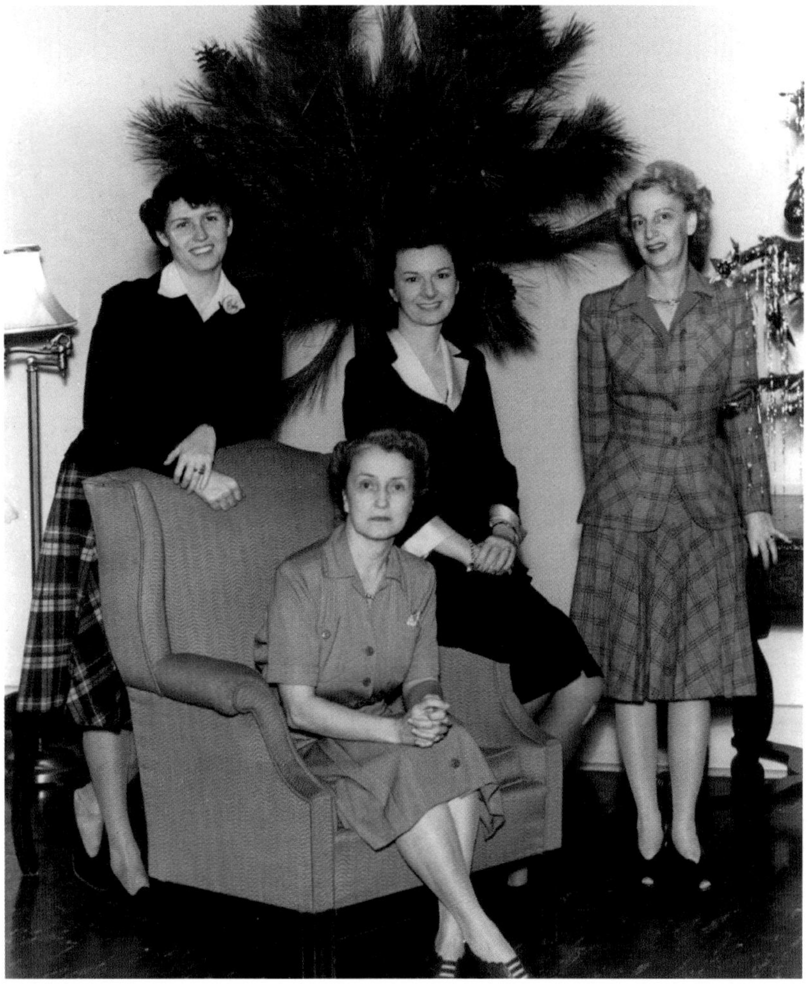

The original Ochsner Clinic receptionists and hostesses gave the facility a reputation for customer service that has endured to the present day.

The partners, meanwhile, began assembling the Clinic's medical staff, which would be the standard by which the institution was judged from then on. Alton Ochsner asked his talented subordinate, Dr. Michael DeBakey, to join the surgical team, which also included old friend Dr. Mims Gage. In addition, Drs. Rudolph Matas, Neal Owens and Dean H. Echols agreed to serve as consultants to the surgery team. Guy Caldwell and Dr. Harry D. Morris constituted the bone and joint surgery staff, and Curtis Tyrone and Dr. John C. Weed made up the OB/GYN team. Duke LeJeune Sr. and Dr. Philip J. Bayon were the Clinic's ear, nose and throat specialists, while Edgar Burns and Dr. W. E. Kittredge were on the Urology staff.[18]

Drs. Thomas Findley and Samuel B. Nadler were the Clinic's original Internal Medicine team, and Dr. John H. Musser, who declined a partnership because of health concerns, and Dr. Julius Wilson served as Internal Medicine consultants. Dr. Edgar H. Little headed the Radiology Department. Before the Clinic even opened its doors, the partners added three more physicians: Dr. William G. Sawitz in Clinical Psychology; Dr. Theodore Soniat in Psychiatry and Neurology; and Dr. Vincent Derbes as a consultant in Dermatology.[19]

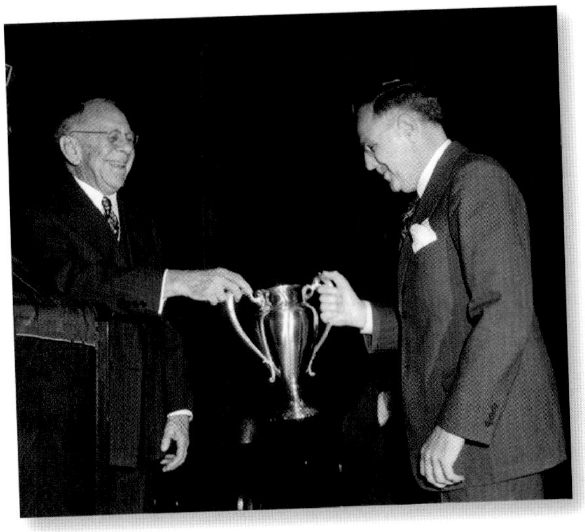

Alton Ochsner receives the Times Picayune Loving Cup in 1947. Ochsner was involved in community and philanthropic affairs for a half-century.

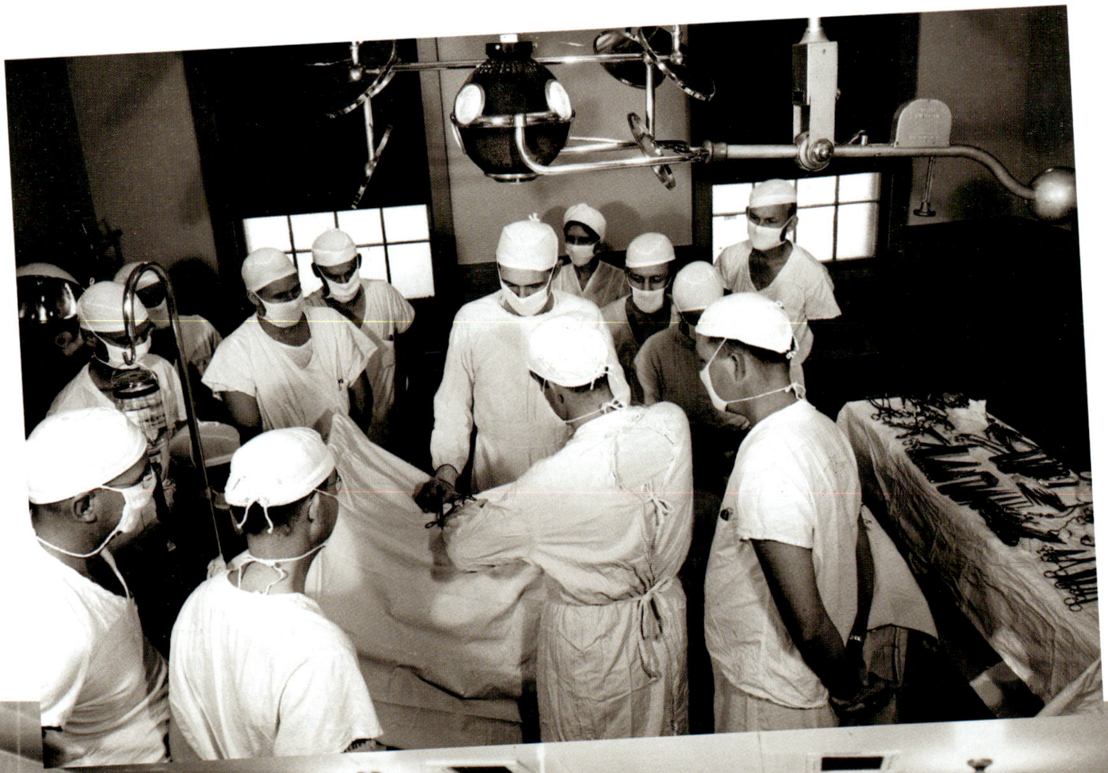

As a teaching hospital, Ochsner Foundation Hospital frequently had an operating room full of medical residents watching the surgeon.

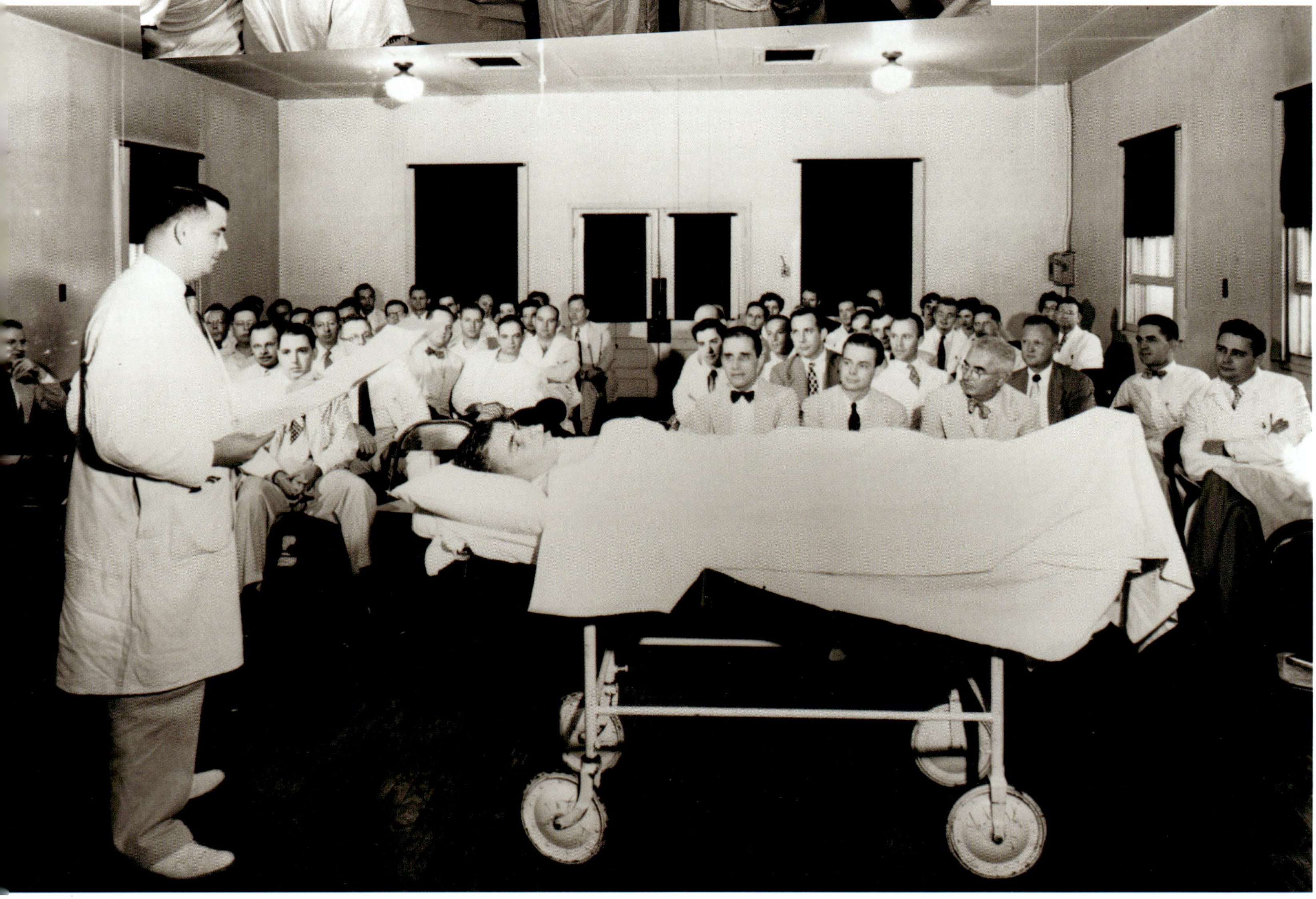

Ochsner staff and medical residents attend a teaching conference in the late 1940s. Alton Ochsner and the founders demanded that the Clinic give as much attention to medical education as to clinical practice and research.

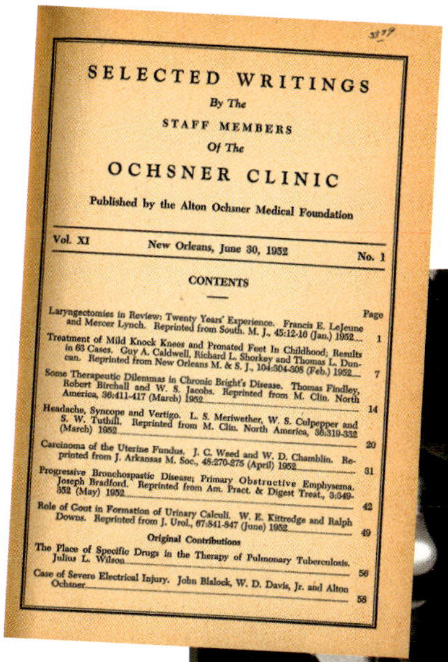
SELECTED WRITINGS
By The
STAFF MEMBERS
Of The
OCHSNER CLINIC

Published by the Alton Ochsner Medical Foundation

Vol. XI — New Orleans, June 30, 1952 — No. 1

CONTENTS

From the start, Ochsner Clinic founders and staff members published their research findings in Clinic publications.

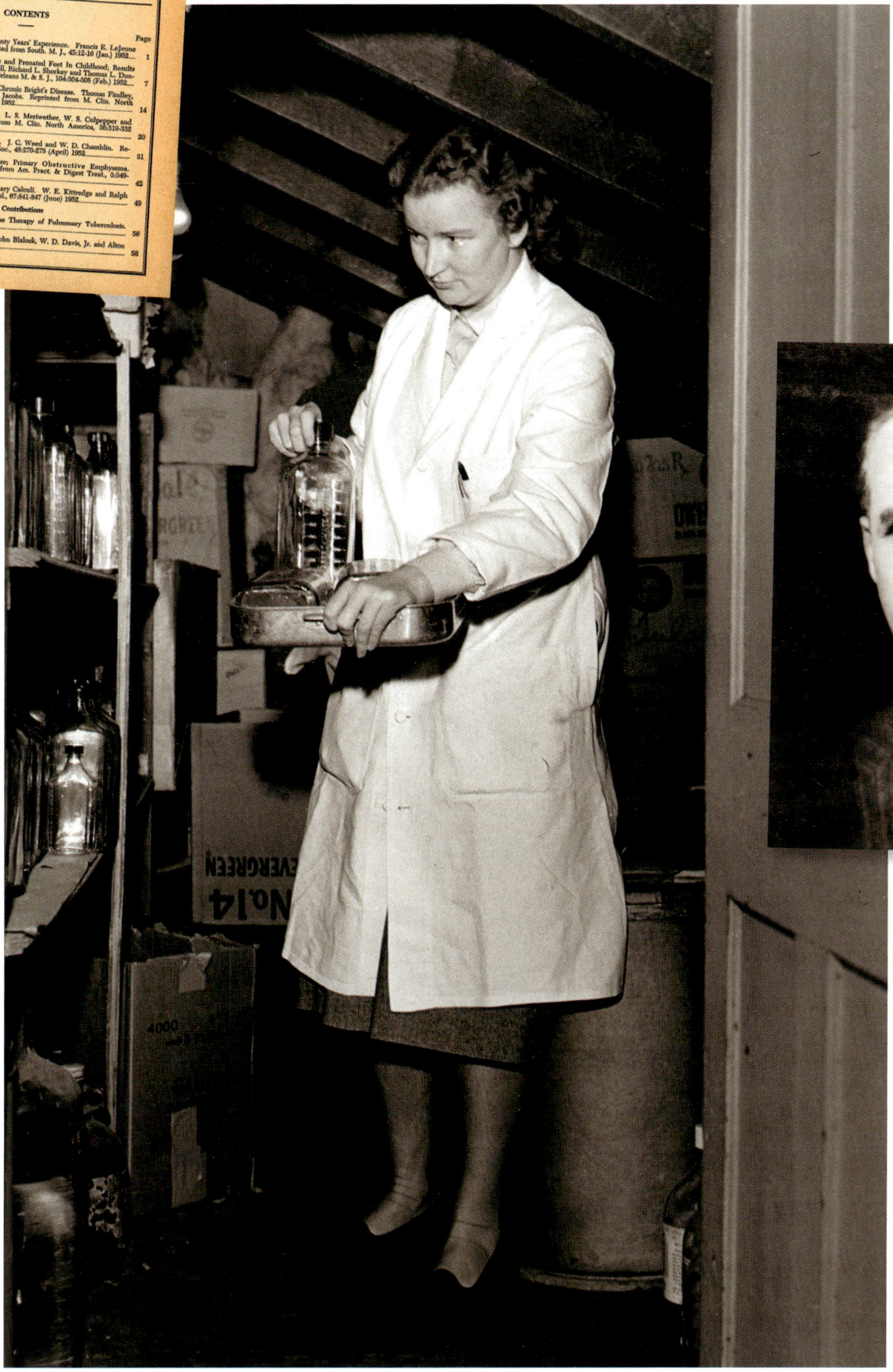

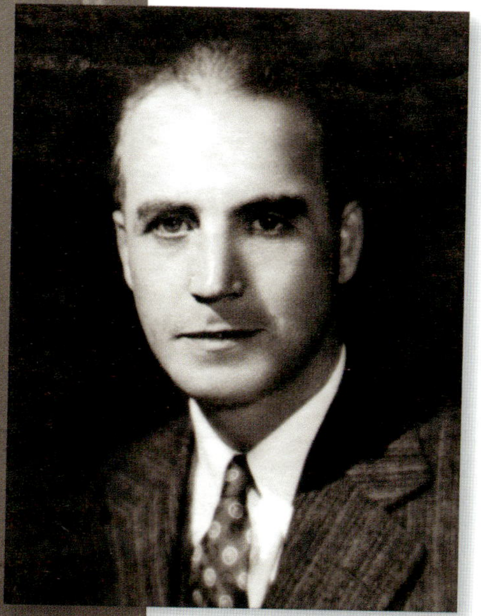

Dean Echols, M.D., sometimes referred to as the "sixth founder," was a Neurosurgeon and a major force in medical education. He oversaw the Clinic's early education efforts.

Research Assistant Nell Taylor tends to chemical supplies in the laboratory on the top floor of the original Clinic where Ochsner was doing research.

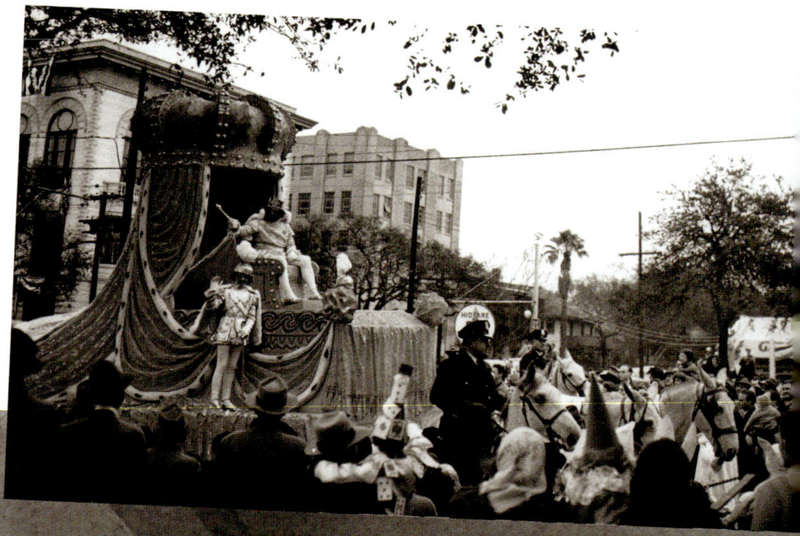

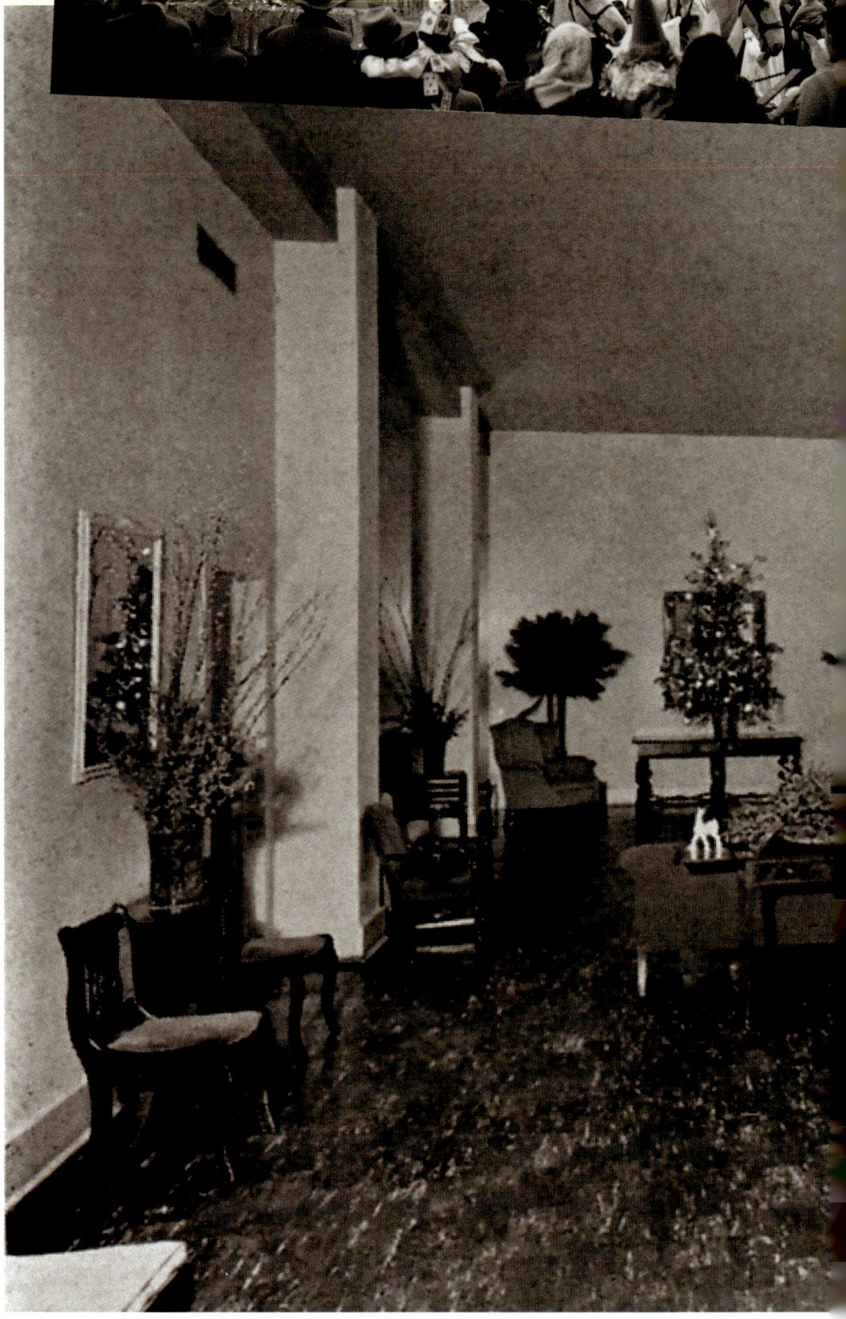

THE CENTRAL AMERICAN GAMBIT

From the start, Alton Ochsner and his partners envisioned that the Clinic would attract private patients from three geographical locales: New Orleans, contiguous areas of Louisiana and Mississippi and from Central and South America.

Ochsner himself was already establishing a reputation in Central America for his surgical prowess. During the spring of 1941, the Santo Tomas Hospital in Panama City invited him to Panama as a visiting professor. Ochsner journeyed south to Panama for two weeks, "gave 28 talks, did 40 operations and saw about 150 people in consultation."[20]

One of the people Ochsner saw during his two weeks in Panama was the former president of the country, Tomas Gabriel Duque. Prime Minister of Panama in 1928, Duque suffered from heart problems. Ochsner noted in his memoirs that he was later personally contacted by U.S. Secretary of State Cordell Hull and asked to go to Panama to operate on Duque.[21] During the war, Ochsner did travel to Panama, operated on Duque, and the former Prime Minister lived for nearly another 25 years.[22]

Ochsner's growing reputation in Central and South America, LeJeune's fluency in Spanish and New Orleans' status as a Latin American port of call all combined to make Ochsner Clinic a preferred destination for Central and South Americans seeking top quality medical care.

OPENING DAY

Ochsner Clinic opened its doors on Friday, January 2, 1942. Less than three weeks before, the United States declared war against Japan following the surprise attack on the U.S. Navy anchorage at Pearl Harbor, Hawaii.

Alton Ochsner and the staff at Ochsner Clinic coped with wartime shortages as they attempted to make the venture a success in the early days. Numerous doctors, nurses and employees answered the call to service during the war, and Ochsner and his colleagues themselves worked closely with the War Department and the Surgeon General on wound infection studies during the period.

The Clinic's main waiting room projected a warm and cheery welcome as New Orleans experienced its second wartime Christmas in 1942. From Guy A. Caldwell's, *Early History of the Ochsner Medical Center - The First Twenty-two Years*, 1965. Courtesy of Charles C Thomas Publisher, Ltd., Springfield, Illinois.

Alton Ochsner as Rex, King of Carnival, in March 1948.

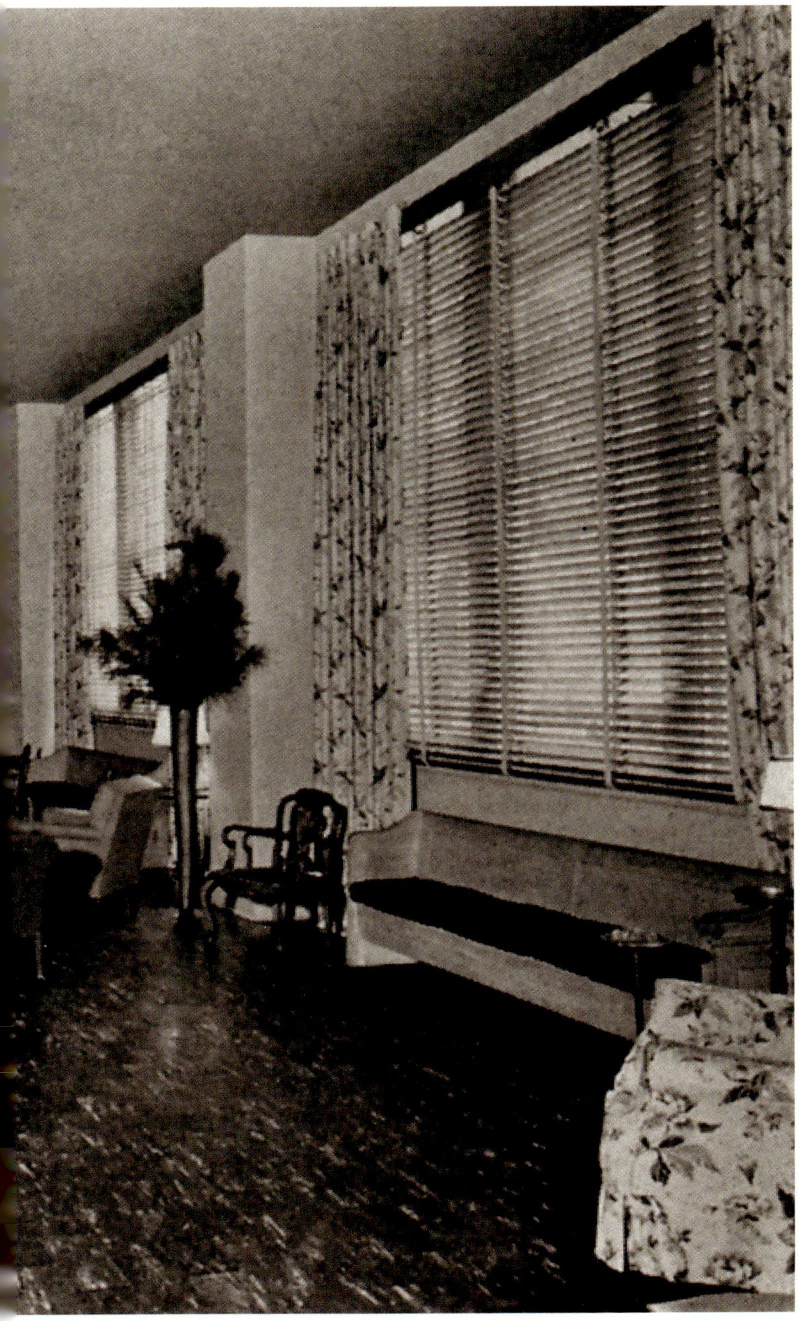

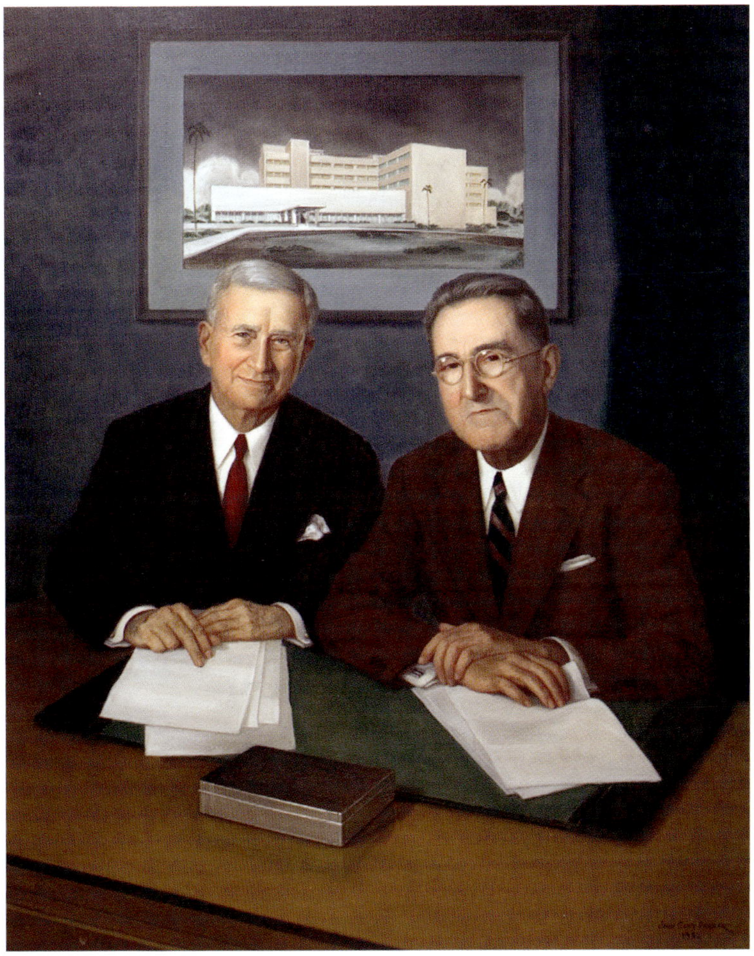

Attorney J. Blanc Monroe and shipping magnate Theodore Brent were the first two non-clinical members of the Alton Ochsner Medical Foundation Board of Trustees.

Perhaps the major organizational change the founders accomplished during the war took place in 1944. Attorney J. Blanc Monroe advised the partners that converting the partnership to an association could pose legal problems in Louisiana. Instead, Monroe suggested the partners consider forming a medical foundation, especially if they envisioned founding a hospital.

They did, and in early 1944, the five founders dissolved the original property-holding corporation and donated its assets to the Alton Ochsner Medical Foundation.[23] "The general purposes of this corporation shall be scientific, educational, literary and charitable," the Foundation's charter noted.[24] The establishment of the Foundation entailed the creation of a seven-member Board of Trustees comprised of the five founders, Monroe and Theodore Brent, the President of the Mississippi Shipping Company.

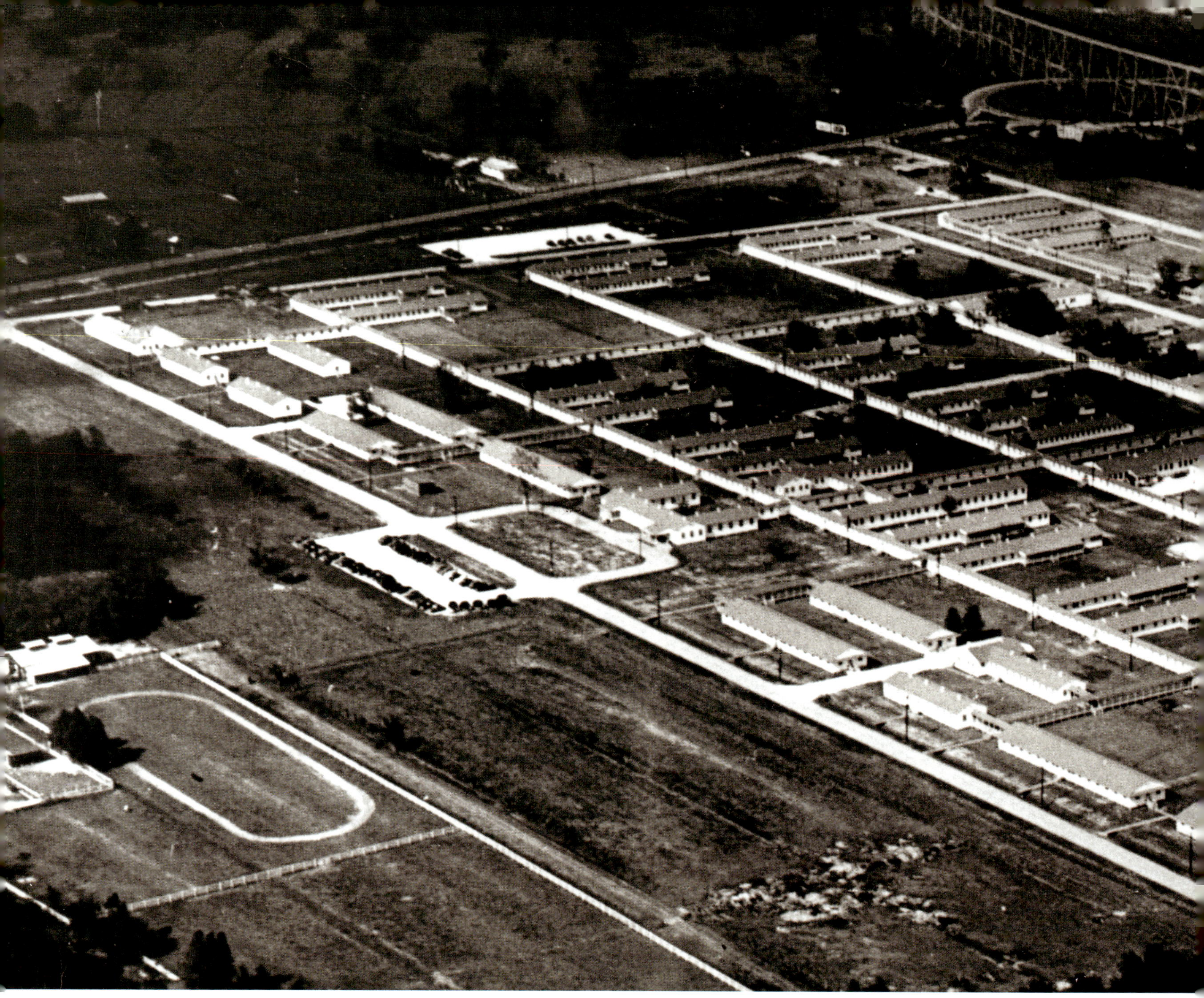

Seen here from the air in 1946, Camp Plauché was the site of the first Ochsner Foundation Hospital, affectionately known as "Splinter Village."

A CRITICAL SHORTAGE OF HOSPITAL BEDS

From the time Ochsner Clinic opened, the medical staff sent Clinic patients requiring hospitalization across the street to Touro Infirmary. The war, however, transformed New Orleans, turning it from a sometimes sleepy port city to a hub of maritime commerce for the defense effort in the Americas. Thousands of soldiers and civilian defense workers flooded the city, and New Orleans found itself bursting at the seams. By 1944, doctors at Ochsner Clinic were coping with a critical shortage of hospital beds.

The Foundation trustees began considering the possibility of establishing the Foundation Hospital as early as the summer of 1944; Brent offered to contribute $100,000 toward the project.[25] Alton Ochsner and most of his colleagues at the Clinic petitioned Tulane to consider building a university hospital. Tulane, however, wasn't interested.

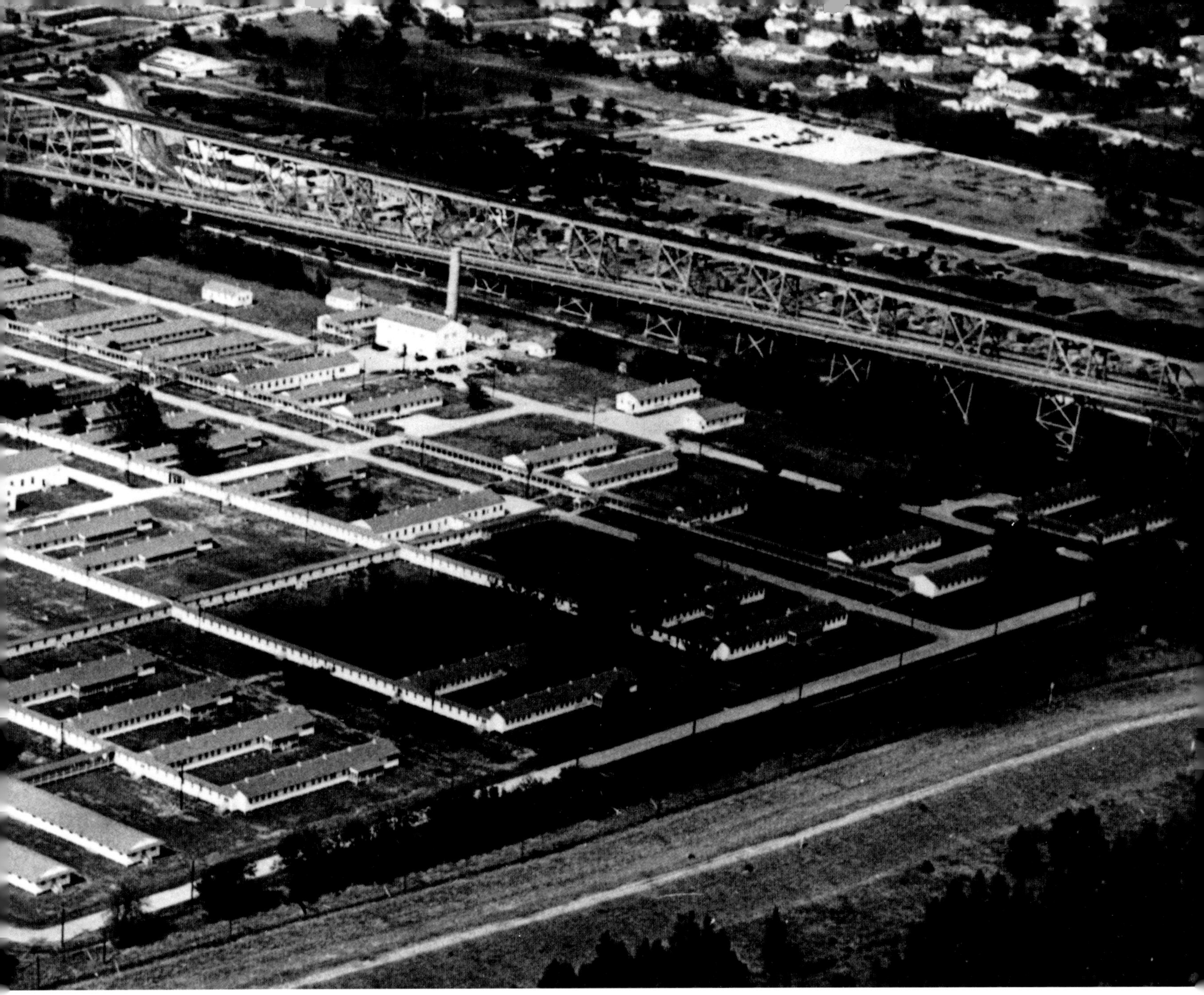

As the war wound down, the shortage of beds in New Orleans accelerated. Ochsner Clinic knew it would have to expand, if nothing else to accommodate the expansion of the medical staff as physicians returned from military service. In March and again in November 1945, the Foundation bought adjacent properties along Foucher Street and St. Charles Avenue as potential hospital sites.

In the end, the Clinic founders and the Foundation trustees opted to pursue converting a military hospital in the New Orleans area to civilian use. The Foundation initially hoped to secure space at the LaGarde Hospital, a 1,000-bed facility on Lake Pontchartrain.[26] The Foundation, however, faced competition for LaGarde, which eventually emerged as a veterans' facility and a private hospital operated by another New Orleans medical foundation.

The Foundation then turned to pursuit of the Station Hospital at Camp Plauché, a somewhat more ramshackle facility at the foot of the Huey P. Long Bridge, which was to become known as the revered "Splinter Village." The price was right. After a spirited bidding war with the same medical foundation that purchased the LaGarde Hospital, the Foundation purchased the Station Hospital from the War Assets Administration for $150,000 in October 1946. Ochsner spent another $50,000 to convert the facilities to civilian use and began operating the hospital in early 1947.[27]

Originally called "Foundation Hospital," the facility and the already established Ochsner Clinic became a force to be reckoned with in medical practice in New Orleans and surrounding areas of Louisiana and Mississippi. The decision to spend $200,000 on the Station Hospital in 1946 was indicative of the founders' willingness to take risks to bring New Orleans world-class medical care.

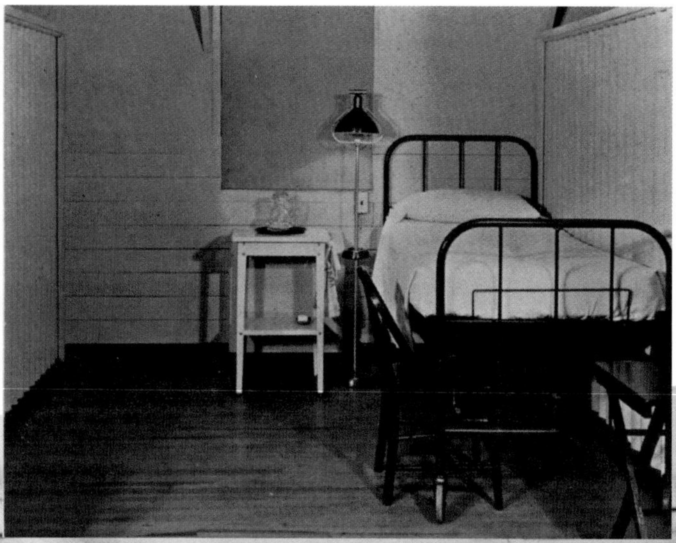

A private room at Camp Plauché, spartan but clean. From Guy A. Caldwell's, *Early History of the Ochsner Medical Center - The First Twenty-two Years*, 1965. Courtesy of Charles C Thomas Publisher, Ltd., Springfield, Illinois.

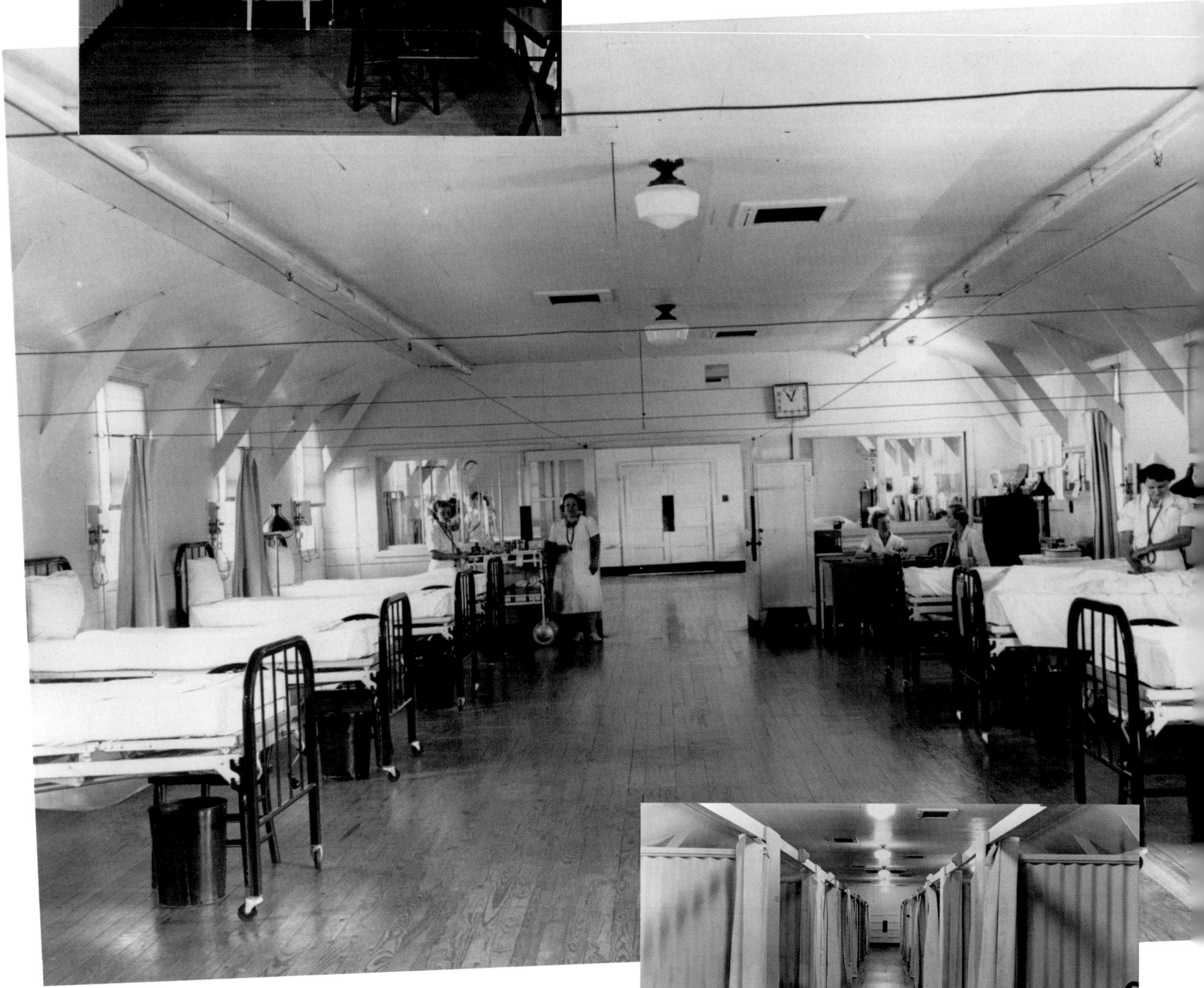

Recovery room at Camp Plauché. Doctors and their families lived in the military barracks attached to the hospital and walked to work.

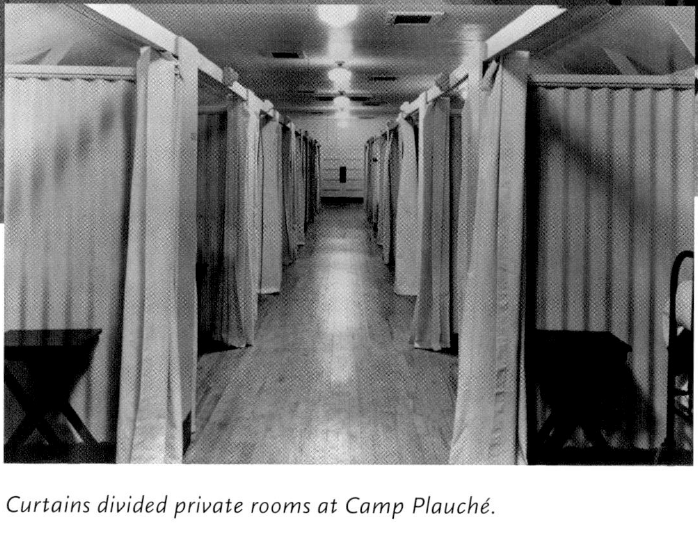

Curtains divided private rooms at Camp Plauché.

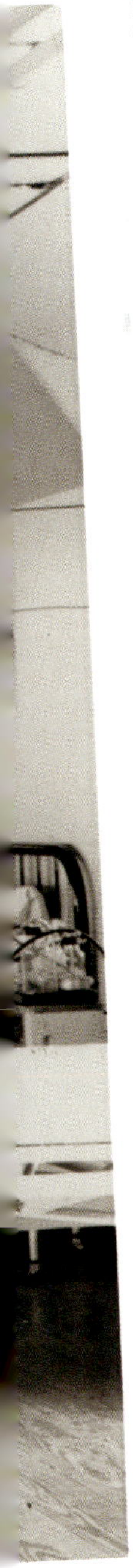

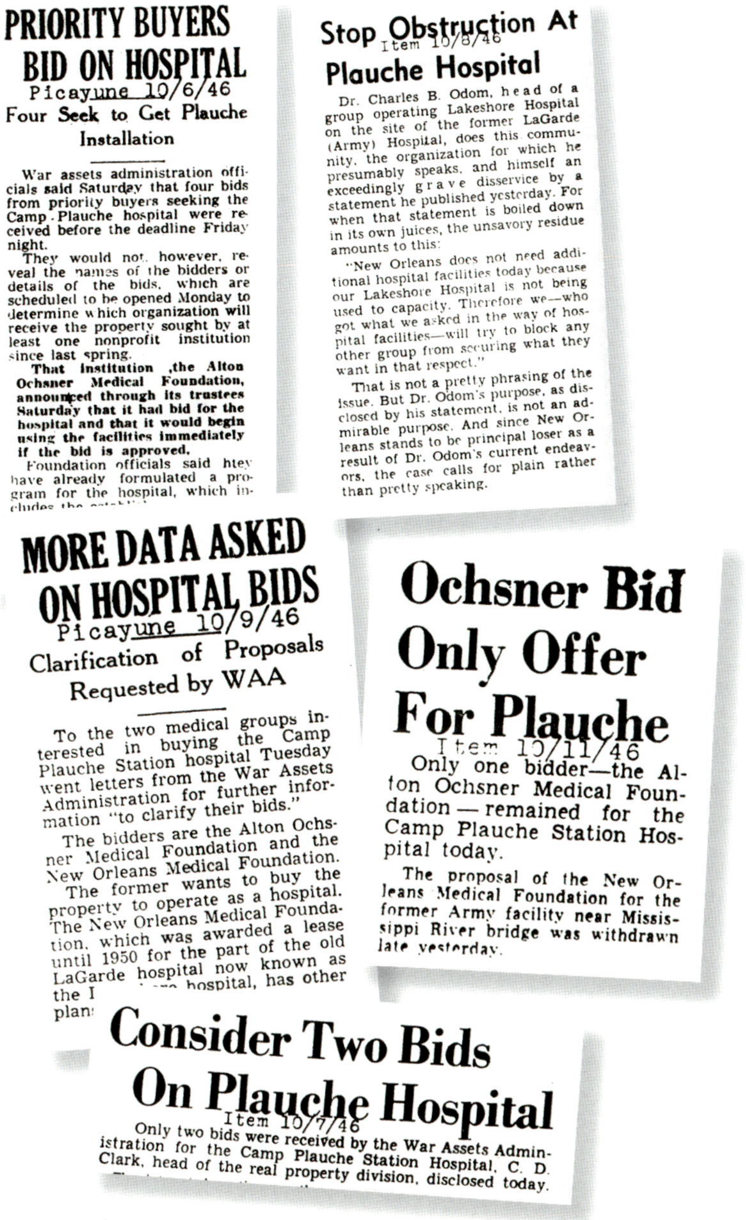

PRIORITY BUYERS BID ON HOSPITAL
Picayune 10/6/46
Four Seek to Get Plauche Installation

War assets administration officials said Saturday that four bids from priority buyers seeking the Camp Plauche hospital were received before the deadline Friday night.
They would not, however, reveal the names of the bidders or details of the bids, which are scheduled to be opened Monday to determine which organization will receive the property sought by at least one nonprofit institution since last spring.
That institution, the Alton Ochsner Medical Foundation, announced through its trustees Saturday that it had bid for the hospital and that it would begin using the facilities immediately if the bid is approved.
Foundation officials said they have already formulated a program for the hospital, which includes the ...

Stop Obstruction At Plauche Hospital
Item 10/8/46

Dr. Charles B. Odom, head of a group operating Lakeshore Hospital on the site of the former LaGarde (Army) Hospital, does this community, the organization for which he presumably speaks, and himself an exceedingly grave disservice by a statement he published yesterday. For when that statement is boiled down in its own juices, the unsavory residue amounts to this:
"New Orleans does not need additional hospital facilities today because our Lakeshore Hospital is not being used to capacity. Therefore we—who got what we asked in the way of hospital facilities—will try to block any other group from securing what they want in that respect."
That is not a pretty phrasing of the issue. But Dr. Odom's purpose, as disclosed by his statement, is not an admirable purpose. And since New Orleans stands to be principal loser as a result of Dr. Odom's current endeavors, the case calls for plain rather than pretty speaking.

MORE DATA ASKED ON HOSPITAL BIDS
Picayune 10/9/46
Clarification of Proposals Requested by WAA

To the two medical groups interested in buying the Camp Plauche Station hospital Tuesday went letters from the War Assets Administration for further information "to clarify their bids."
The bidders are the Alton Ochsner Medical Foundation and the New Orleans Medical Foundation.
The former wants to buy the property to operate as a hospital. The New Orleans Medical Foundation, which was awarded a lease until 1950 for the part of the old LaGarde hospital now known as the L... hospital, has other plan...

Ochsner Bid Only Offer For Plauche
Item 10/11/46

Only one bidder—the Alton Ochsner Medical Foundation—remained for the Camp Plauche Station Hospital today.
The proposal of the New Orleans Medical Foundation for the former Army facility near Mississippi River bridge was withdrawn late yesterday.

Consider Two Bids On Plauche Hospital
Item 10/7/46

Only two bids were received by the War Assets Administration for the Camp Plauche Station Hospital, C. D. Clark, head of the real property division, disclosed today.

The Foundation had competition on its 1946 bid for the Camp Plauché Hospital.

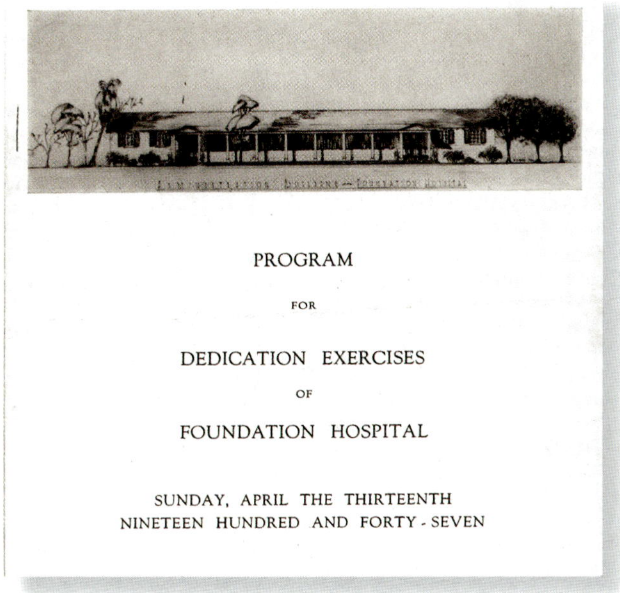

PROGRAM

FOR

DEDICATION EXERCISES

OF

FOUNDATION HOSPITAL

SUNDAY, APRIL THE THIRTEENTH
NINETEEN HUNDRED AND FORTY - SEVEN

Program for the 1947 dedication of the Camp Plauché Hospital.

SPLINTER VILLAGE

Dr. Francis Xavier LeTard, his wife, Evelyn, and their son, Frank Jr. moved into converted civilian housing at the former Station Hospital at Camp Plauché in the shadow of the Huey P. Long Bridge in 1948. The Alton Ochsner Medical Foundation had purchased the facility from the government less than two years before, and most on the staff referred to the sprawling complex of wooden buildings as the Foundation Hospital.

The residents called it "Splinter Village," because it was so hot that the nurses frequently took off their shoes and got splinters in their stocking feet from the wood floors. The Foundation Hospital occupied the facility for more than seven years, however, and medical staff, nurses and employees developed a fondness for Splinter Village that transcended the sometimes primitive conditions.

"Nobody had any money," Evelyn LeTard recalled of the five years she and her family lived at Splinter Village. Her husband, Frank, served as the Hospital's first Anesthesiology resident, and LeTard said he "would put on his scrubs and walk down to the operating room."[28]

Residents of Splinter Village received free utilities, and the Hospital provided maintenance for the living units.[29] The families of the doctors all socialized together, and Evelyn LeTard recalled Alton Ochsner telephoning to ask for her chicken dumpling recipe. Curtis Tyrone delivered the great majority of the children born in Splinter Village, and several of the residents formed a hospitality club to welcome the wives of new doctors to the Village. "If the wife wasn't happy," LeTard said, "the doctor wasn't going to be happy. There was such a wonderful feeling when the Hospital was so small."[30]

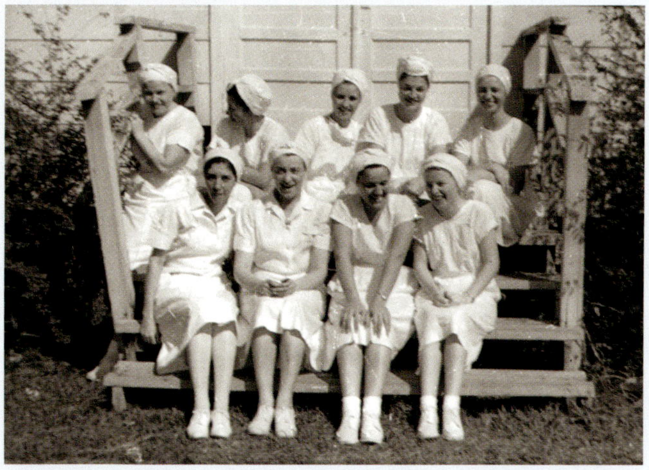

Nurses nicknamed Camp Plauché "Splinter Village" because they often got splinters in their stocking feet from the wood floors.

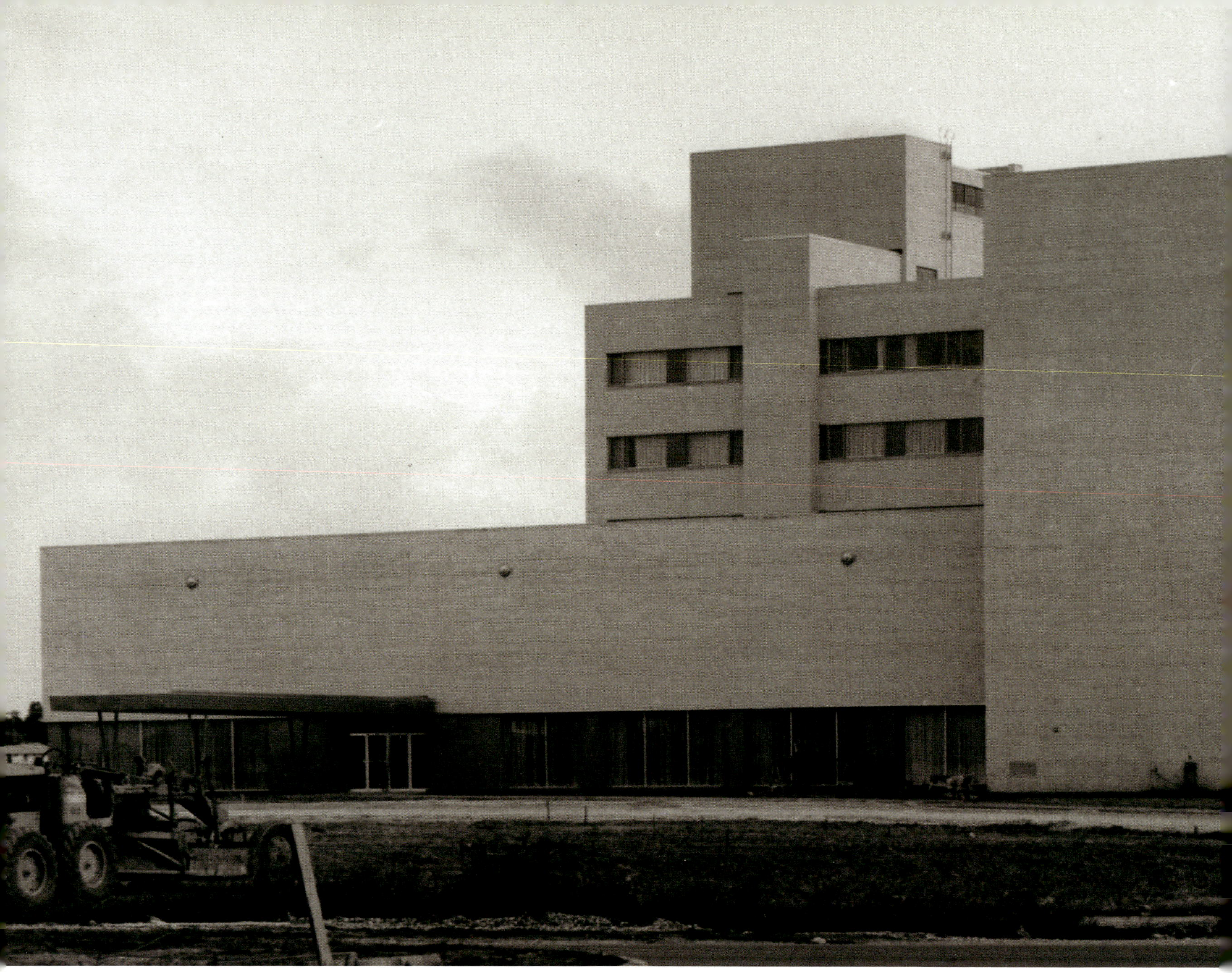

CHAPTER 3:

BUILDING A HOSPITAL

THE SUCCESS OF OCHSNER CLINIC and the rapid growth of the Foundation Hospital, the legendary "Splinter Village," led the founders to consider expanding their services during the early 1950s. The Clinic and the Foundation selected a site on Jefferson Highway for a new hospital, which opened in 1954. Ochsner was able to fulfill its role as a teaching hospital, and the Foundation decided late in the decade to open a research building at that site.

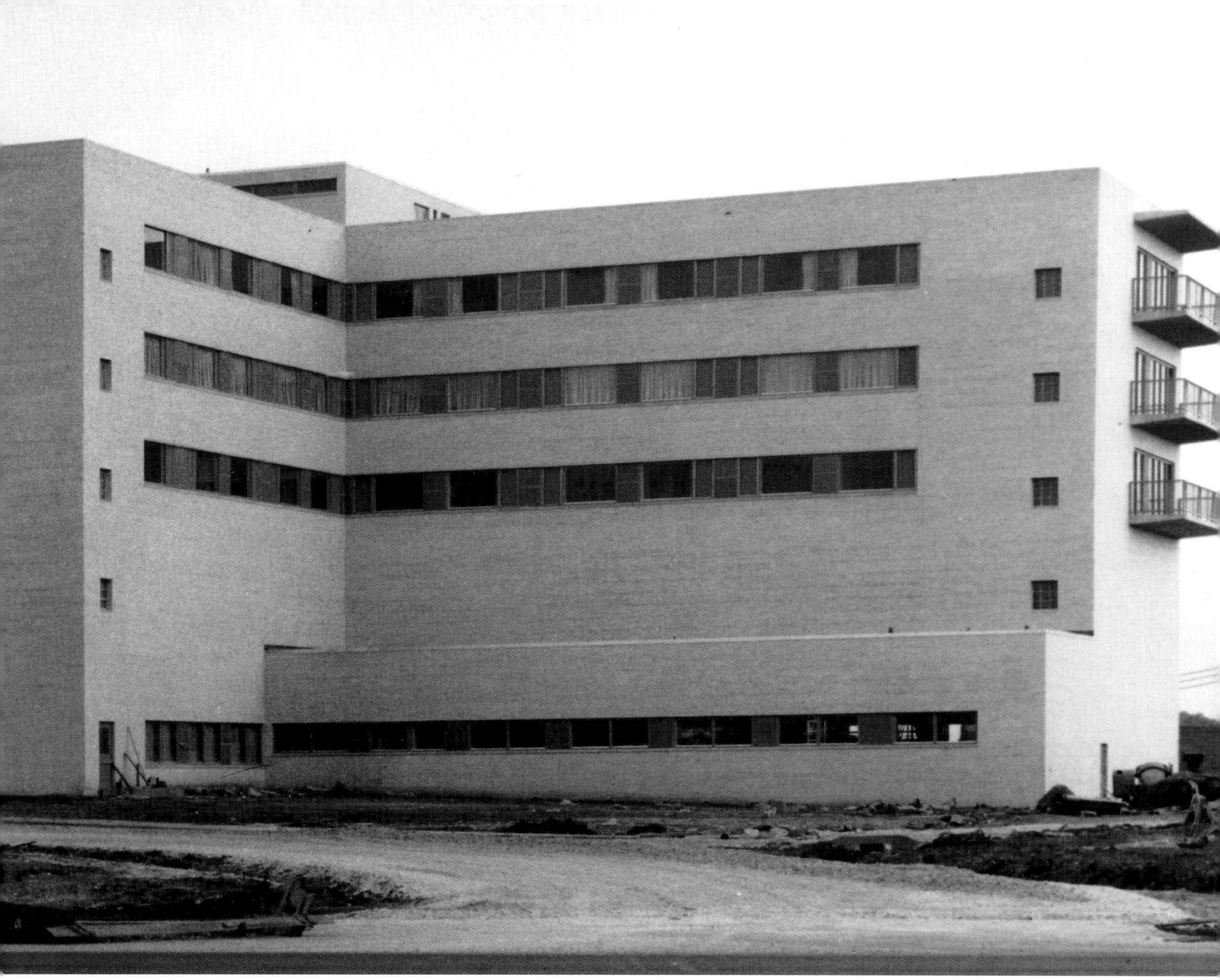

The Foundation Hospital ready to receive patients on June 12, 1954.

Ochsner's reputation transcended the New Orleans area. The Clinic and Hospital treated such notable Americans as golfer Ben Hogan and actor Gary Cooper. Alton Ochsner flew to Buenos Aires to treat Argentine President Juan Peron. Increasingly, researchers in the medical community were coming to the same conclusion reached by Alton Ochsner a decade earlier: cigarette smoking caused a host of fatal medical conditions, including lung cancer, emphysema and cardiovascular disease.

YEARS OF NEGOTIATIONS

By 1949, the Hospital at Camp Plauché had 250 beds and a medical staff that was known throughout the Gulf South. The Hospital had come through the September 1947 hurricane with the loss of only a few roof shingles. Ochsner Clinic fared less well. The storm, which killed more than 50 people in Florida, made a second landfall in southeastern Louisiana and hit the New Orleans area particularly hard. The Clinic building at Prytania and Aline streets sustained major water damage on the first floor.

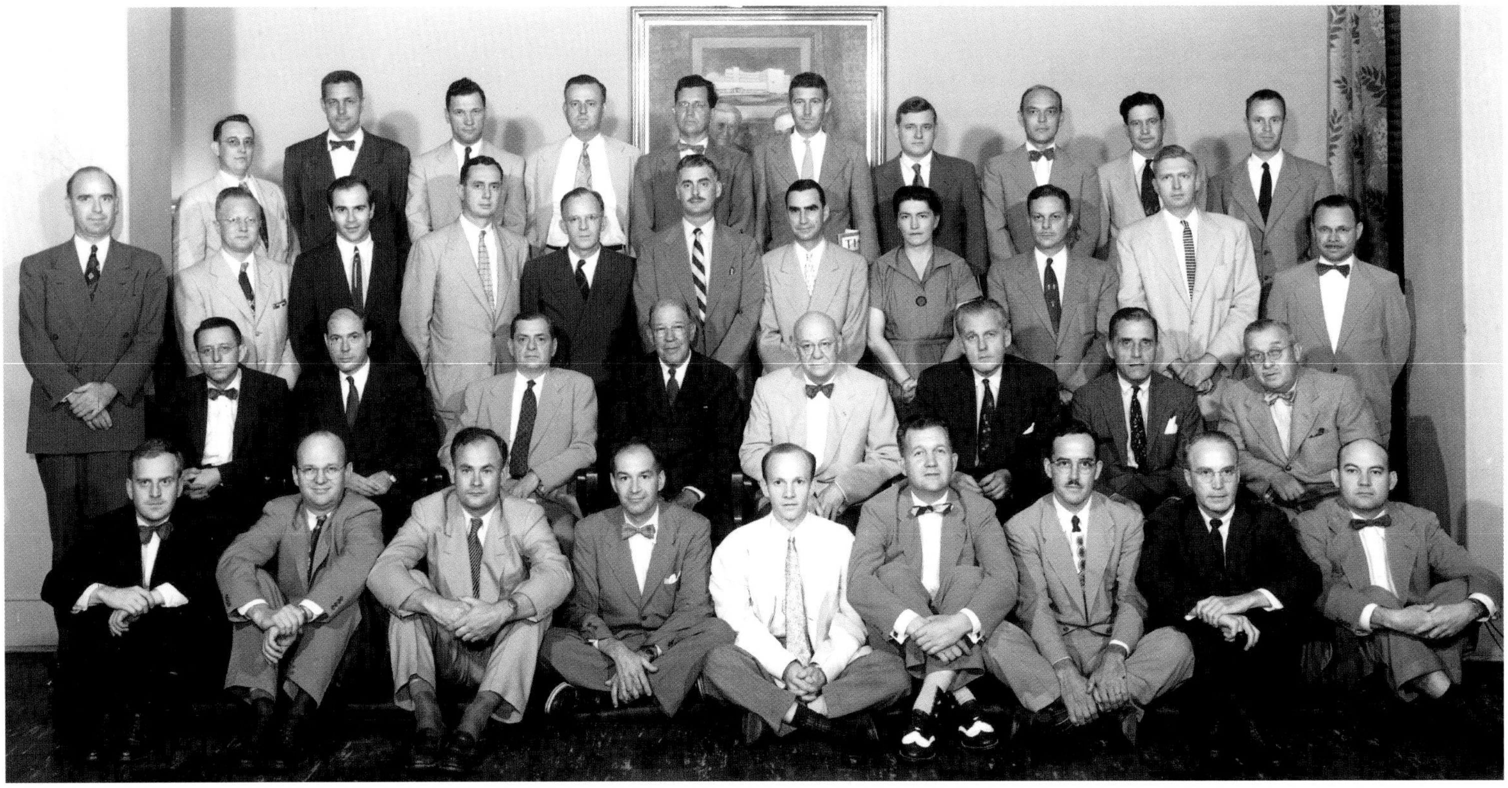

A group photo of members of the Foundation Hospital staff in 1953. The new facility was a vast improvement over the antiquated Splinter Village.

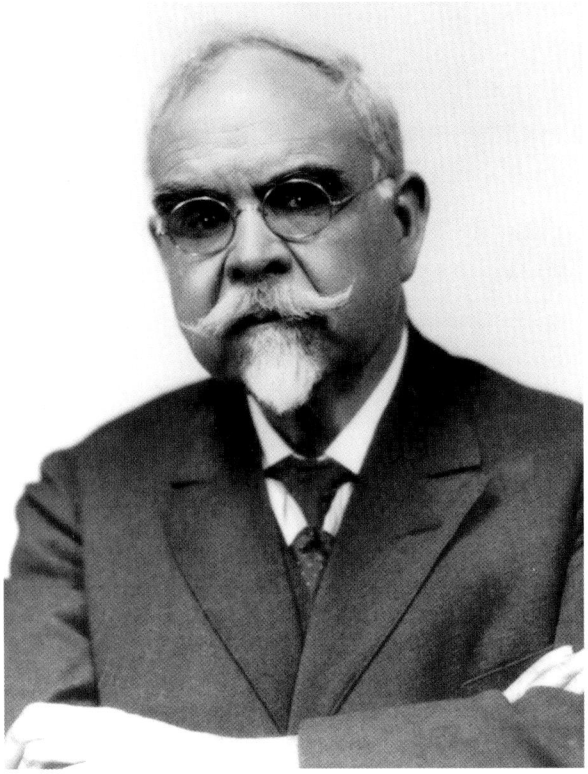

Ninety-year-old Rudolph Matas, senior member of the New Orleans medical community, was the honorary chairman of the Foundation Hospital's fund-raising campaign to replace Camp Plauché.

Those Clinic staff members who made it to work during the peak of the storm greeted patients who refused to let gusts of 110 mph and sheets of rain deter them from seeing their favorite physicians.[1]

During the late 1940s, the Alton Ochsner Medical Foundation made plans to locate a site for a completely new hospital. Foundation trustees hoped that Tulane's Board of Administration would join them as partners in the search for a site that would accommodate a new 250-bed hospital. As in 1940 and 1941, however, the university was noncommittal about a formal partnership. Tulane had already rejected a proposal to create an Ochsner/Tulane wing at Touro Infirmary, so there was little precedent to expect closer ties between the Foundation and the university.

Meanwhile, the Foundation trustees narrowed potential sites to three possibilities: four square blocks of land off Carrollton Avenue in Uptown New Orleans, an island in Bayou St. John near the City Park golf course, and a 21-acre plot owned by the Illinois Central Railroad in Jefferson Parish between Jefferson Highway and the Mississippi River.[2]

For various reasons, the first two sites proved to be impractical as hospital locations. During the spring of 1948, negotiations resumed with Tulane, Touro Infirmary and Ochsner about a three-way partnership that would essentially double the beds at Touro and convert it into a Tulane hospital.

The three-way partnership foundered on the rocks of opposition from the Touro medical staff. This reinforced the conviction of the Clinic founders that they needed an Ochsner-only hospital. The Foundation trustees also held talks with the trustees of Southern Baptist Hospital about building a separate Ochsner wing at the New Orleans hospital.[3]

'NOT SURPASSED ANYWHERE IN THE COUNTRY'

In the end, Alton Ochsner, his colleagues and the Foundation trustees realized that the Clinic and the Foundation would have to go it alone and build a new facility. Foundation trustees estimated fund-raising would take four years and require $4 million to build a new hospital from scratch.

Fund-raising got underway in early 1950. Ben Hogan, one of the greatest golfers to ever play the game, served as chairman of the fund drive. Rudolph Matas, then 90 years old, served as honorary chairman.

Alton Ochsner had gotten to know Hogan the previous year. Hogan nearly died in a 1949 head-on collision with a Greyhound bus on a fog-shrouded west Texas highway, and Ochsner, one of the nation's best-known specialists in embolisms, rushed to Hogan's bedside in El Paso to prevent additional, potentially lethal, pulmonary emboli.[4]

Thanks in part to Ochsner's treatments, Hogan survived and left the hospital 59 days after the accident. Orthopedic surgeons at the Texas hospital cautioned Hogan he might never walk again. When he appeared at the Roosevelt Hotel to initiate the Foundation Hospital fund drive in early June 1950, Hogan was the picture of health. Just 10 days later, he won the U.S. Open title at Merion Golf Club outside Philadelphia.[5]

Hogan attributed his recovery to Alton Ochsner. "These doctors have an ideal of medical practice which is not surpassed anywhere in the country," Hogan told the audience at the Roosevelt Hotel that June day. "Furthermore, they are personally contributing to the maintenance of a hospital, to a program of medical research, and to a program of training in the specialties which ultimately will benefit the whole South."[6]

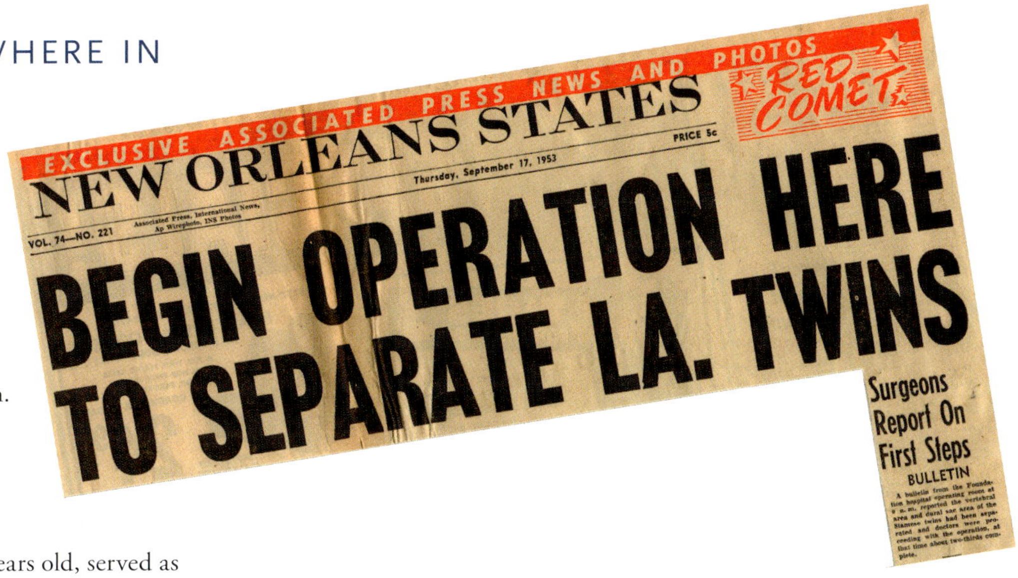
EXCLUSIVE ASSOCIATED PRESS NEWS AND PHOTOS

RED COMET

NEW ORLEANS STATES

VOL. 74—NO. 221 Associated Press, International News, Ap Wirephoto, INS Photos

Thursday, September 17, 1953

PRICE 5c

BEGIN OPERATION HERE TO SEPARATE LA. TWINS

Surgeons Report On First Steps

BULLETIN

A bulletin from the Foundation hospital operating room at 9 a.m. reported the vertebral area and dural sac area of the Siamese twins had been separated and doctors were proceeding with the operation, at that time about two-thirds complete.

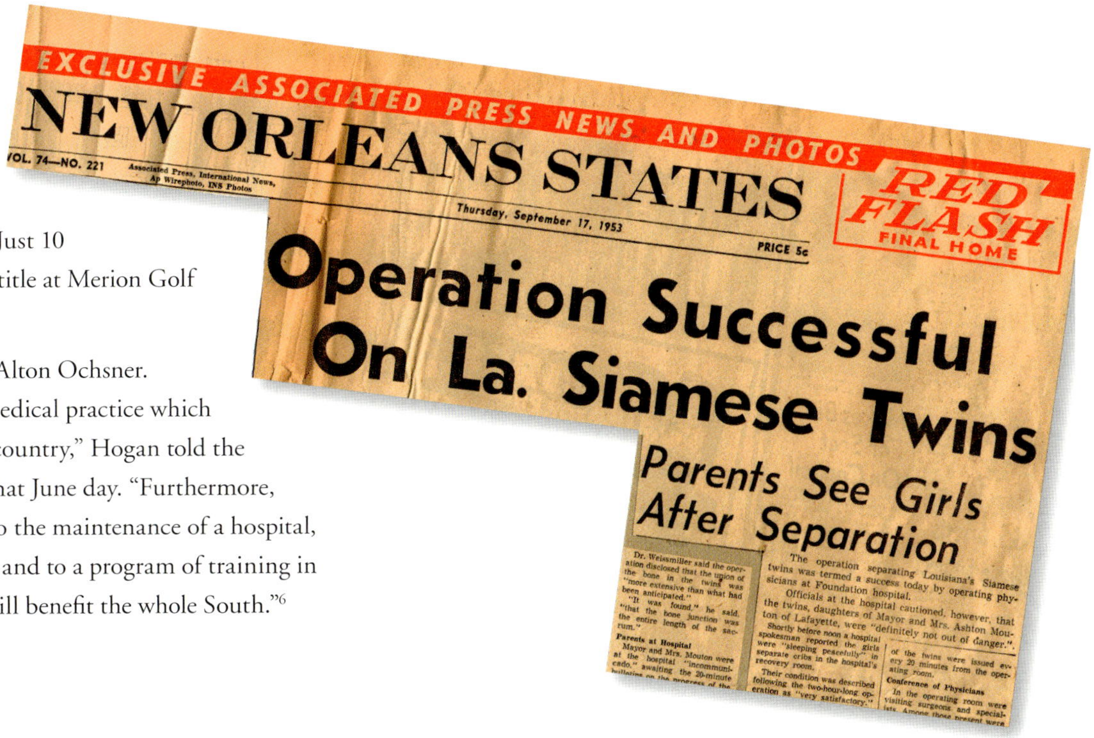
EXCLUSIVE ASSOCIATED PRESS NEWS AND PHOTOS

NEW ORLEANS STATES

VOL. 74—NO. 221 Associated Press, International News, Ap Wirephoto, INS Photos

Thursday, September 17, 1953

PRICE 5c

RED FLASH FINAL HOME

Operation Successful On La. Siamese Twins

Parents See Girls After Separation

The operation separating Louisiana's Siamese twins was termed a success today by operating physicians at Foundation hospital.

Officials at the hospital cautioned, however, that the twins, daughters of Mayor and Mrs. Ashton Mouton of Lafayette, were "definitely not out of danger."

Shortly before noon a hospital spokesman reported the girls were "sleeping peacefully" in separate cribs in the hospital's recovery room.

Their condition was described following the two-hour-long operation as "very satisfactory."

... of the twins were issued every 20 minutes from the operating room.

Conference of Physicians

In the operating room were visiting surgeons and specialists. Among those present were

Dr. Weissmiller said the operation disclosed that the union of the bone in the twins was "more extensive than what had been anticipated."

"It was found," he said, "that the bone junction was the entire length of the sacrum."

Parents at Hospital

Mayor and Mrs. Mouton were at the hospital "incommunicado," awaiting the 20-minute bulletins on the progress of the

Alton Ochsner's separation of conjoined twins was front-page news in 1953.

PERON, SOMOZA AND GARY COOPER

The renown of Ochsner Clinic and the Foundation Hospital spread well beyond the New Orleans area during the late 1940s and 1950s. Movie star Gary Cooper checked into the Foundation Hospital in March 1952 on the advice of his friend, Hogan. Alton Ochsner surgically repaired a hernia for the star, who was in the process of filming *High Noon*. Nurses and patients scurried to get a glimpse of the Hollywood heartthrob during his weeklong stay at the Hospital. In 1954, Ochsner flew to Paris to repair a second Cooper hernia. On another visit, the actor stayed with Alton and Isabel Ochsner while undergoing a routine checkup at the Foundation Hospital at Splinter Village.[7]

Another famous patient was General Claire Lee Chennault, the Louisiana native who rose to fame with his command of the Flying Tigers during World War II.[8]

The Foundation Hospital and the Clinic attracted a huge clientele from Central and South America during the 1950s and 1960s. "Twelve percent of their patients came from Central and South America," said Dr. John Ochsner. "New Orleans had daily flights to South America, and Delta had flights to Caracas, Venezuela three times a week."[9] John Ochsner recalled that some patients from Latin America "flew in on their private planes. They spent more money at the Clinic than the Super Bowl, Mardi Gras and Spring Fiesta put together."[10]

Wealthy residents of Latin America would fly to New Orleans for a week or two of shopping and sightseeing wrapped around a visit to Ochsner Clinic. "One day, 67 people showed up without appointments," said John Ochsner, describing the Clinic's Latin American clientele. With all of the international patients showing up unannounced, it made for a very chaotic day at the Clinic.

Active in the Inter-American Section of the American College of Surgeons, Alton Ochsner enjoyed a reputation in Central and South America as the continent's most accomplished physician. Besides Tomas Duque, his patient list included Anastasio Somoza, the President of Nicaragua.

In 1955, Ochsner flew to Buenos Aires to treat Argentine President Juan Peron for a thrombosis in his leg. Ochsner took the trip under such secrecy that most of his colleagues suspected he was flying to the Vatican to treat an ailing Pope Pius XII. Ochsner advised Peron to quit smoking and told the Argentine leader that he would have to fly to New Orleans to have surgery at the new Foundation Hospital. Peron promised to follow Ochsner to New Orleans, but later was ousted in a *coup d'etat* and left for exile in Spain.[11]

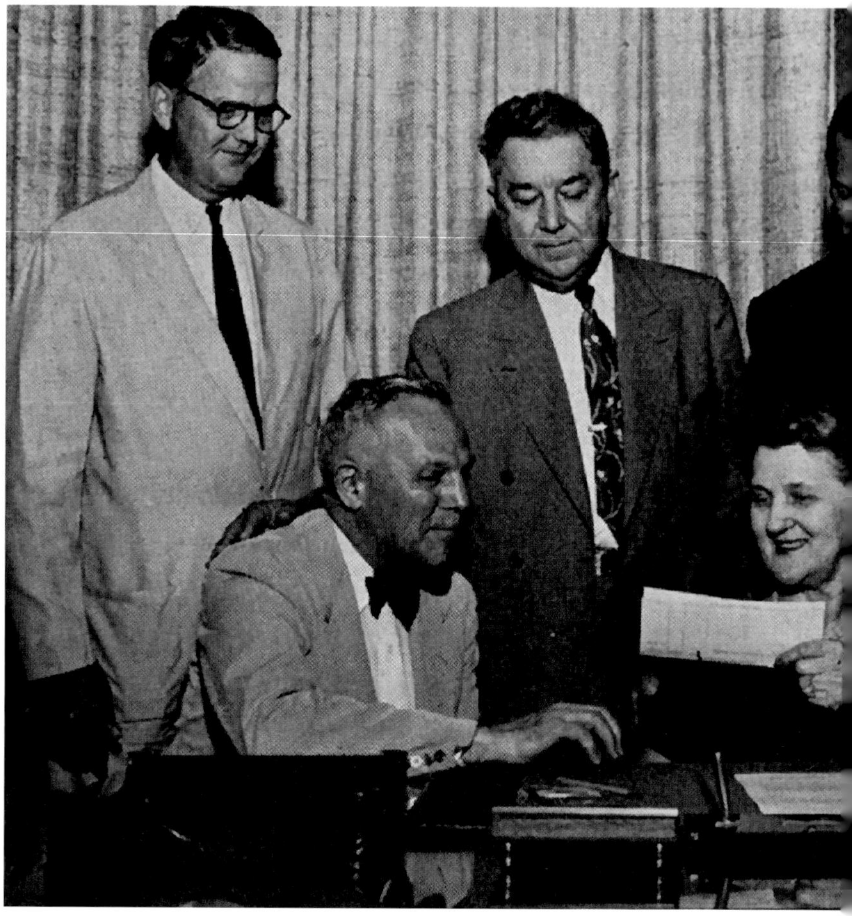

GROUNDBREAKING

With the fund-raising program underway, plans rapidly developed for the new Ochsner Foundation Hospital. By the spring of 1951, New Orleans, Louisiana and Gulf South residents had contributed nearly $1 million to the hospital building campaign, a measure of the high esteem in which the community held the Clinic and Foundation Hospital. The Crosby family, a Mississippi dynasty with extensive holdings in timber and newsprint, donated the lion's share of the Hospital's first $1 million. Alton Ochsner began treating L. O. Crosby, the family's patriarch in the mid-1940s, and his three sons each donated $100,000 to the initial Hospital fund.[12]

The strong start to fund-raising allowed the Foundation trustees to purchase the property fronting Jefferson Highway it had identified several years before. The site of a former riding academy, the property had attracted the eye of Foundation trustees as far back as 1947. At the time, a lack of sewers threatened to torpedo the property's use as a hospital site. Jefferson Parish, however, installed sewers to serve the property. In late 1951, Guy Caldwell, Theodore Brent and J. Blanc Monroe signed papers transferring the property from Illinois Central Railroad to the Alton Ochsner Medical Foundation.[13]

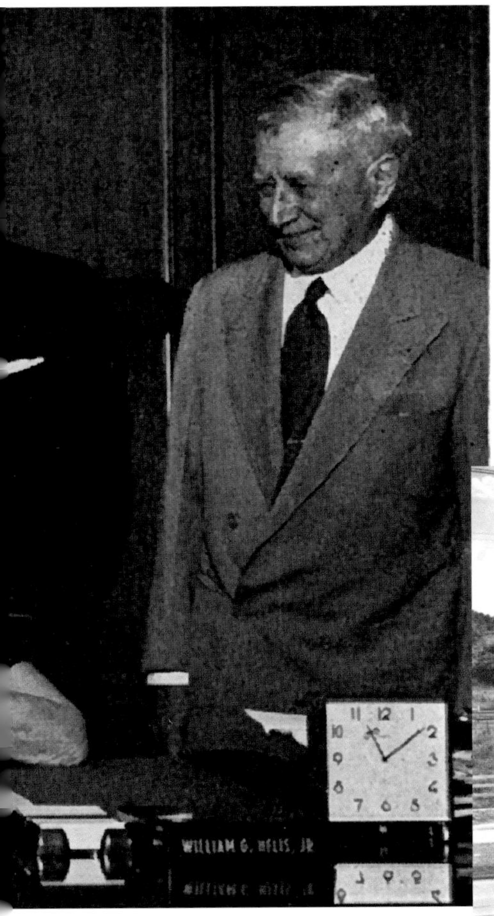

Mrs. William G. Helis of the Helis Foundation presents a $250,000 check to Alton Ochsner for the new hospital. Mrs. Helis was just one of dozens of local donors who contributed to the Ochsner building fund during the 1940s and 1950s. From Guy A. Caldwell's, *Early History of the Ochsner Medical Center - The First Twenty-two Years*, 1965. Courtesy of Charles C Thomas Publisher, Ltd., Springfield, Illinois.

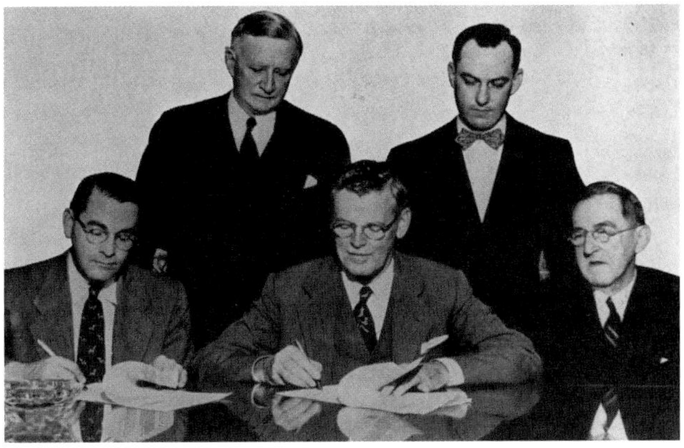

Guy Caldwell, center, signs sales documents for the Foundation's purchase of the riding academy site at 1514 Jefferson Highway in December 1951. From Guy A. Caldwell's, *Early History of the Ochsner Medical Center - The First Twenty-two Years*, 1965. Courtesy of Charles C Thomas Publisher, Ltd., Springfield, Illinois.

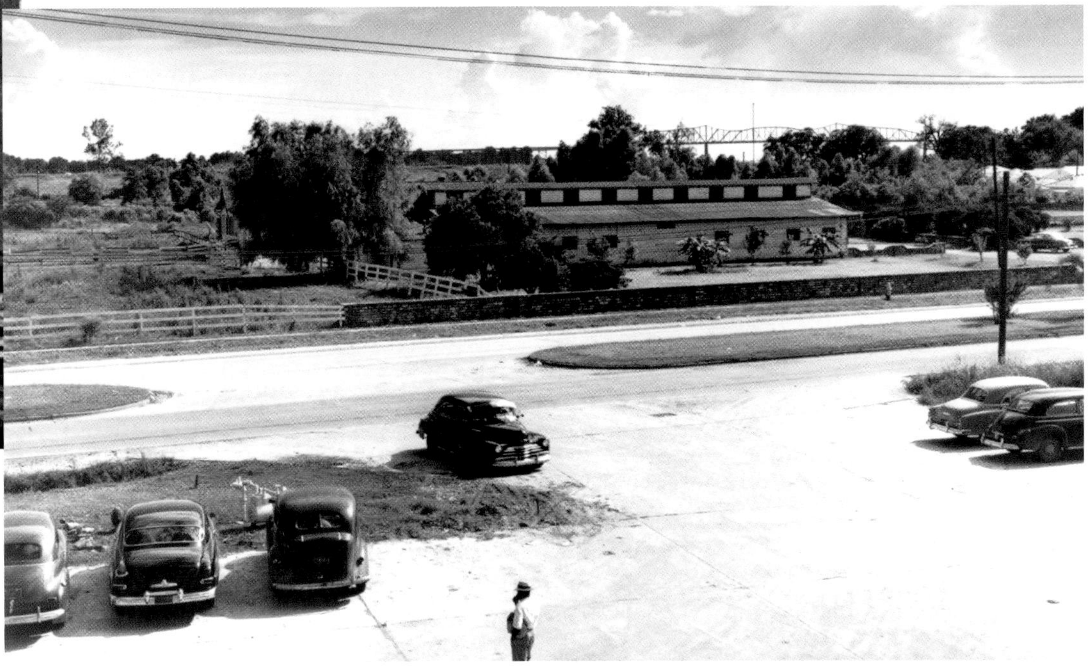

The Foundation purchased the 21-acre riding academy site from the Illinois Central Railroad for $126,000.

In March 1952, the trustees took out a $1 million loan from New Orleans' Pan American Life Insurance Company. The Foundation also qualified for federal funding through the Hospital Survey and Construction Act of 1946. Better known as the Hill-Burton Act, the legislation provided money to the states to help them reach a level of 4.5 hospital beds per 1,000 residents.[14]

With the federal funding and loan money in hand, the trustees engaged the services of the New Orleans firm of Farnsworth and Chambers as the general contractor for the new Hospital. Six weeks later, on July 2, 1952, crews drove the first pilings for the Hospital's foundation in a gala groundbreaking.[15] Over the next 60 years, the Foundation Hospital would emerge as one of the region's best healthcare facilities.

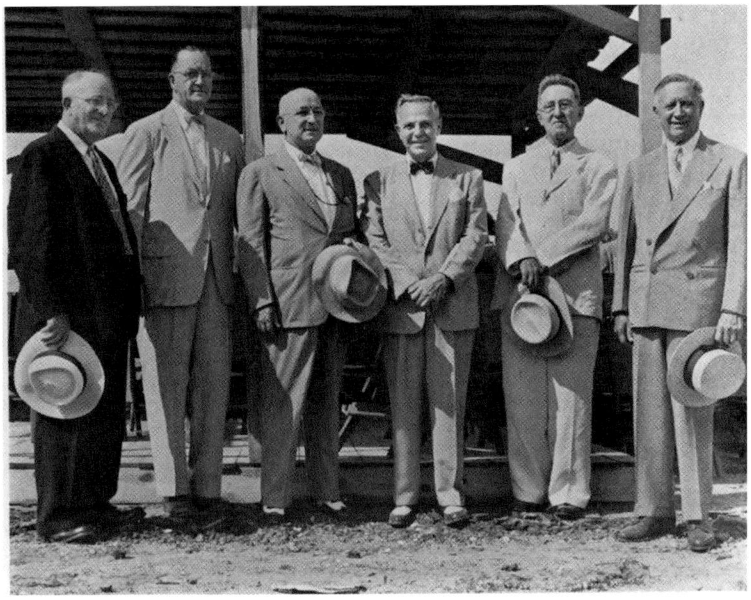

Alton Ochsner flanked by founders and supporters at the July 1952 groundbreaking for the new Foundation Hospital. From Guy A. Caldwell's, *Early History of the Ochsner Medical Center - The First Twenty-two Years*, 1965. Courtesy of Charles C Thomas Publisher, Ltd., Springfield, Illinois.

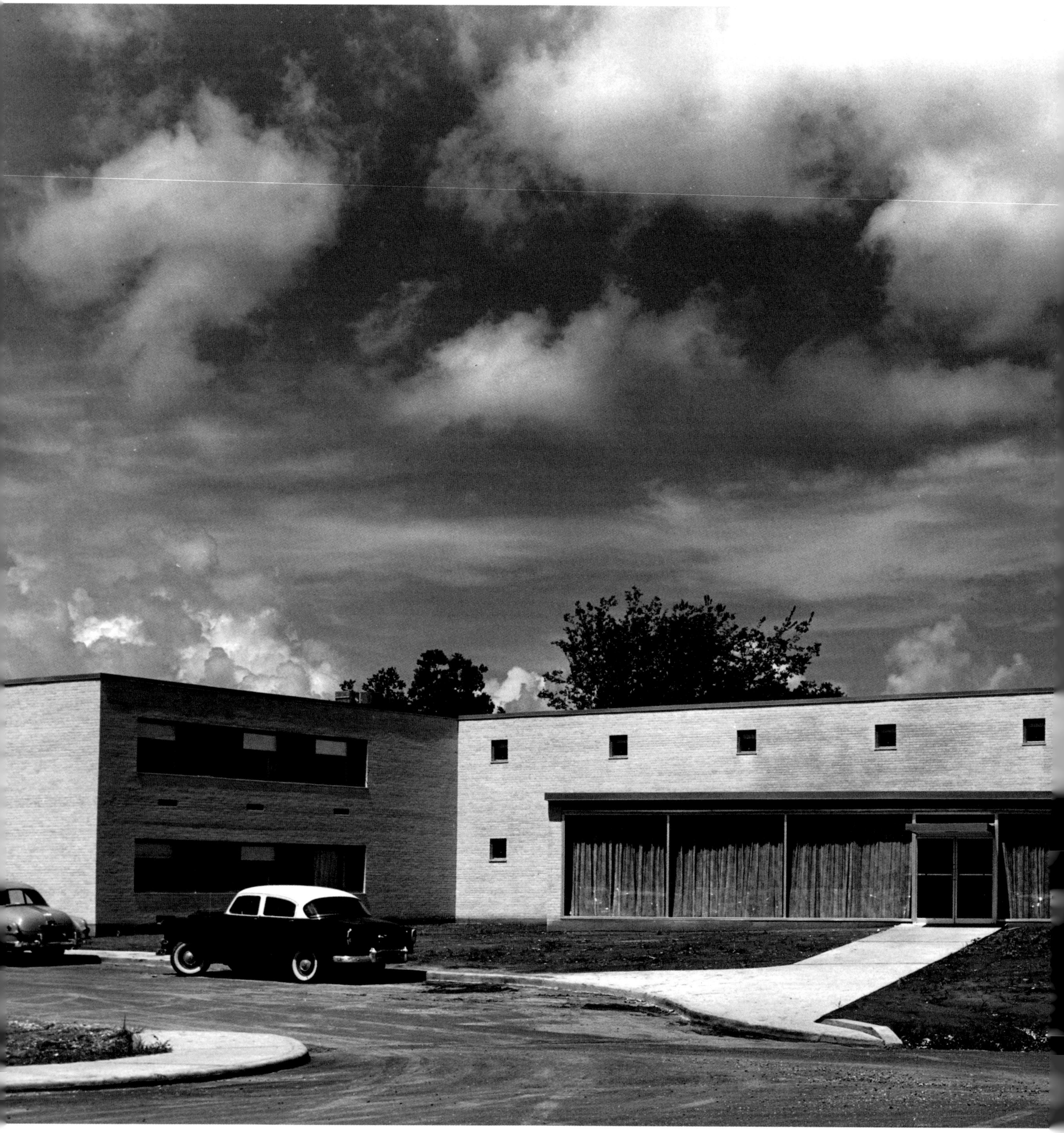

The Libby Dufour Residence housed Ochsner nurses and house staff in an era when the Jefferson Highway campus was considered to be in the far suburbs of New Orleans.

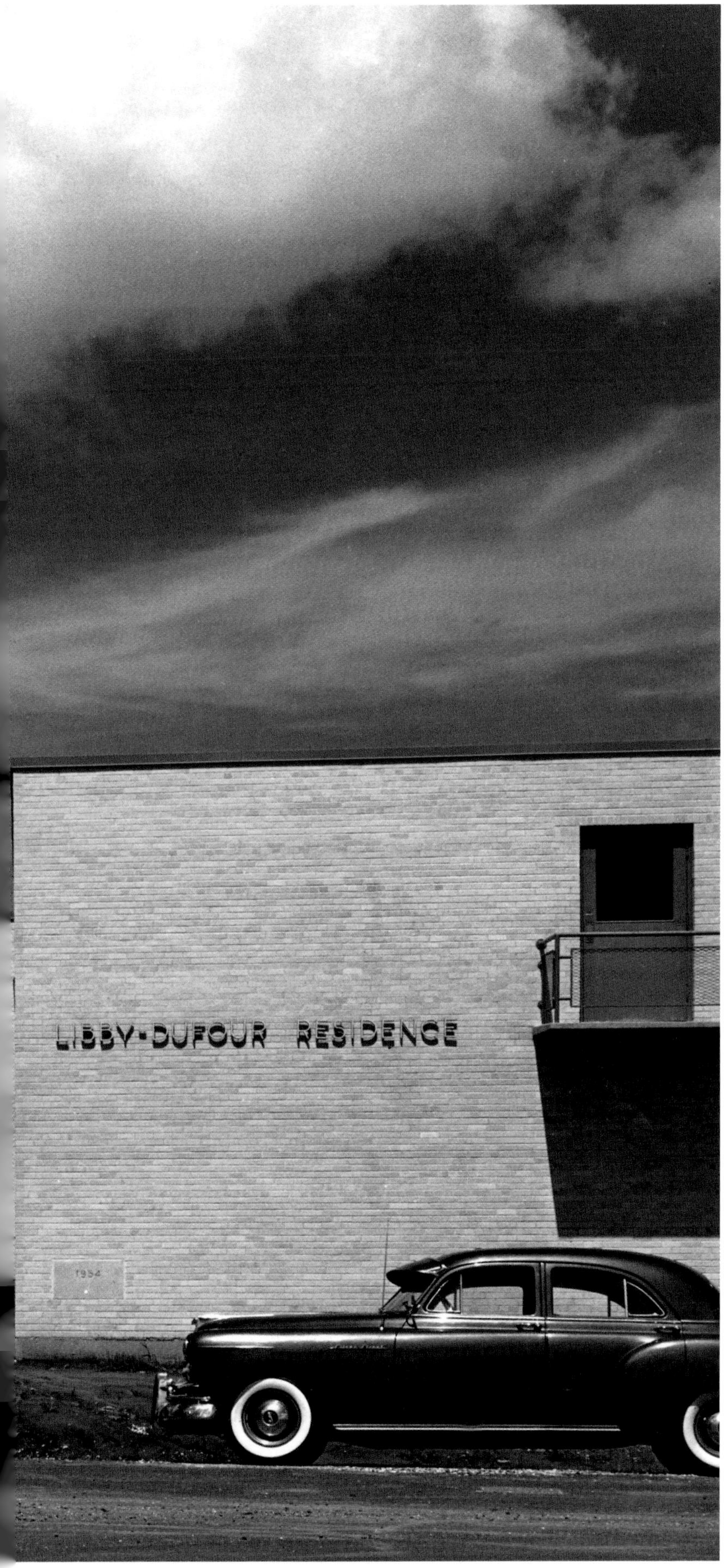

THE CAPTAINS AND THE KINGS DEPART

With the new Hospital under construction, and donations flooding in, the trustees broadened the scope of their mission to provide quality medical care to the people of New Orleans. In early 1953, the trustees asked Ellerbe and Company, the Hospital's architects, to provide estimates for an adjacent Clinic and research building on the riding academy site. Ellerbe quickly reported back that the two buildings could be built and equipped for no more than $2.5 million.[16] In March 1953, the trustees asked Ellerbe to proceed with plans for the two buildings, which would be constructed in the year following completion of the new Hospital.

Two other buildings arose on the Hospital site during the construction phase in 1953–1954. Crews built a $300,000 nurses' residence—later known as the Libby Dufour Residence. Because Jefferson Parish was considered the far suburbs in 1953, and because the trustees expected patients and their families to come to the new Hospital from across Louisiana, Mississippi and east Texas, they decided to build a modern hotel on the Jefferson Highway side of the property.[17]

When Trustee Theodore Brent died in June 1953, his fellow trustees suggested naming the soon-to-be-completed hotel after the New Orleans shipping magnate. Accordingly, the Brent House Hotel has been part of the Ochsner campus ever since.[18] Brent left the bulk of his estate, estimated at more than $1 million, to the Foundation, the largest such bequest in Ochsner history. In a larger sense, Brent's death marked the mid-point of a decade in which some of the more important players in establishing the Clinic and building the Foundation Hospital passed from the scene.

Michael DeBakey's departure was an important loss to the professional staff of Ochsner. The son of a Lebanese immigrant, DeBakey studied under Alton Ochsner at Tulane Medical School during the 1930s and joined the staff of Ochsner Clinic soon after it opened in 1942. After serving as a Colonel in the U.S. Army Medical Corps during World War II, DeBakey returned to New Orleans and Ochsner Clinic in 1945. He had worked closely with Alton Ochsner establishing a link between cigarette smoking and lung cancer and routinely performed surgery at the Foundation Hospital after it opened at Camp Plauché in 1947.[19]

DeBakey's reputation as one of the finest surgeons in the South made him an attractive catch for university hospitals seeking to augment their staffs in postwar America. In 1948, DeBakey agreed to join the faculty of Baylor University Medical School. Baylor was in the process of moving its College of Medicine from Dallas to Houston, and DeBakey had free rein to develop a Cardiovascular Surgery specialty in his new Texas home.[20]

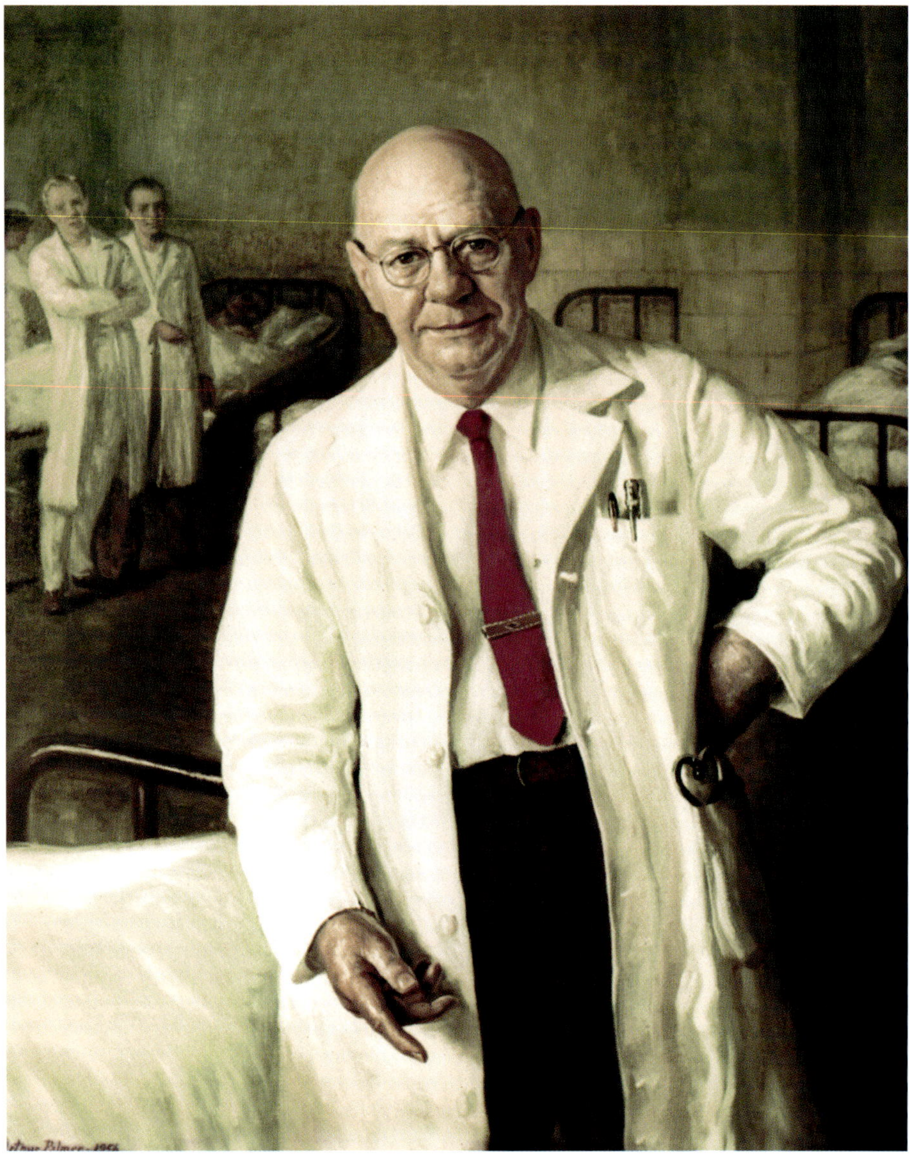

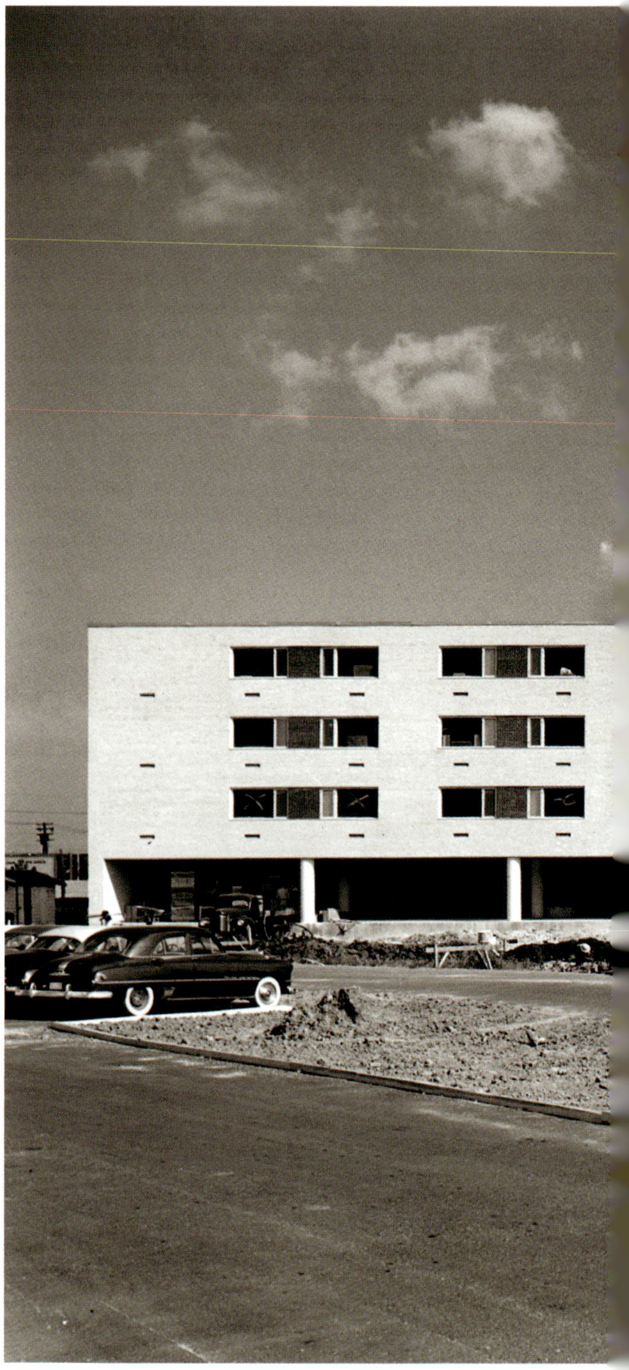

Mims Gage was the first of the original generation of Clinic staffers to pass away, in 1957. His death hit Alton Ochsner particularly hard.

DeBakey, however, never forgot his New Orleans roots. John Ochsner earned his medical degree in 1952 and later went to Houston to train under DeBakey and Denton Cooley, another Texas heart surgery legend. "It was an opportunity to be in the front row of American heart surgery," Ochsner said.[21]

When John Ochsner was growing up, Alton Ochsner's student was always "Mike" DeBakey. When John Ochsner arrived in Houston, it was "Dr. DeBakey," he said, "and I didn't say anything to him but 'yes, sir' and 'no sir.' He was a real taskmaster. He was also the smartest man that I ever knew in my life."[22]

The third Ochsner loss during this period was Alton Ochsner's closest friend. Mims Gage died the week before Christmas 1957 at the young age of 64. Gage befriended Alton Ochsner shortly after he arrived at Tulane in 1927, and the two were inseparable surgical colleagues for 30 years. Gage possessed legendary diagnostic skills and could frequently diagnose a patient's illness just from reading the charts. Proud of his service in both wars, Gage shaped the careers of hundreds of medical students during the 40 years he devoted to Tulane Medical School.[23]

• WHAT OCHSNER MEANS TO ME •

"Ochsner means everything to me. Being here has given me the OPPORTUNITY to work, to serve and to achieve things I otherwise would not have done. I'm eternally grateful."

Betty Wells, Environmental Services, Ochsner Medical Center

To watch the full interview with Betty Wells, visit **ochsner.org/history**.

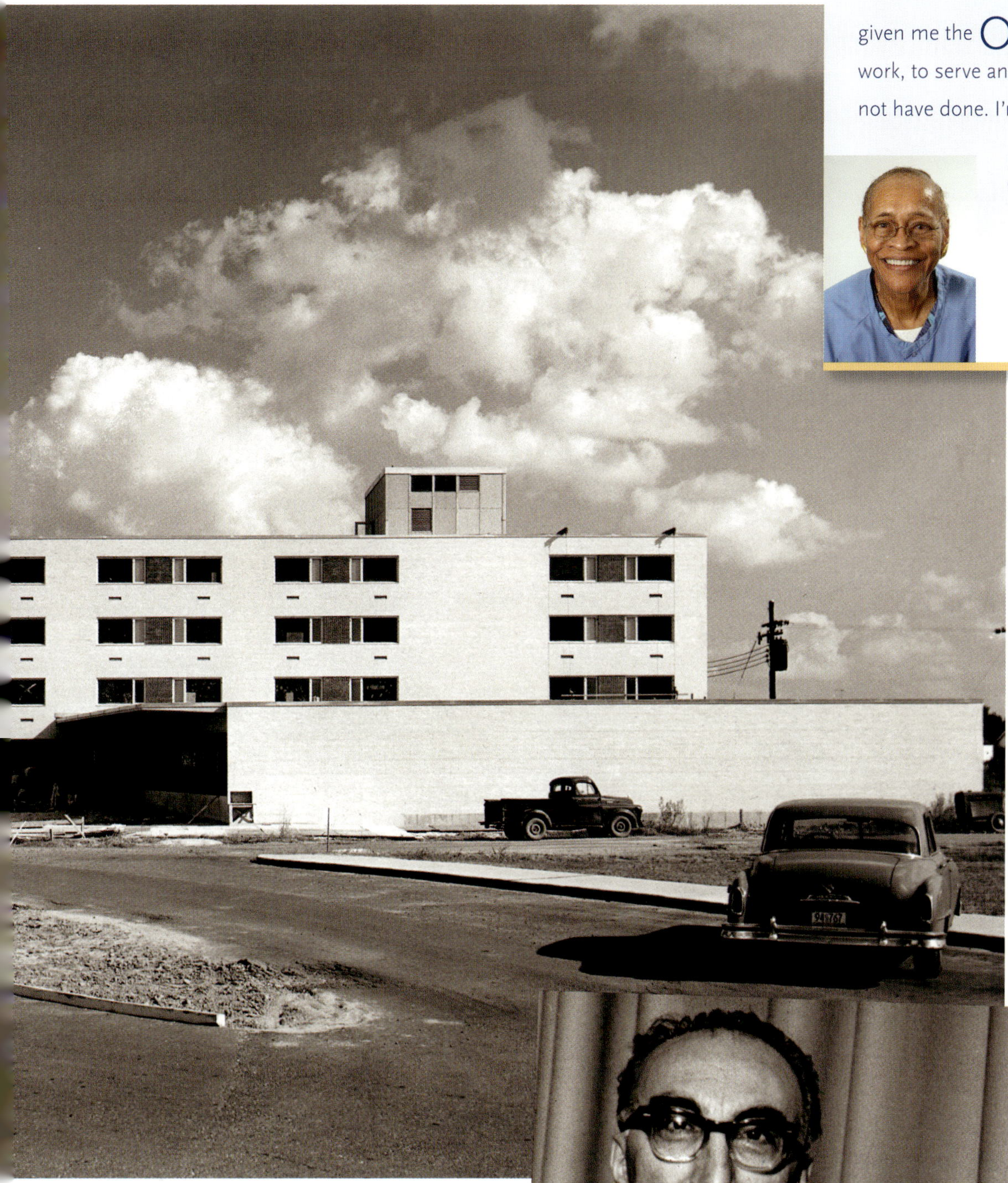

The Brent House Hotel offers first class accommodations for long-term patients and their families, many of whom come from Central and South America.

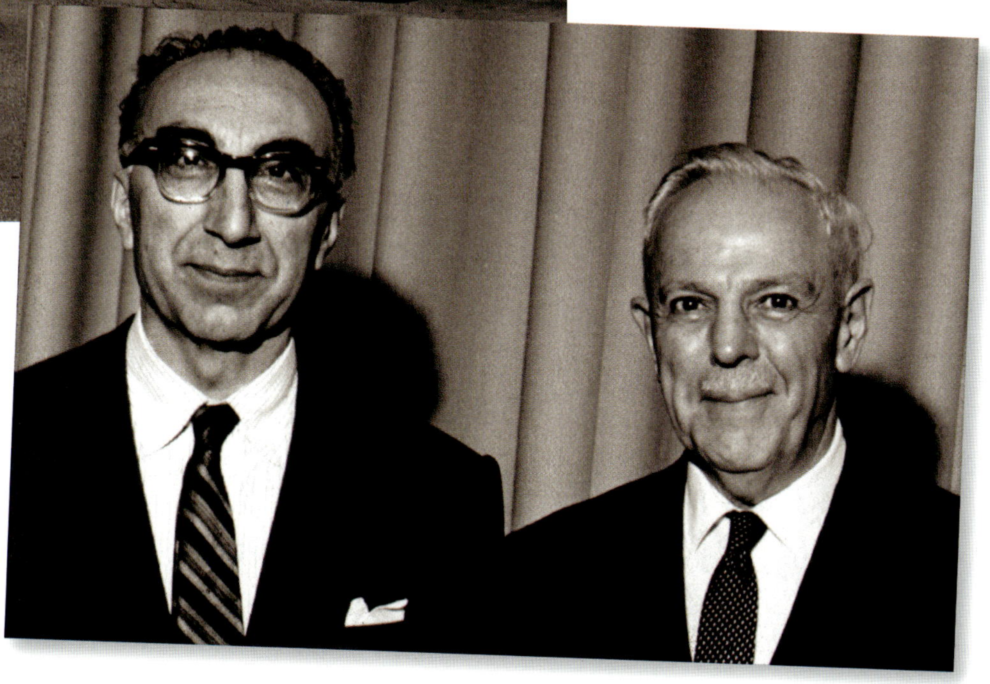

Alton Ochsner was a mentor to Michael DeBakey (pictured left), who went on to establish a reputation as one of America's preeminent heart surgeons and later trained John Ochsner.

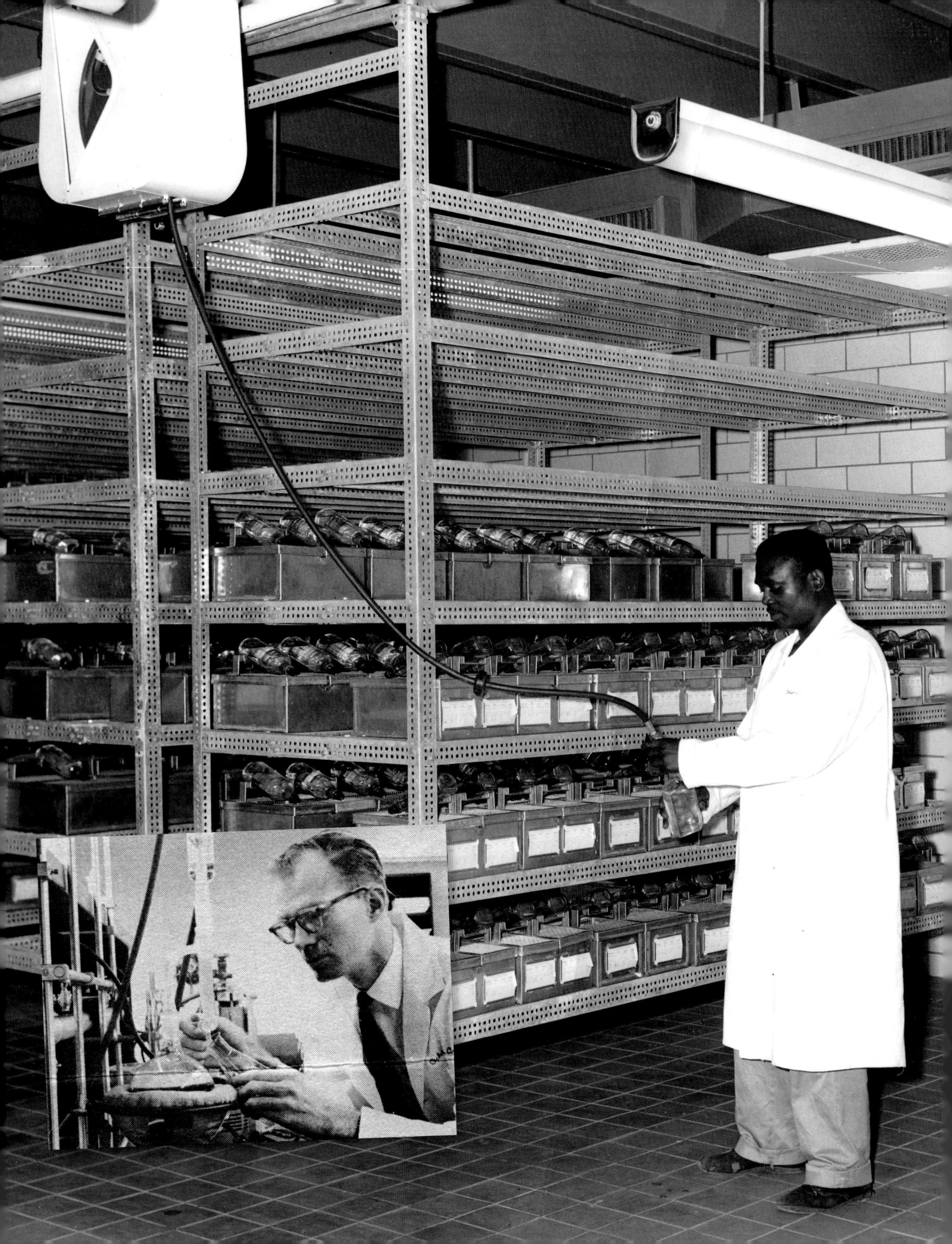

OCHSNER FOUNDATION HOSPITAL

Mims Gage lived long enough to see a modern medical center rise from the scrubland squeezed between Jefferson Highway and the Mississippi River levees. Nurses, medical staff and patients moved to the new Ochsner Foundation Hospital on June 12, 1954. A whirlwind of construction activity transformed the former riding academy property during the next five years.

The Libby Dufour Residence for nurses opened later that summer, providing housing for approximately 92 nurses.[24] In the fall of 1955, Ochsner opened its $750,000 research building, immediately adjacent to the Foundation Hospital. The new building included significant facilities to house small animals for medical research.[25]

After completion of the Brent House Hotel in 1956, two additional floors were added to the structure in 1957. As soon as the addition was completed, the Foundation leased the extra space to Ochsner Clinic, which immediately transferred the General Surgery, Neurosurgery, Orthopedic Surgery, Neurology, Psychiatry, Pediatrics, Allergy and Pulmonary Departments.[26]

The new Research Building on the Jefferson Highway campus in 1959 allowed Ochsner to intensify its research efforts in breast cancer and hypertension. Pictured is a technician.

Inset: Ochsner's research laboratories were an integral part of the organization's mission in the 1950s. Pictured is R. Bruce Gabbard, Ph.D.

FIRST HELIPORT IN THE REGION

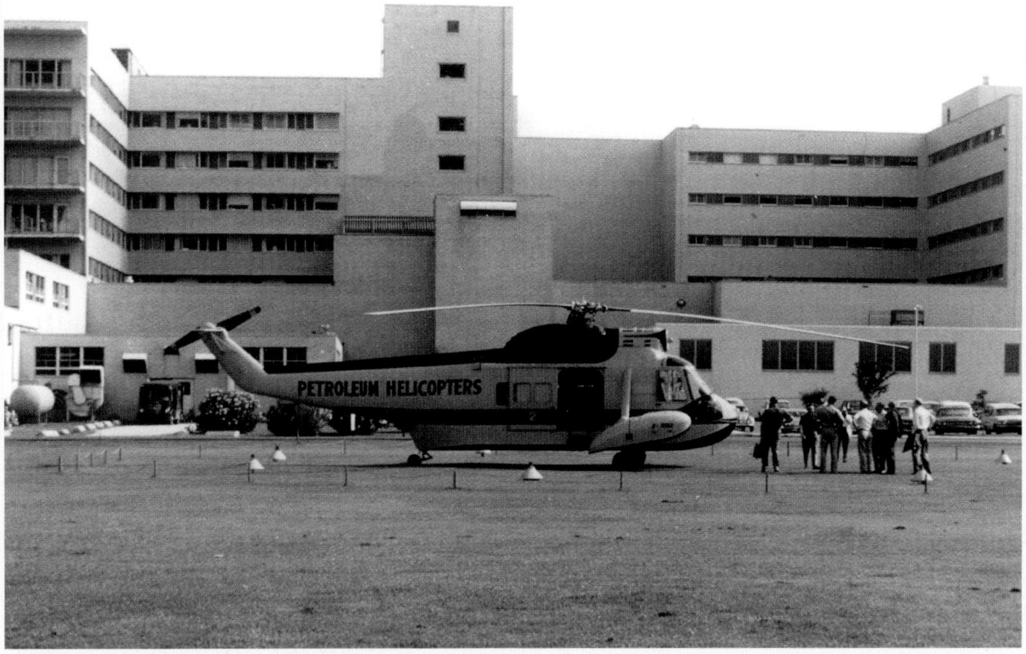

The heliport at the rear of the new Hospital was the first such facility in the New Orleans area.

The Foundation Hospital boasted a first when it opened in 1954: a heliport on the grassy strip between the Hospital and the Mississippi River levee. The U.S. military pioneered the use of helicopters in combat in Korea from 1950 to 1953, and civilian contractors were quick to realize the potential of a type of aircraft that did not need a runway to take off and land.

Companies servicing offshore oil and gas platforms were among the first firms to take advantage of a helicopter's ability to hover and land in tight, confined spaces. Oil and gas rigs in the Gulf of Mexico offshore from Louisiana and Texas used helicopters to ferry crews and supplies back and forth from the mainland to the oil and gas platforms.

Petroleum Helicopters, Inc. approached the Foundation Hospital about the possibility of constructing a heliport behind the facility. The firm offered to pay for construction of the heliport and agreed to station a helicopter at the Hospital.[27]

Events quickly proved the wisdom of the establishment of the heliport. On October 15, 1958, a flash fire broke out on Offshore Drilling Platform 45-E in the West Delta Block, Gulf of Mexico, south of New Orleans. Operated by Continental Oil Company, the steel platform housed a crew of 29 men.[28]

The explosion and resulting fire killed one man outright and blew six crew members into the water, none of whose bodies were recovered. The remaining 22 crew members evacuated the platform aboard helicopters to the heliport behind the Foundation Hospital. The helicopter crew radioed ahead, and emergency staff awaited the injured. All of the injured platform crew received treatment for injuries within 90 minutes of the explosion.[29] The establishment of the heliport was a signal to the community the Foundation Hospital intended to stress innovation when delivering medical care to New Orleans.

As research continued, the first edition of *Ochsner Clinic Reports* came out in 1955.

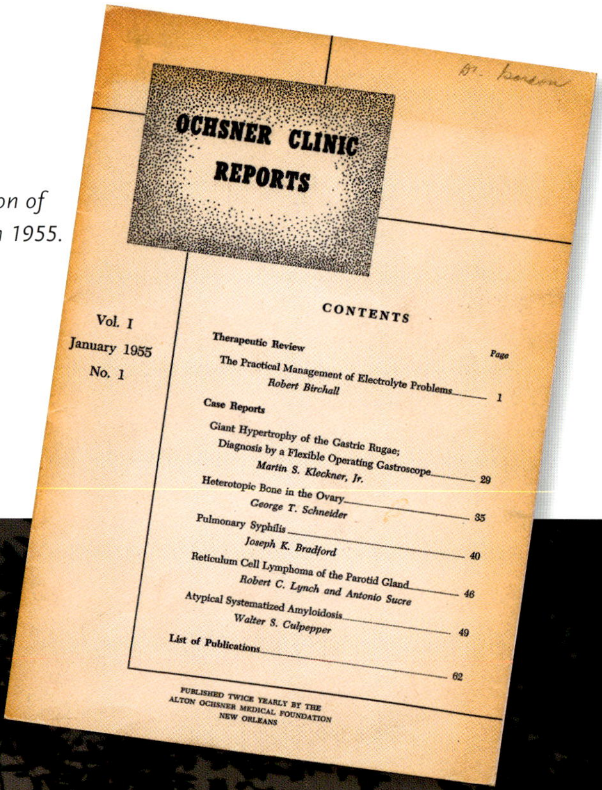

OCHSNER CLINIC
REPORTS

Vol. I
January 1955
No. 1

CONTENTS

Therapeutic Review — Page
The Practical Management of Electrolyte Problems — 1
Robert Birchall

Case Reports
Giant Hypertrophy of the Gastric Rugae; Diagnosis by a Flexible Operating Gastroscope — 29
Martin S. Kleckner, Jr.
Heterotopic Bone in the Ovary — 35
George T. Schneider
Pulmonary Syphilis — 40
Joseph K. Bradford
Reticulum Cell Lymphoma of the Parotid Gland — 46
Robert C. Lynch and Antonio Sucre
Atypical Systematized Amyloidosis — 49
Walter S. Culpepper
List of Publications — 62

PUBLISHED TWICE YEARLY BY THE
ALTON OCHSNER MEDICAL FOUNDATION
NEW ORLEANS

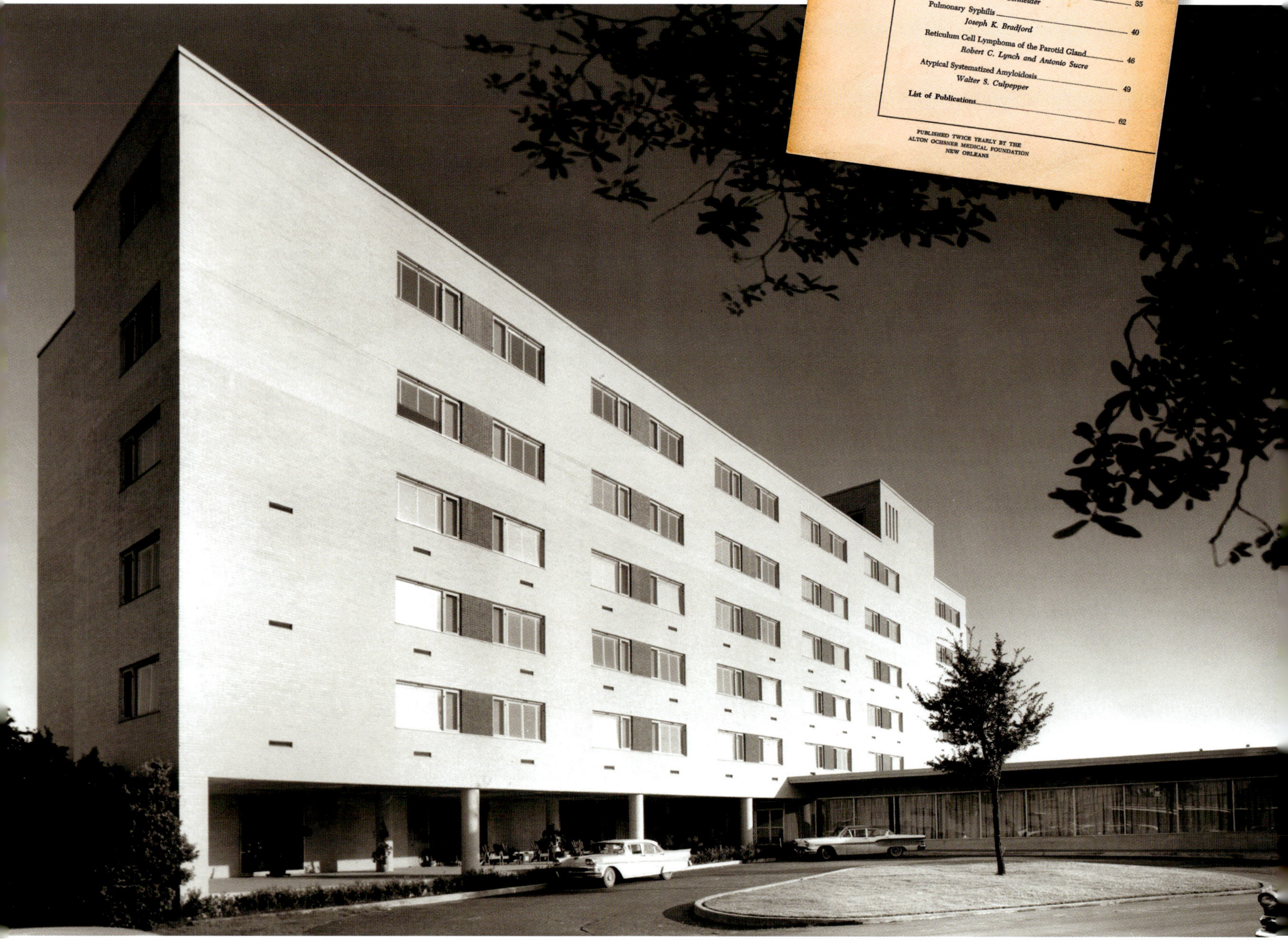

The Brent House Hotel added two floors in 1957 and leased them to Ochsner Clinic, which used the space for physicians' offices.

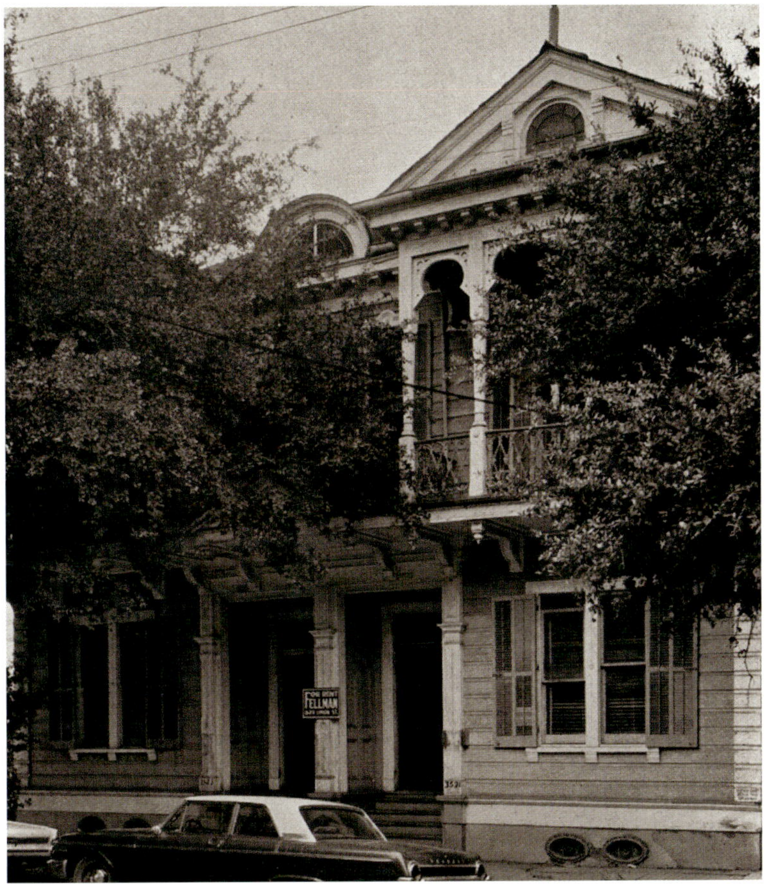

Ochsner Clinic leased the former Rudolph Matas office at 3521 Prytania Street for record storage. From Guy A. Caldwell's, *Early History of the Ochsner Medical Center - The First Twenty-two Years*, 1965. Courtesy of Charles C Thomas Publisher, Ltd., Springfield, Illinois.

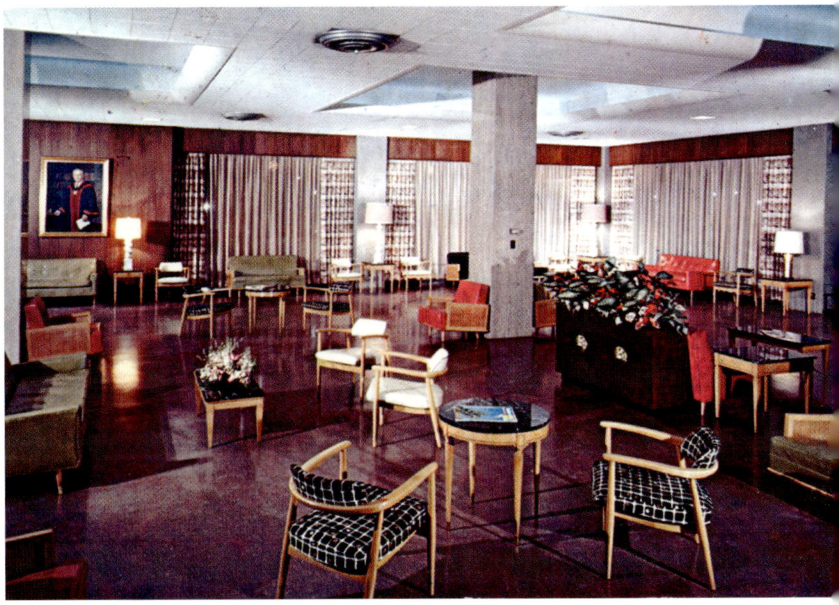

The Foundation Hospital lobby was a brightly lit, welcoming place in 1955.

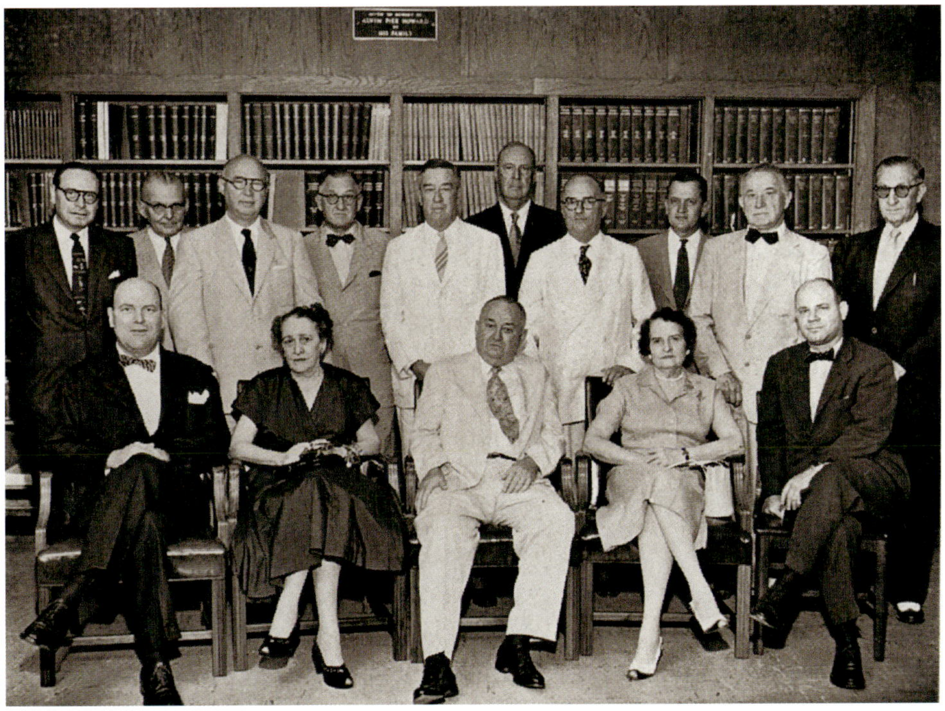

The First Board of Governors of the Ochsner Foundation Hospital. From Guy A. Caldwell's, *Early History of the Ochsner Medical Center - The First Twenty-two Years*, 1965. Courtesy of Charles C Thomas Publisher, Ltd., Springfield, Illinois.

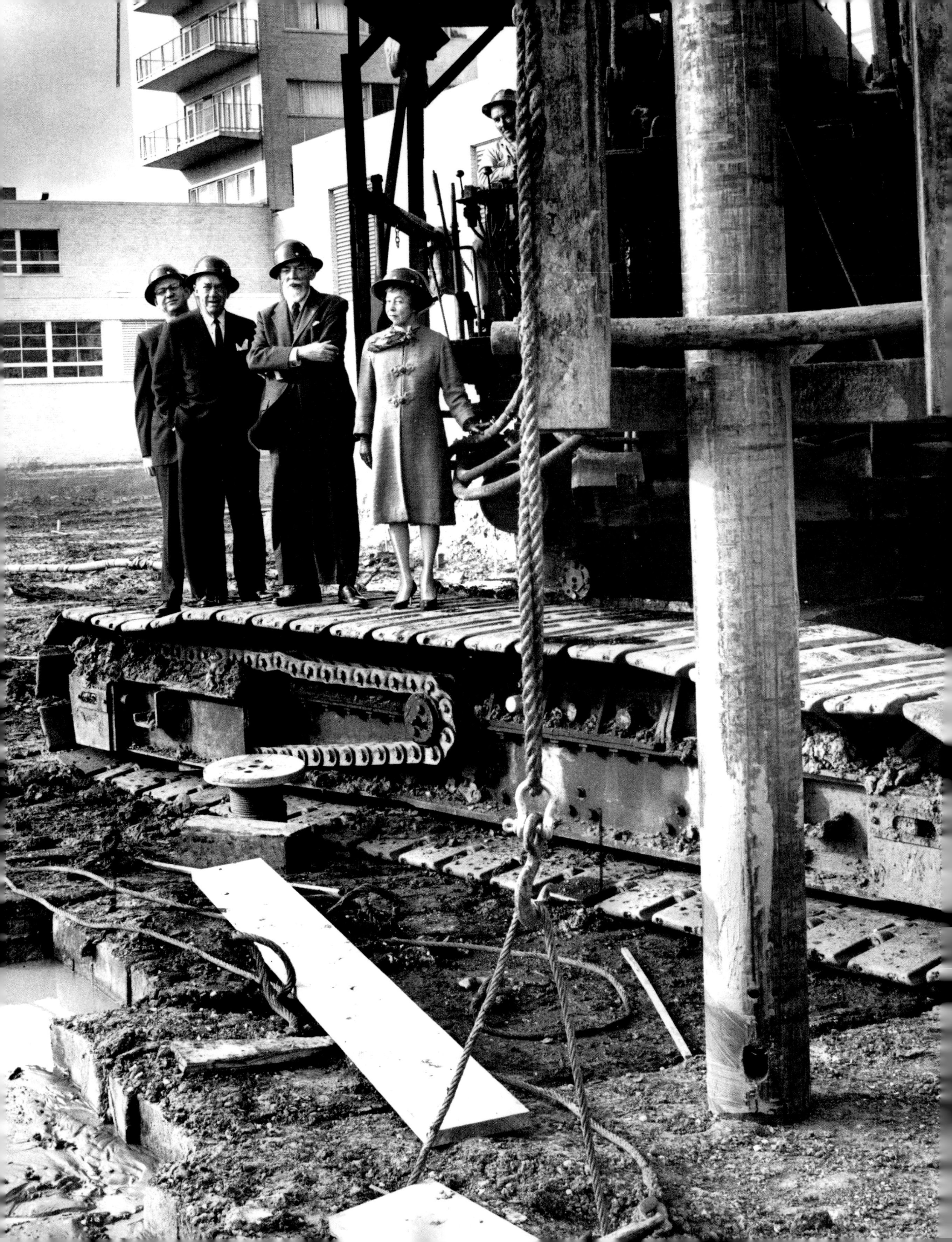

CHAPTER 4:

EXPANDING THE ART OF HEALING

THE OPENING OF THE OCHSNER FOUNDATION HOSPITAL during the mid-1950s on a site fronting Jefferson Highway spurred a flurry of development in the east end of Jefferson Parish. Worries that the hospital would be too far removed from New Orleans evaporated as businesses developed along a stretch of U.S. 90 that had once been considered a country highway.

Buoyed by the community's welcoming reception, Foundation trustees expanded the Jefferson Highway campus by building a research building, nurses' residence, hotel and other facilities. The campus took one of its most important steps in 1959 when the Clinic trustees committed to building a new Clinic building adjacent to the Foundation Hospital. The move of Ochsner Clinic to the Jefferson Highway campus created a full-service medical complex that catered to patients from New Orleans, much of south Louisiana and as far away as Texas and the Mississippi Gulf Coast.

Ochsner Clinic and Ochsner Foundation Hospital pioneered advanced medicine in south Louisiana during the 1960s and 1970s. Ochsner physicians began performing heart valve replacements, a technique that would lead to developing the Hospital's expertise in coronary artery bypass surgery during the following decade. Radiation Oncologists used one of the South's first rotational cobalt therapy units to treat tumors. Ochsner became synonymous with medical excellence in the Gulf South region.

Mrs. Rawley M. Penick, the widow of the distinguished surgeon whose name graces the Rawley M. Penick Memorial Pavilion, at the 1966 groundbreaking for the Pavilion.

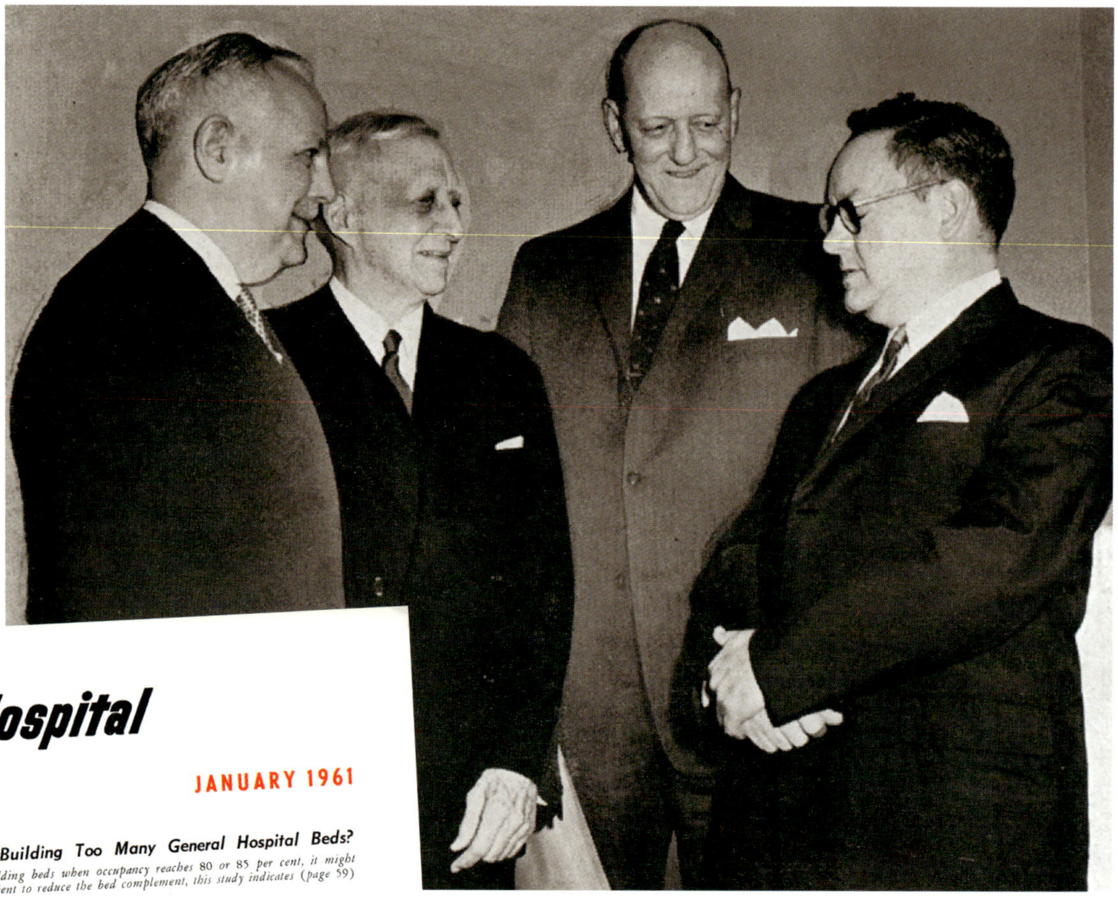

Alton Ochsner confers with colleagues at the dedication of the Research Building in 1959; Ochsner and the founders had long believed that research along with patient care and education was an integral part of Ochsner Clinic. From Guy A. Caldwell's, *Early History of the Ochsner Medical Center - The First Twenty-two Years*, 1965. Courtesy of Charles C Thomas Publisher, Ltd., Springfield, Illinois.

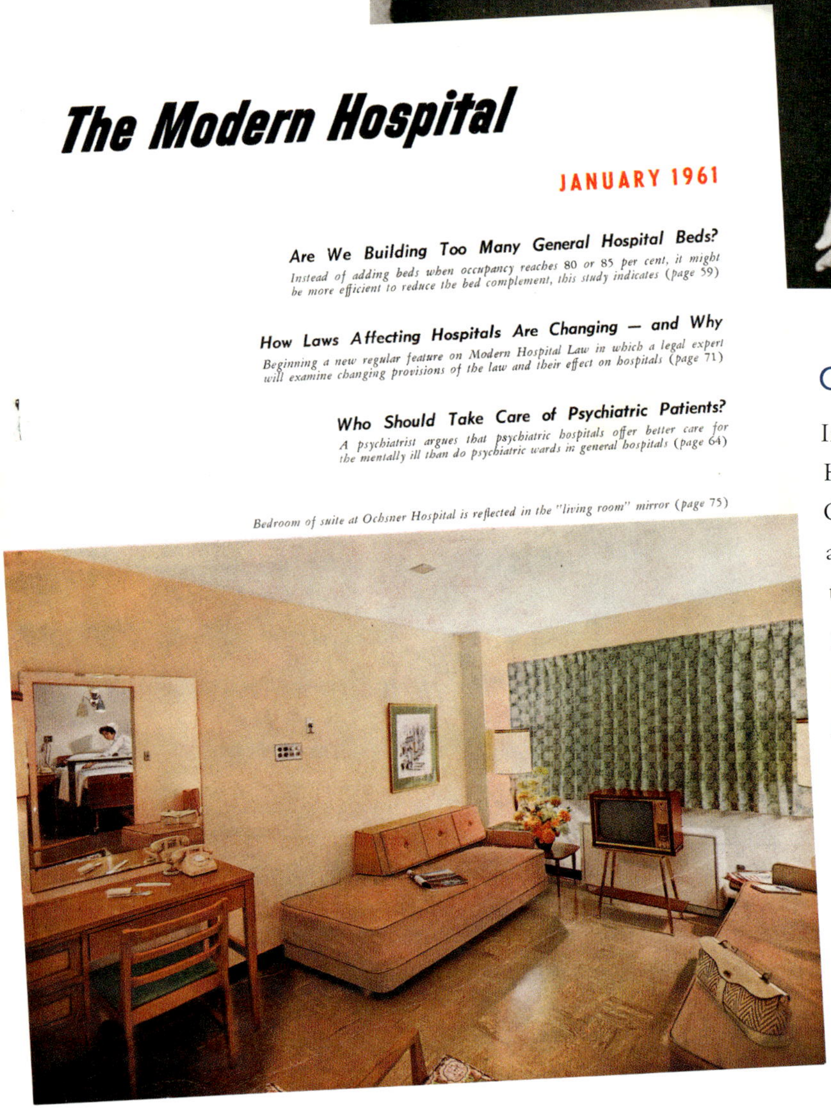

The Modern Hospital

JANUARY 1961

Are We Building Too Many General Hospital Beds?
Instead of adding beds when occupancy reaches 80 or 85 per cent, it might be more efficient to reduce the bed complement, this study indicates (page 59)

How Laws Affecting Hospitals Are Changing — and Why
Beginning a new regular feature on Modern Hospital Law in which a legal expert will examine changing provisions of the law and their effect on hospitals (page 71)

Who Should Take Care of Psychiatric Patients?
A psychiatrist argues that psychiatric hospitals offer better care for the mentally ill than do psychiatric wards in general hospitals (page 64)

Bedroom of suite at Ochsner Hospital is reflected in the "living room" mirror (page 75)

ONE MAJOR DISADVANTAGE

In late 1960, the Foundation added two floors to the 1954 Hospital, bringing the total number of beds to 362. Guy Caldwell successfully petitioned the federal government for a grant of 25 percent of the $1.8 million construction cost through the use of Hill-Burton funds.[1]

By 1961, Ochsner Foundation Hospital trailed only Touro Infirmary and Southern Baptist Hospital in size among local private hospitals. Ochsner, however, labored under one major disadvantage compared to the other two: it did not have an attached medical office building to house doctors' offices.

A suite at the Foundation Hospital appears on the cover of the January 1961 issue of The Modern Hospital.

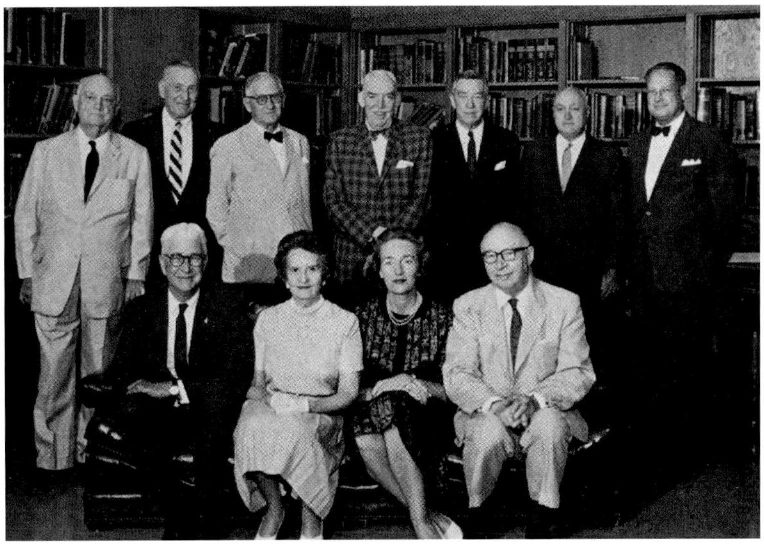

The Board of Governors of the Foundation Hospital in 1964 was responsible solely for the operation of the Hospital. The divided nature of Clinic, Foundation and Hospital governance would cause organizational challenges for Ochsner for years. From Guy A. Caldwell's, *Early History of the Ochsner Medical Center - The First Twenty-two Years*, 1965. Courtesy of Charles C Thomas Publisher, Ltd., Springfield, Illinois.

Alton Ochsner and several departments of Ochsner Clinic moved into the top two floors of the Brent House Hotel in 1957, but the addition of more than 100 beds at the Foundation Hospital created more of a demand for Clinic physicians. The decision to more closely align the offerings of the Hospital and the Clinic represented a sizable risk on Ochsner's part, but one that would be rewarded by growing community support for both the Hospital and the Clinic.

Foundation trustees awarded a nearly $3.5 million bid for construction of a six-story Clinic building adjacent to the Foundation Hospital in May 1961.[2] Ochsner Clinic doctors practiced great medicine, but they did not make much money. That had been a fact of life since the Clinic opened in 1942. The difficulty of non-competitive salaries caused a minor revolt among junior Clinic physicians in the mid-1950s. As a result, the Clinic broadened the original partnership in 1957. The five founders retained half of the ownership of the Clinic and agreed to phase out their ownership over a period of years. Physicians who had accumulated five years of service were eligible to buy a partnership share.[3]

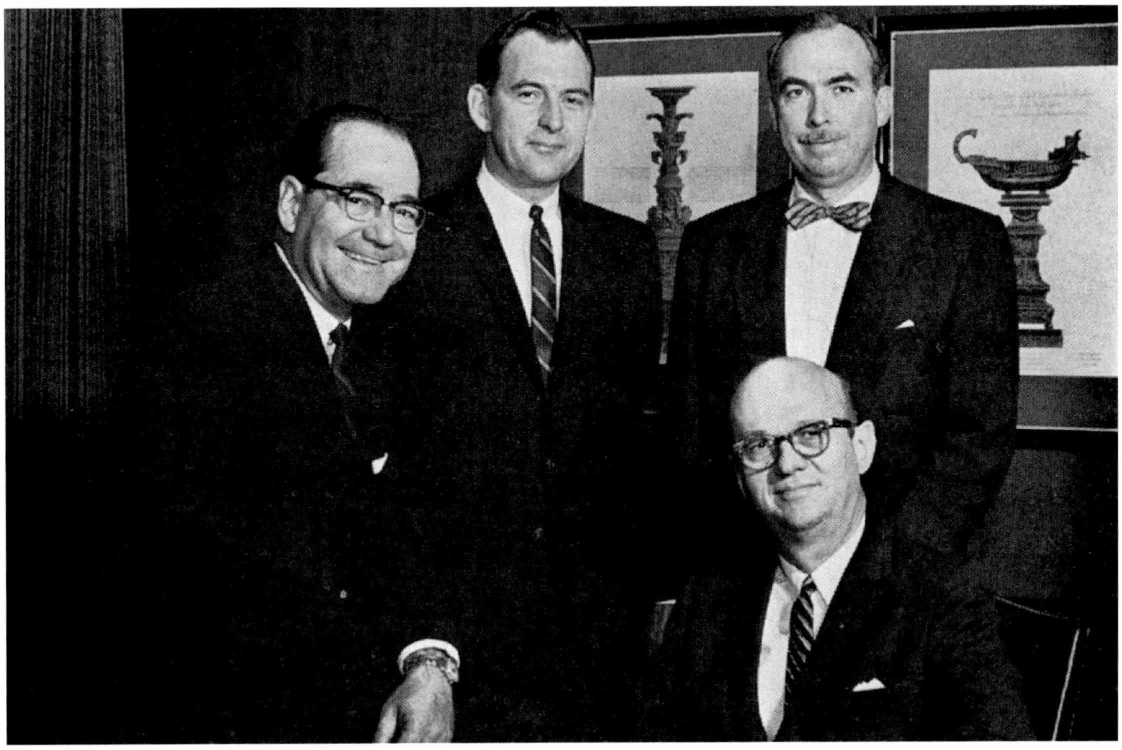

The administrative officers of Ochsner Clinic in 1963. Former FBI Agent Edgar J. Saux helped guide the Clinic's affairs for years. From Guy A. Caldwell's, *Early History of the Ochsner Medical Center - The First Twenty-two Years*, 1965. Courtesy of Charles C Thomas Publisher, Ltd., Springfield, Illinois.

THE EDGAR SAUX LEGACY

Finding the nearly $3.5 million needed to build a new Clinic building at the Jefferson Highway campus posed huge problems for the trustees. The only money the Foundation could put together for a down payment was the revenue from the sale of the old Clinic building, and that was estimated to be less than $700,000.

Clinic administrator Edgar Saux reported that the Clinic's revenue could increase to as much as $5 million a year in a new facility on the Jefferson Highway campus, which would allow the Foundation to borrow for a new building.[4] Saux, a former FBI agent appointed Clinic Business Manager in 1951, capably oversaw the Clinic's financial affairs for nearly 30 years. At his interview, he told Duke LeJeune Sr. he couldn't even pronounce "Otolaryngologist," but Saux quickly learned the ins and outs of the medical business and proved to be one of the best hires the Clinic ever made.[5]

Francis LeJeune Sr. (third from left) accepts a check for $2.675 million to close the loan for the new Clinic building, already under construction on the Jefferson Highway campus.

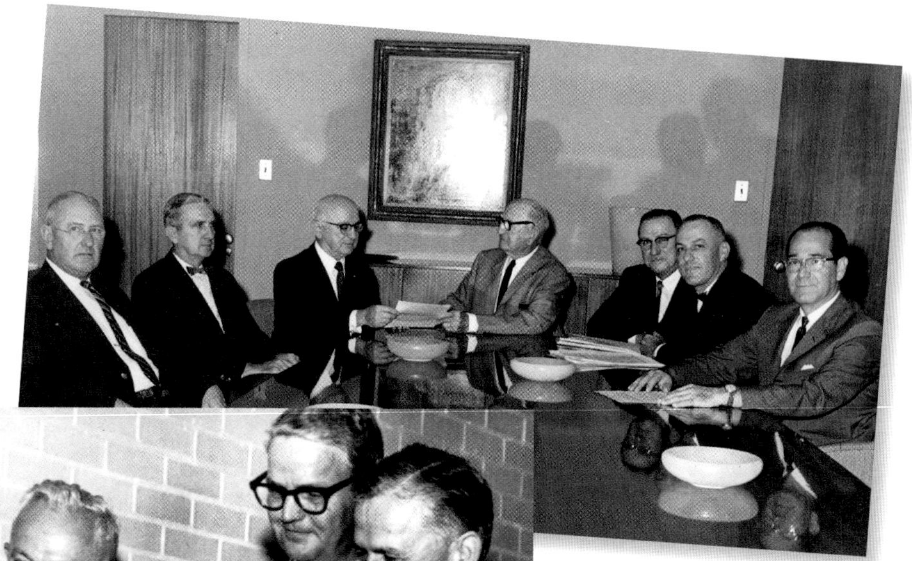

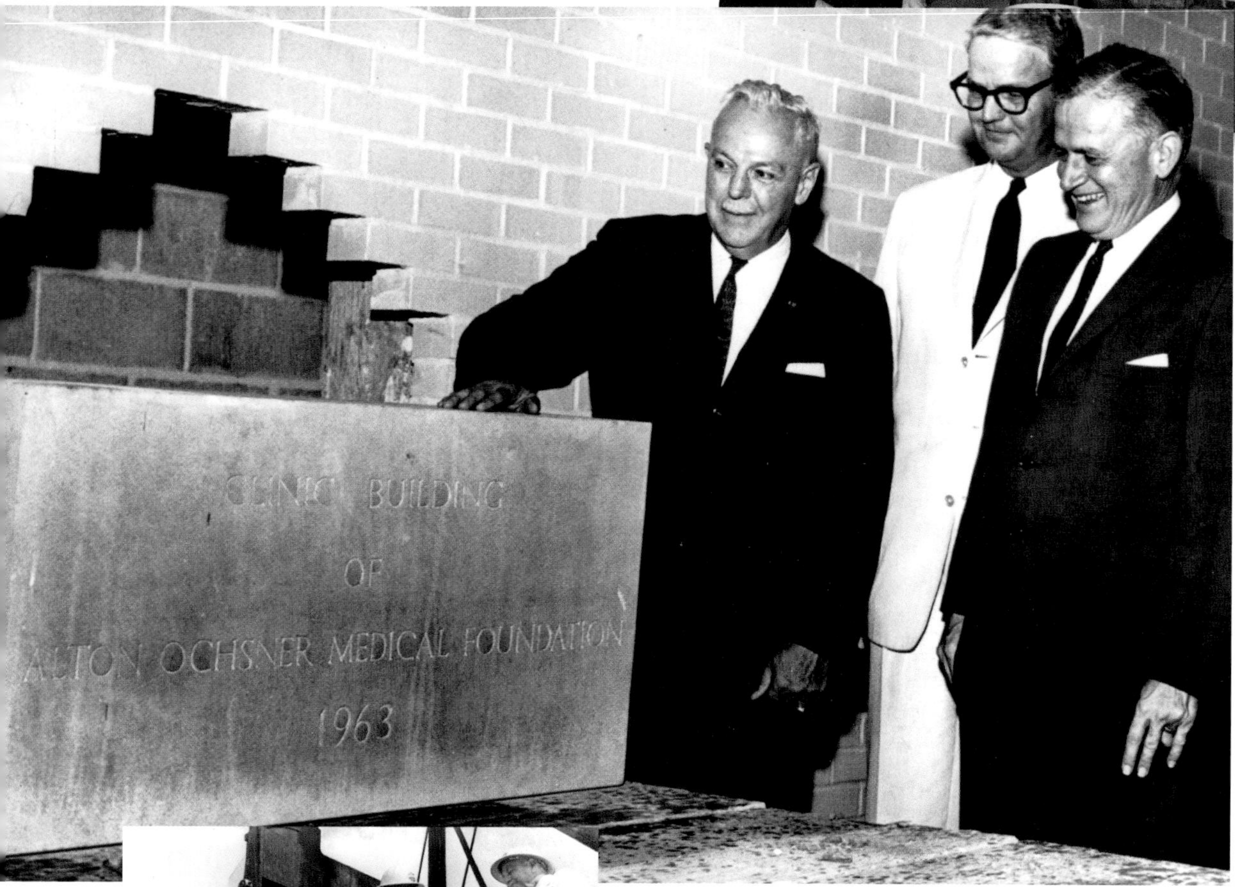

Alton Ochsner, Richard Freeman Sr. and Malcolm Monroe examine the cornerstone for the new Clinic building at the 1961 groundbreaking.

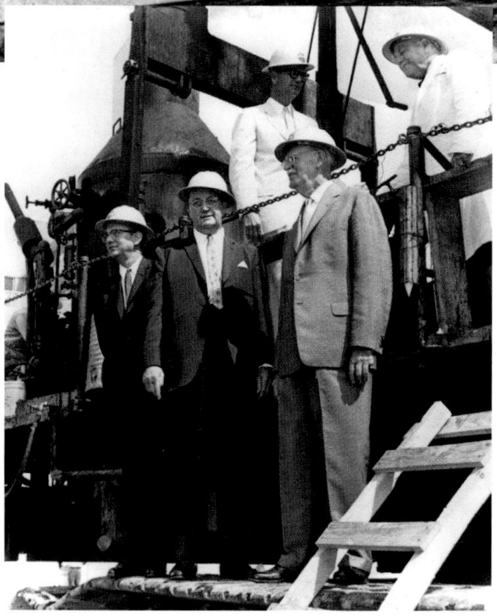

Alton Ochsner, top right, oversees driving the first piling for the new Clinic building.

RACE TO COMPLETION

Guy Caldwell, whose aptitude for business made him the *de facto* Clinic Manager, had tapped into a group of Texas oilmen through his treatment of Dallas oil tycoon Clint Murchison. Murchison and his associates, including Sid Richardson and Perry R. Bass, donated a West Virginia horseracing track to help fund the new Clinic.

Pan American Life Insurance Company stepped in with a mortgage loan for the new Clinic building, and the founders helped place the cornerstone of the new building in September 1961, 20 years after buying the Physicians and Surgeons Building on the corner of Prytania and Aline streets.[6]

Eighteen months later, on March 18, 1963, the new Clinic opened for business. Movers spent the previous week loading and unloading five moving vans each day, working from dawn until 10:30 at night. The 19 people on the staff of the Clinic when Alton Ochsner and the other founders opened for business in January 1942 had nearly quintupled by 1963.

Ochsner Clinic opened its new facilities at the Jefferson Highway campus in 1963, joining the Foundation Hospital that had opened in Jefferson Parish the decade before.

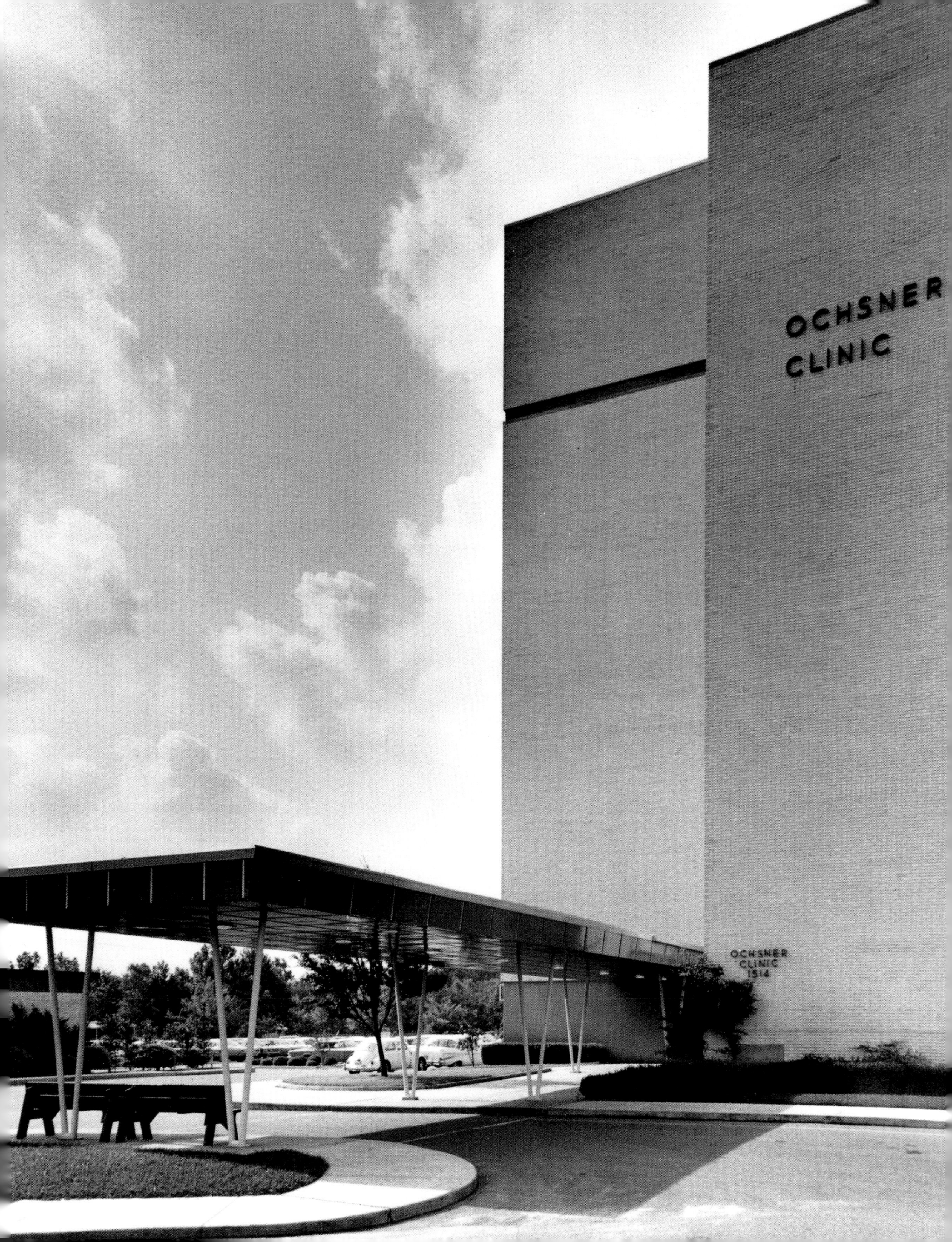
OCHSNER
CLINIC
OCHSNER
CLINIC
1514

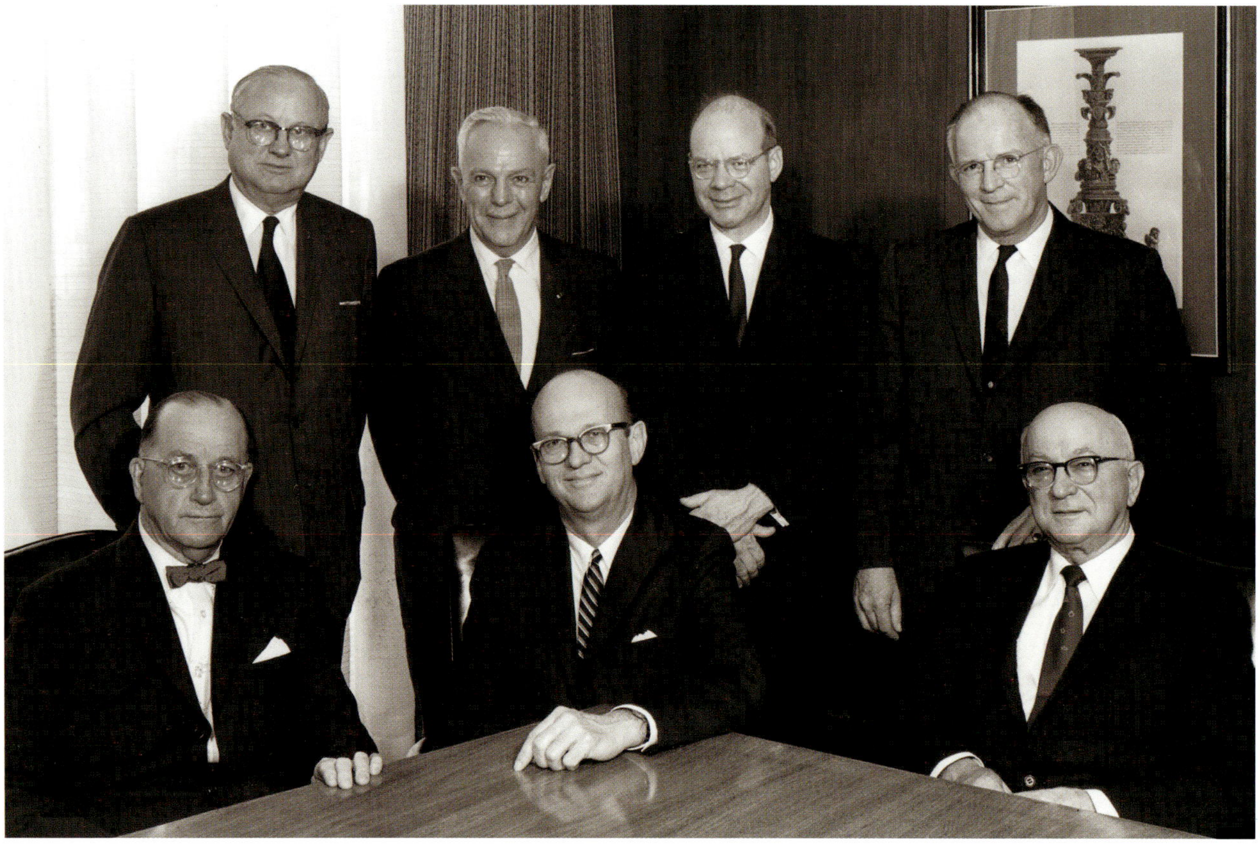

The Clinic Board of Management in 1963. Seated left to right are Burns, Hines and Francis LeJeune Sr. Standing left to right are Tyrone, Ochsner, William Davis and William Arrowsmith.

• WHAT OCHSNER MEANS TO ME •

"Over the past several years, I've become involved with mission programs in which Ochsner physicians SERVE in other countries like Central and South America and Africa. Despite what some people feel are inadequacies in the U.S. healthcare system, my experience has made me realize just how fortunate we are to have this advanced level of care."

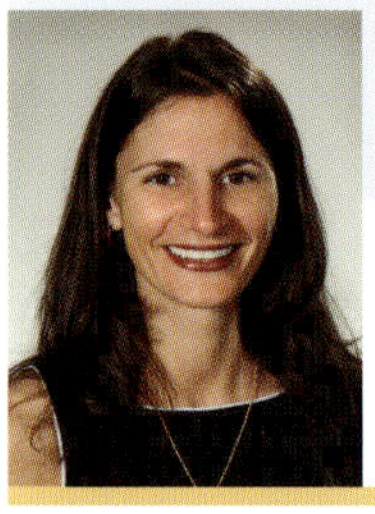

Dr. Lisa Bazzett-Matabele, Gynecologic Oncologist, Ochsner Medical Center

To watch the full interview with Dr. Lisa Bazzett-Matabele, visit **ochsner.org/history**.

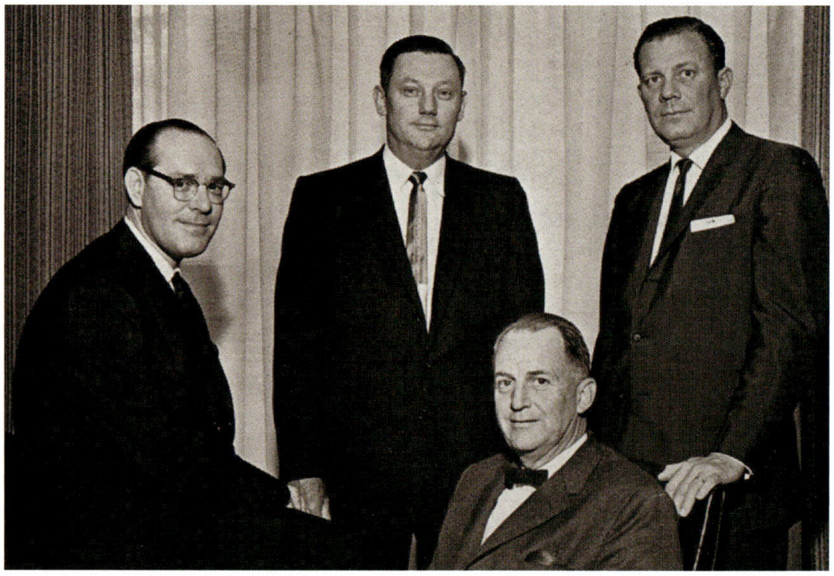

Horace E. Hamilton, Director of the Ochsner Foundation Hospital (seated at center), is surrounded by his administrative staff in 1963. From Guy A. Caldwell's, *Early History of the Ochsner Medical Center - The First Twenty-two Years*, 1965. Courtesy of Charles C Thomas Publisher, Ltd., Springfield, Illinois.

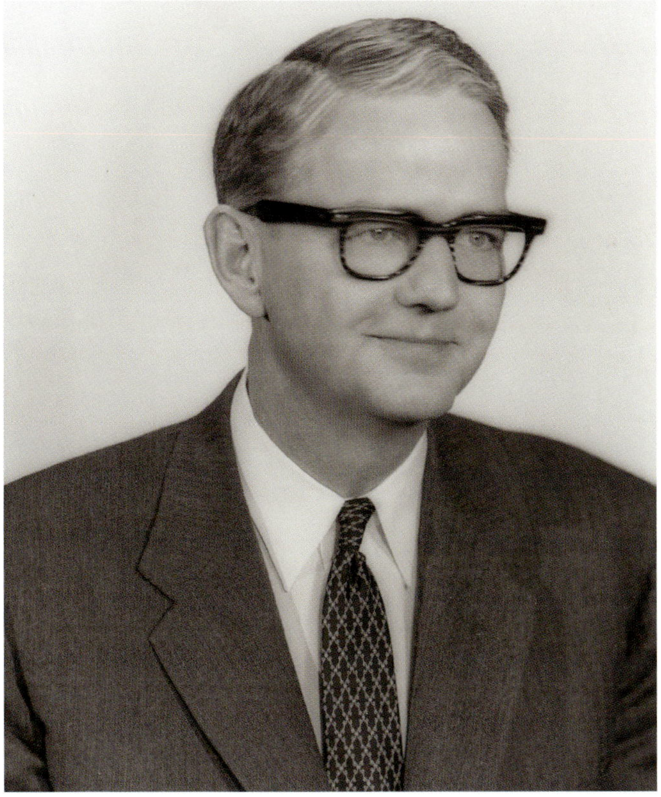

Richard "Dick" Freeman Sr.'s business acumen as Chairman of the Foundation Board of Trustees and Head of Finance helped Ochsner during the expansion years of the 1960s and 1970s.

OLD BLOOD AND SECOND GENERATION

Several veterans of the Ochsner institutions were not around to see the Clinic and the Foundation Hospital united on the Jefferson Highway campus. J. Blanc Monroe, whose steady hand had helped guide the Foundation since its inception in 1944, died in New Orleans at the age of 80 in 1960.[7]

Mercer Lynch, who joined the Clinic's then Department of Otorhinolaryngology following his return from military duty in 1946, died at the young age of 52 in February 1960. Edward Leveroos, who accepted the position of Director of the Foundation Hospital in 1956, passed away in June 1960, one week past his 50th birthday.[8] Edmund E. Richardson, a member of the Hospital's Board of Governors, died in March 1962.[9]

New Orleans attorney Malcolm L. Monroe succeeded his father, J. Blanc Monroe, on the Board of Trustees of the Alton Ochsner Medical Foundation during the spring of 1960. Richard W. "Dick" Freeman Sr., who had succeeded Theodore Brent on the Board of Trustees, emerged as a solid leader. Chairman of the Louisiana Coca-Cola Bottling Company, Freeman guided the Foundation with a capable hand during the 1960s.[10]

Guy Caldwell's retirement as Ochsner Clinic Medical Director in 1960 brought another second-generation leader to the fore. Dr. Merrill Hines studied under Alton Ochsner at Tulane during the 1930s and returned to Ochsner Clinic following service in World War II. He helped the Clinic develop its Colon and Rectal Surgery Department during the late 1940s and became a leader nationally in the emerging field of Proctology. Hines revealed his capacity for clinic administration in 1954 when he was named Clinic Assistant Medical Director. Six years later, he succeeded Caldwell as Clinic Medical Director, a position he held for the next 15 years.[11]

Alton Ochsner's three sons joined their father in practice at the Clinic during the early 1960s. Alton Jr. "Akky," John and Mims Ochsner all elected to return to New Orleans. John reluctantly told Michael DeBakey in 1961 that he was going to leave Houston and go home. "My wife didn't want to leave," he said. "I was making $38,000 a year on DeBakey's staff."[12]

John Ochsner did return to New Orleans and never regretted a minute. "I put in more hours at less money," he said. "It was the most fun I ever had in my life. Everything was new. Every operation that we did was new."[13] John Ochsner brought with him DeBakey's expertise in cardiovascular surgery. During the 1960s, Ochsner and the Foundation Hospital developed a reputation for skill in repairing heart valves. A surgical proficiency in open heart surgery led to advances in coronary bypass operations at the Hospital by the early 1970s that allowed local residents to receive top quality cardiology care close to home.

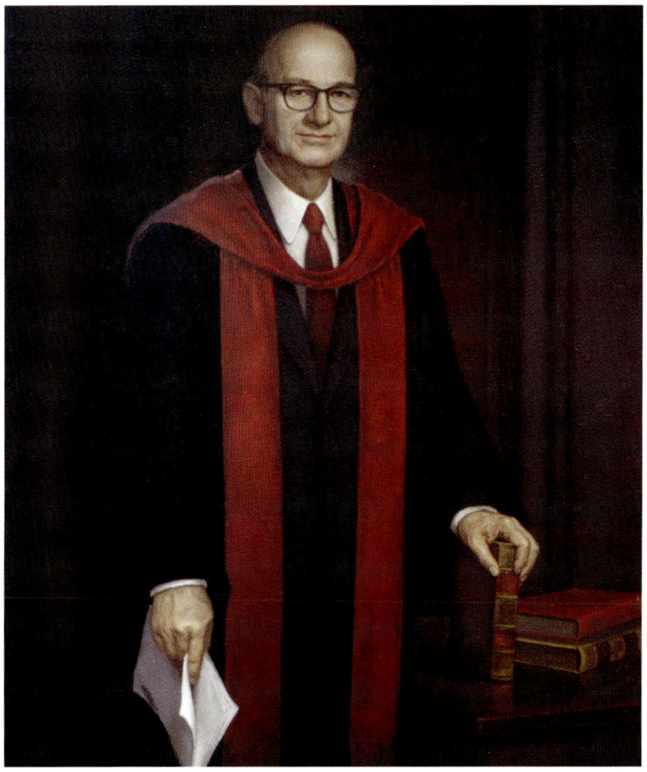

Merrill Hines was Medical Director of Ochsner Clinic from 1959–1975 and later served as Chairman of the Foundation's Board of Trustees and President of the Foundation.

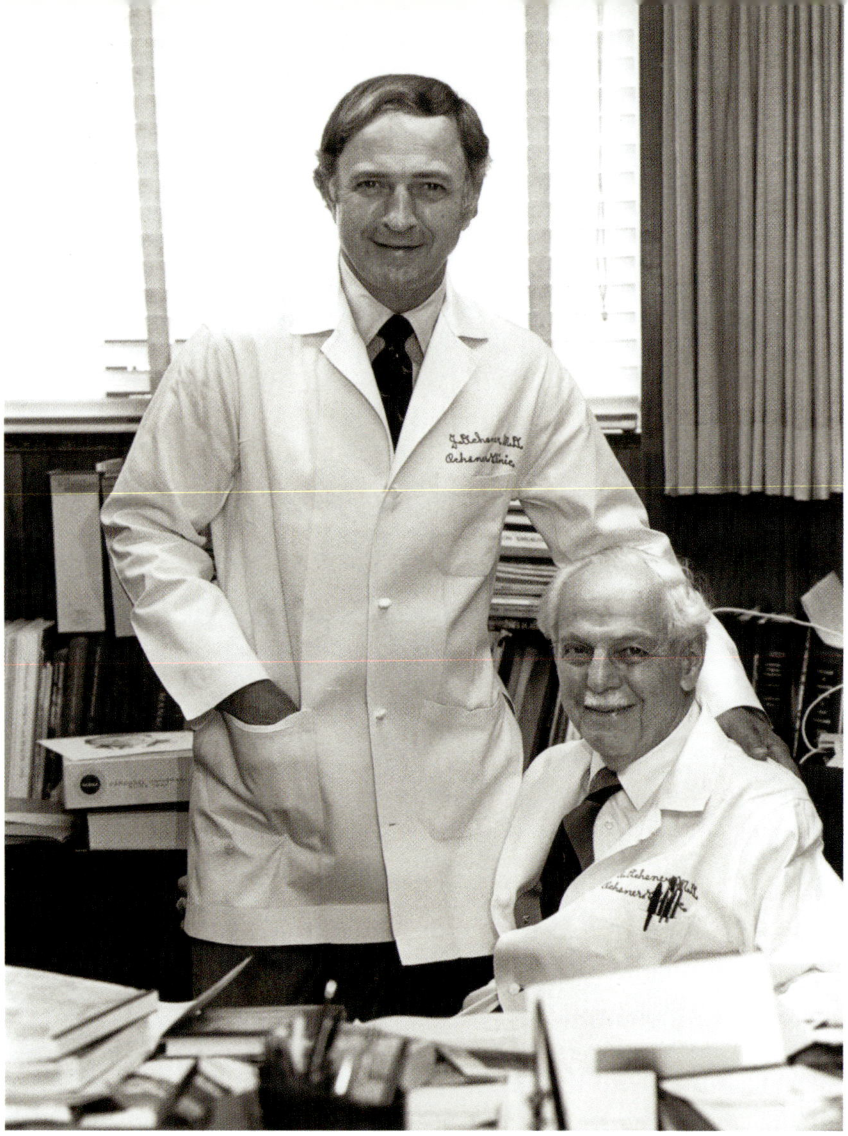

John L. Ochsner and his father in 1965, after the younger Ochsner completed his training under Michael DeBakey.

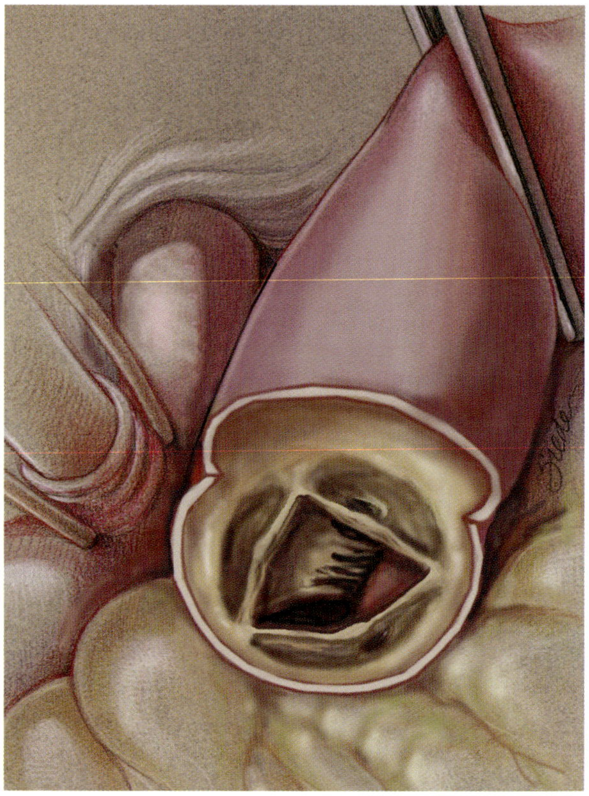

Ochsner Cardiovascular Surgeons began performing heart valve replacements during the late 1960s, as depicted by Barbara Siede, Ochsner's longtime Medical Illustrator.

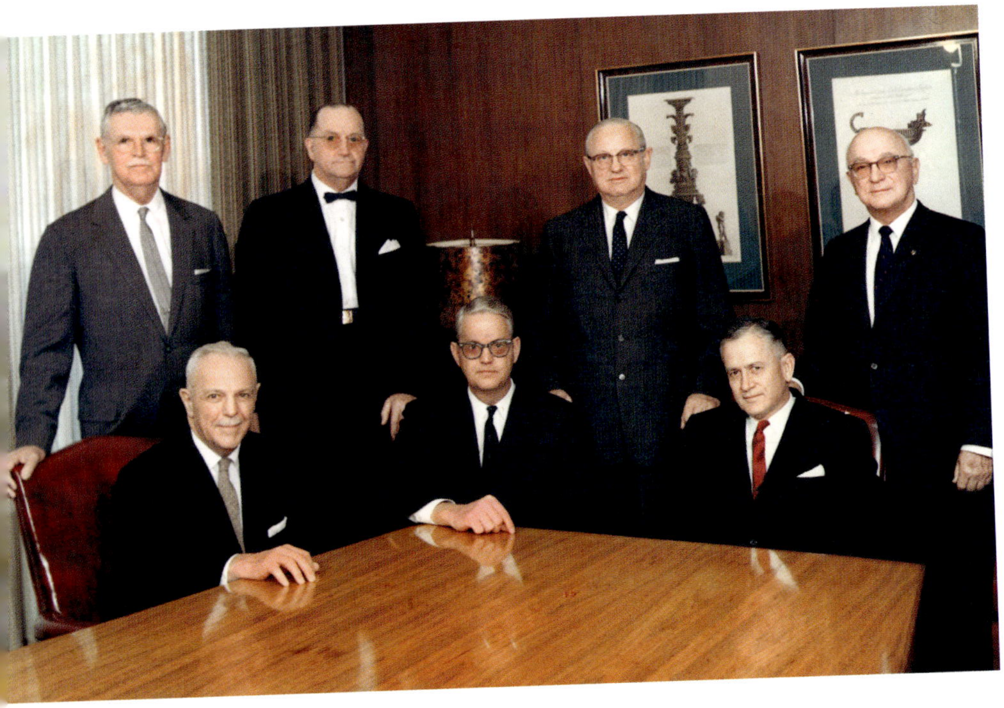

The Board of Trustees of the Foundation during the 1960s consisted of the five founders, Richard "Dick" Freeman Sr. and Malcolm Monroe. Seated left to right are Alton Ochsner, Freeman and Monroe. Standing left to right are Caldwell, Burns, Tyrone and Francis LeJeune Sr.

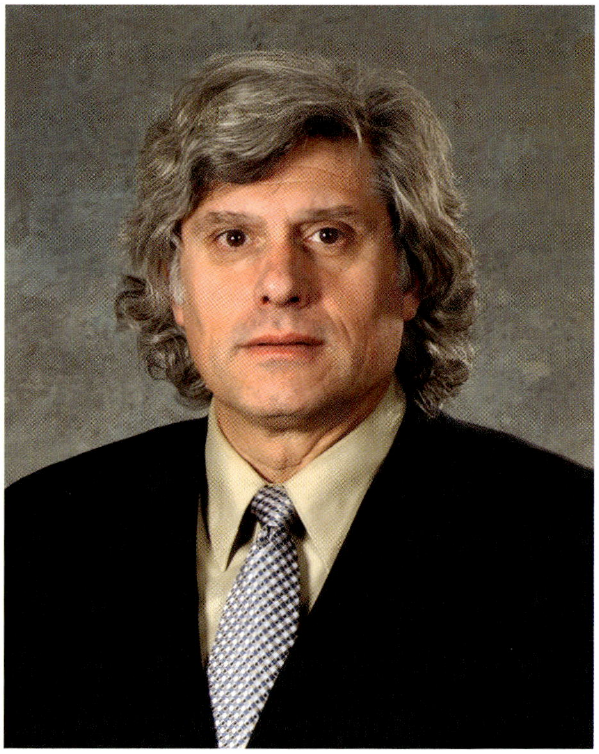

Hector Ventura is both physician and educator. Section Head, Cardiomyopathy and Heart Transplantation, Ventura is deeply involved in post-graduate medical education.

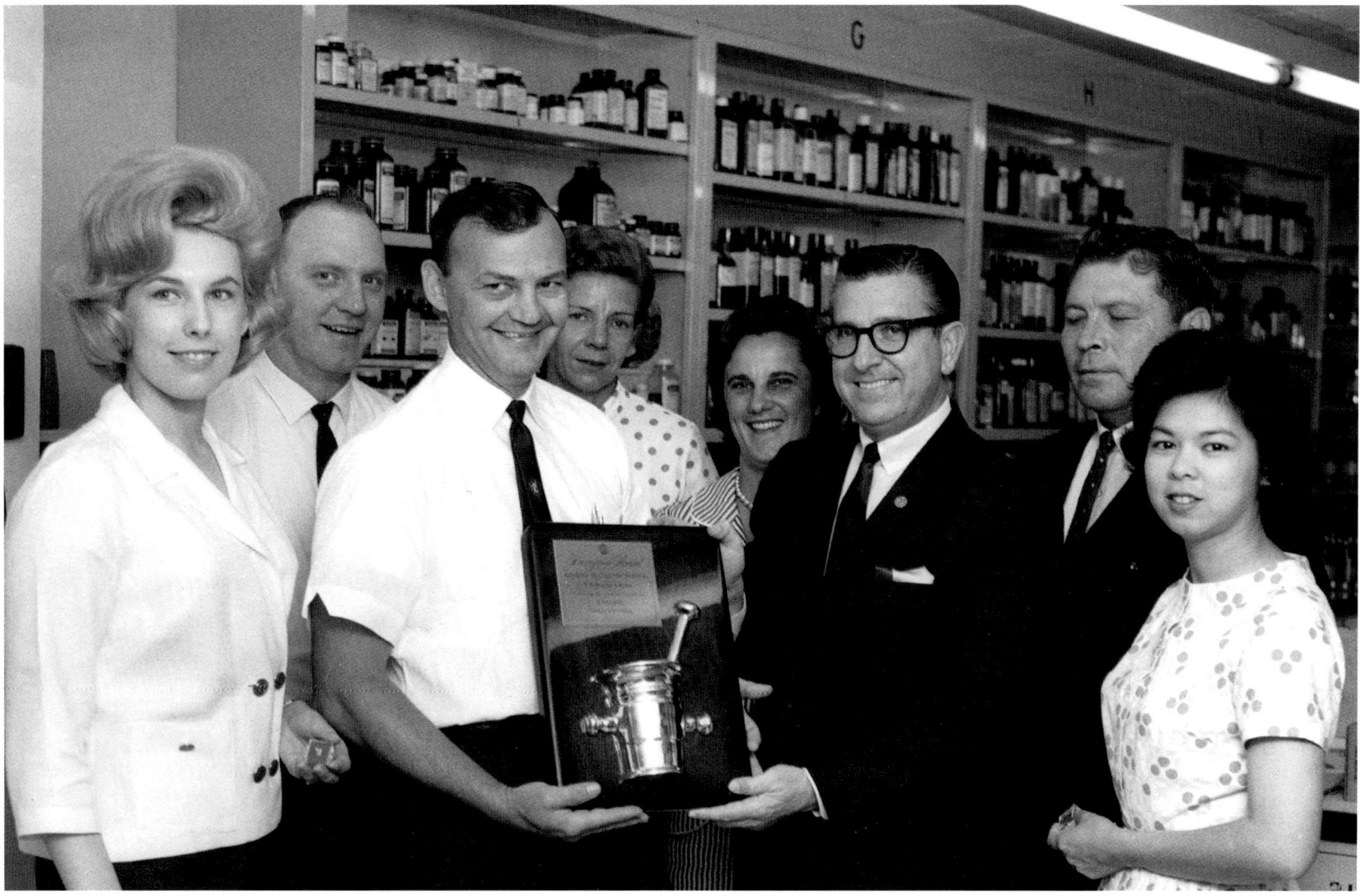

Ochsner filled its two-millionth prescription at the Hospital pharmacy in 1964.

WORD OF MOUTH

When Frank Riddick arrived at Ochsner Clinic as an Internal Medicine physician in 1961, work was less hectic than it later became. "You could almost tell who was going to work out at Ochsner and who wasn't by the way they developed in their initial years here, by the relationship they developed with the appointment desk," Riddick said. "If one was very picky, and gave the appointment desk a list as long as his arm of things he would not do, it usually meant this was not the place for him."[14]

Riddick arrived at Ochsner Clinic from Barnes Hospital in St. Louis, Missouri, where he had been chief resident. A specialist in Endocrinology, Riddick enjoyed the challenge of clinical medicine and took pleasure in teaching at Washington University in St. Louis. He was not enchanted with laboratory work.

"I wasn't sure my skills lay in that line of work," he said. "Academic medicine success then, as now, depended on your skill at getting research grants."[15]

Riddick joined a cohesive staff of three Endocrinologists practicing at Ochsner Clinic and made the move to the new building at the Jefferson Highway campus in 1963. He quickly learned the importance of getting along with the appointment desk staff. "You got patients by word of mouth," he said. "The ladies at the appointment desk as well as the senior staff physicians really could control the direction your practice went. The surgeons would refer patients to internists. If you did a good job, you would all of a sudden start having patients steered to you. Dr. Ochsner used to send a large number of patients."[16]

MEDICARE AND THE TULANE AFFILIATION

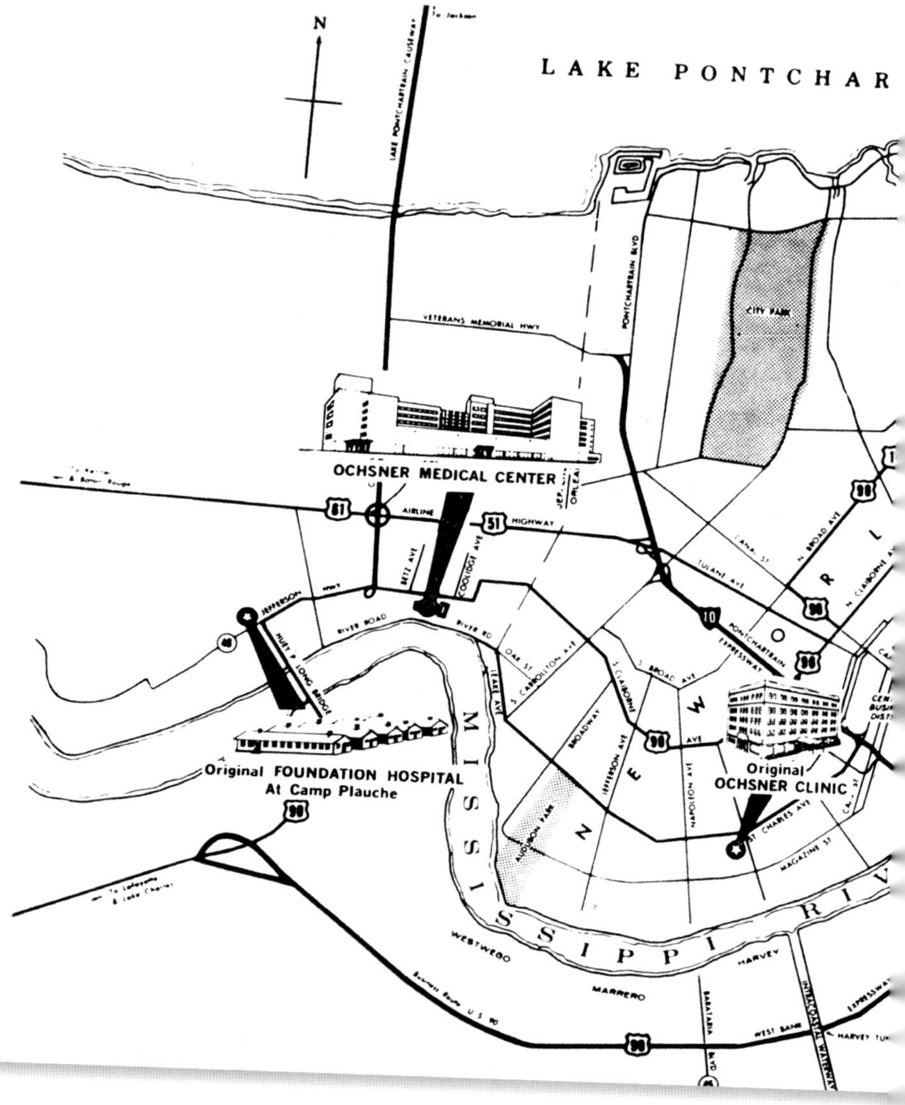

Alton Ochsner's dream since 1927 included an affiliation between Ochsner Clinic and Tulane. The time, however, never proved appropriate for the Clinic and the university to come together in a joint project, although the idea of combining had come up several times since the Clinic opened in 1942.

When the idea surfaced again in 1965, the Foundation was receptive. Alton Ochsner and the other founders still believed that an affiliation made sense. The Foundation committed substantial resources to research, and the Board of Trustees realized that the federal government dictated growth of medical research through its funding support. Increasingly during the 1950s and early 1960s, federal research money went to medical schools.

Tulane, meanwhile, would benefit from an association with Ochsner. The Foundation brought a thriving teaching Hospital, a well-respected Clinic and donor lists that had been instrumental in building both the Hospital and the Clinic.

Talks began in early 1965, and Tulane secured a $250,000 grant to pay for a feasibility study. The talks, however, revealed the same fault lines that had thwarted earlier attempts to merge. Clinic partners feared that Tulane would reap the benefits of a business they had long labored to build. Tulane faculty worried that Clinic staff would dominate the merged entity.[17]

In late 1966, Hines and Edgar Saux traveled to Washington, D.C. for a briefing on federal healthcare policy. President Lyndon B. Johnson had signed Medicare legislation the year before—the most sweeping healthcare legislation in the nation's history. One message Hines and Saux carried back to New Orleans was that the federal government intended to reexamine its funding support of university hospitals, since they only treated about 1 percent of the U.S. population.[18]

At a Christmas week meeting in 1966, the two sides agreed to cancel the merger negotiations. Less than 18 months later, the Louisiana State Legislature began debating a bill to establish the Health Education Authority of Louisiana (HEAL) and create a vehicle that would allow the issuance of tax-free revenue bonds for hospital construction. Ochsner would use HEAL bonds to help finance a major expansion during the 1970s.

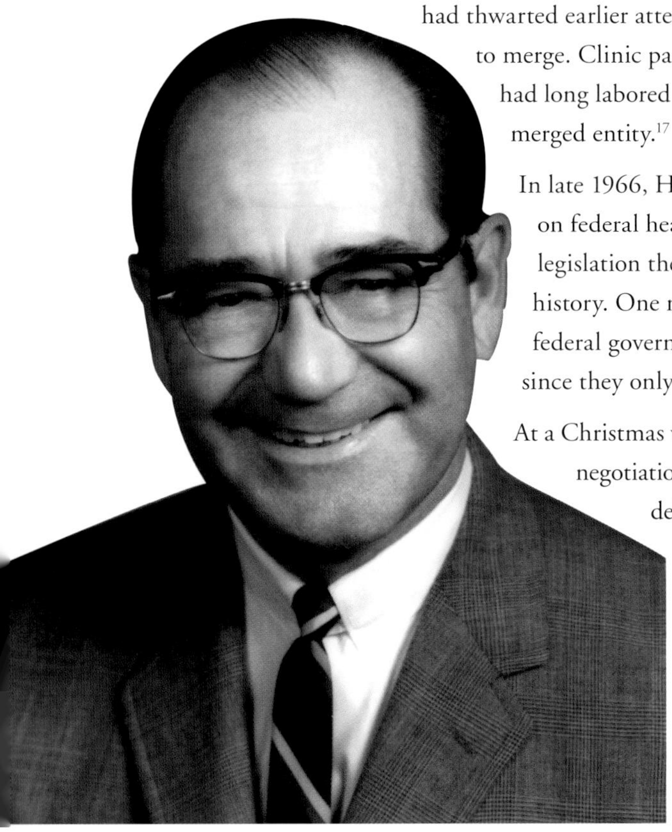

Clinic Manager Edgar J. Saux, a former FBI Special Agent, orchestrated the 1963 move of the facility from Prytania Street to the Jefferson Highway campus.

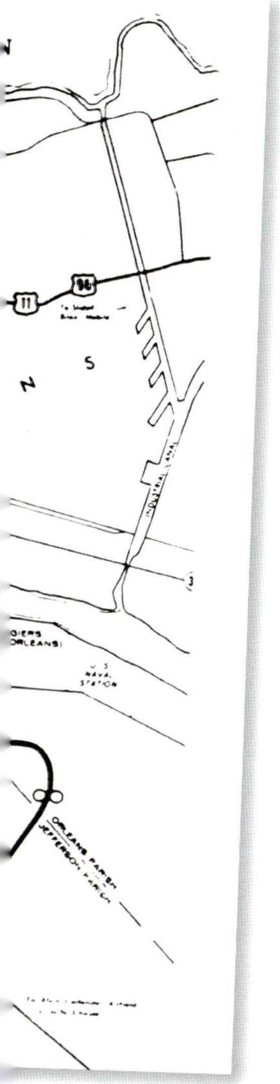

A map of the various sites Ochsner has occupied since 1942.

THE PENICK PAVILION

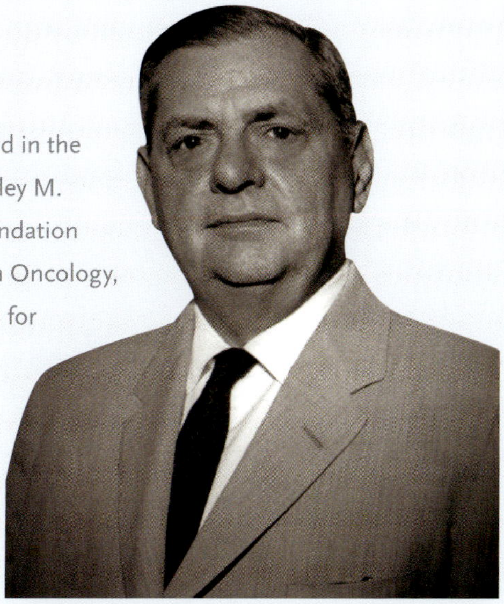

Rawley M. Penick Jr., M.D., succeeded Alton Ochsner as the Chief of Surgery and was on the Clinic staff from 1942 until his death in 1963.

Advances in technology during the 1950s and 1960s resulted in the Foundation building a major new pavilion in 1965. The Rawley M. Penick Memorial Building, opened in 1967, housed the Foundation Hospital's first rotational cobalt unit for advanced Radiation Oncology, Nuclear Medicine laboratories and a new Emergency Room for the Hospital.[19]

Construction of what quickly became known as the "Penick Pavilion" began in early 1966. The 20,000-square-foot, two-story building interconnected the Hospital and Clinic. The cobalt unit and Nuclear Medicine labs occupied about 60 percent of the space in the building, and the modern Emergency Room took most of the first floor.[20]

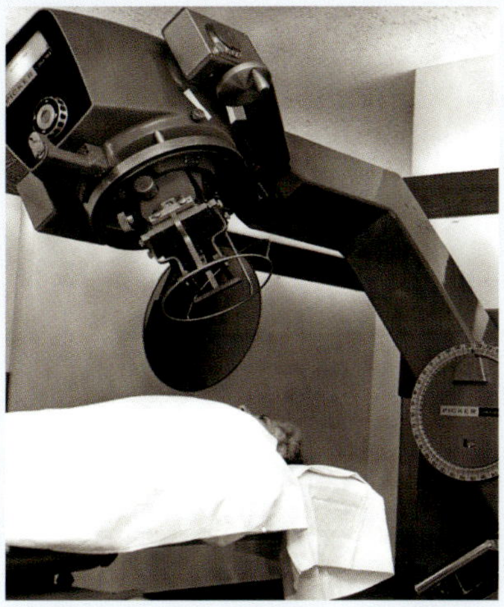

A rotational cobalt radiation therapy unit treating an Ochsner cancer patient in 1967 in the Penick Pavilion

Cobalt radiotherapy units, a technological advance stemming from U.S. atomic research during World War II, improved the ability of Radiation Oncologists to treat tumors.[21] The Penick Pavilion included space for installation of a second cobalt unit at a future date and propelled Ochsner into the forefront of radiation oncology practice in the region.

The new building honored one of the Clinic's pioneers, Rawley M. Penick, who died in early 1963. He had joined Ochsner Clinic shortly after it opened in 1942.[22] Penick, who taught clinical surgery at Tulane for 12 years, also helped start the Tumor Registry at Charity Hospital. He succeeded Alton Ochsner as head of the Department of Surgery at Ochsner Clinic and served as one of the two non-founders on the Clinic's Board of Management. Memorial donations in Penick's name helped fund much of the $1.5 million construction cost for the new pavilion.[23]

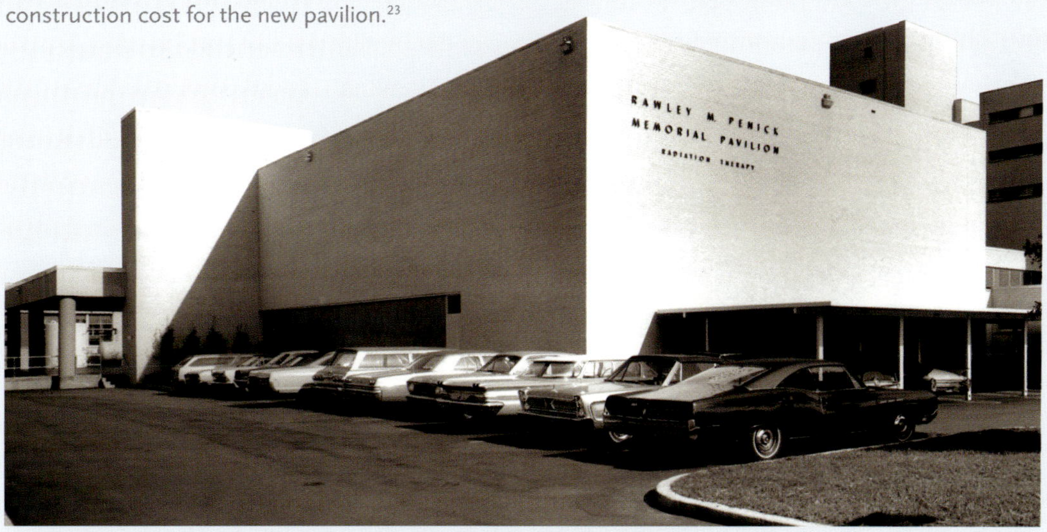

The Rawley M. Penick Memorial Pavilion shortly after it opened in 1967 to treat cancer patients.

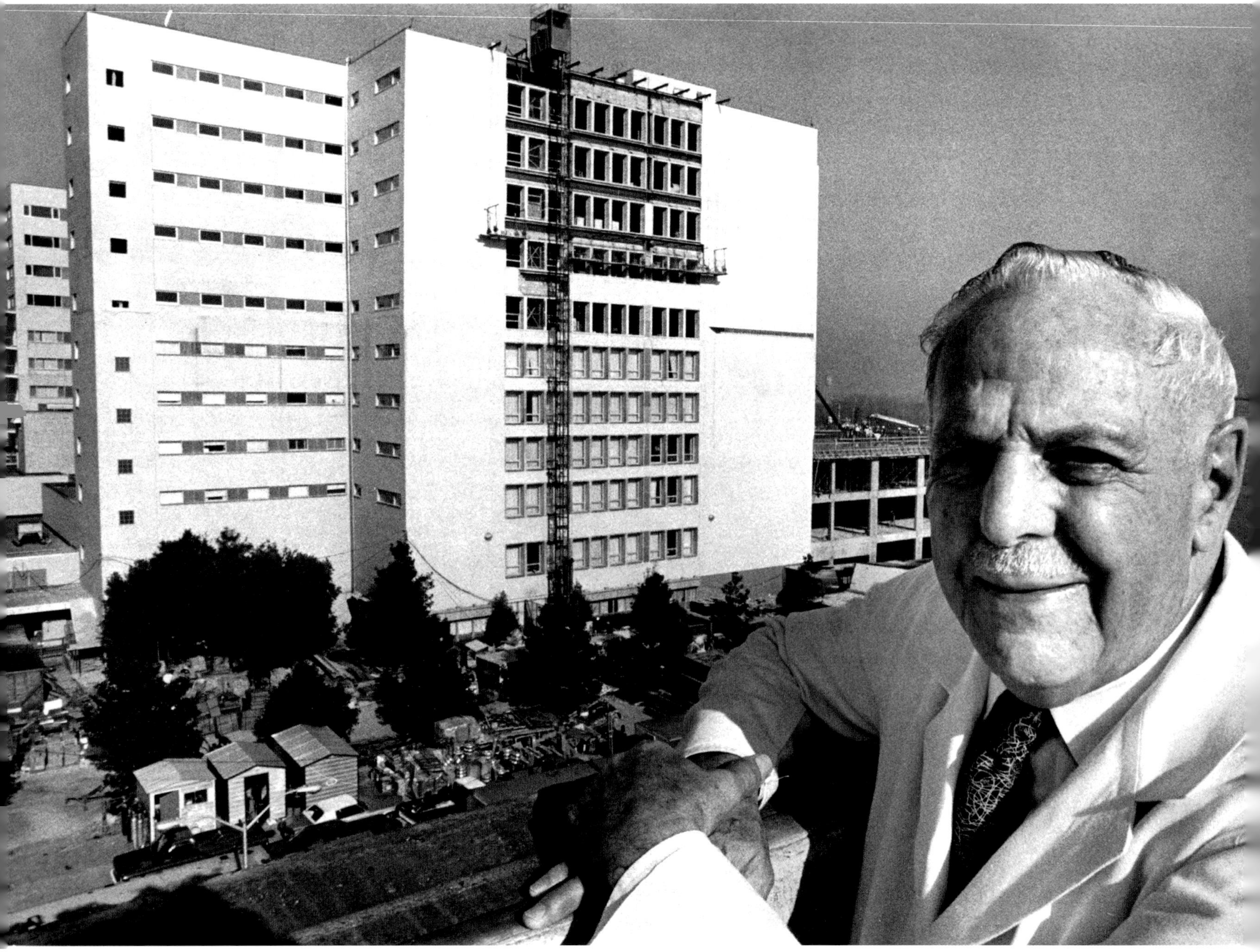

CHAPTER 5:

THE FRUITS OF INNOVATION

On January 9, 1970, Dr. John Ochsner made medical history at Ochsner Foundation Hospital when he led the surgical team that performed the first heart transplant in the Gulf South region. The younger Ochsner, who had trained under Dr. Michael DeBakey in Houston, Texas, who in turn had been mentored by Dr. Alton Ochsner, would go on to perform hundreds of heart transplants at Ochsner Foundation Hospital. In 1974, a surgical team headed by John Ochsner pioneered pediatric heart surgery when it implanted a pacemaker into an infant only 18 hours old.

John Ochsner's work in cardiac surgery during the 1970s was but one facet of the medical firsts pioneered by Ochsner physicians and just another example of the organization's focus on treating patients and not just disease. Dr. Terry D. King and Dr. Noel L. Mills invented an umbrella device that they implanted by catheter in the heart of a 17-year-old patient in 1975. The King-Mills Umbrella Device, used for non-surgical closure of congenital interatrial septal defects, won the two Ochsner physicians the Young Investigator Award of the Cardiology Section of the American Academy of Pediatrics.

Dr. Albert Segaloff's studies gave Ochsner a strong reputation in the field of breast cancer research during the 1950s, 1960s and 1970s. In 1975, the National Cancer Institute (NCI) recognized Segaloff's contributions when it awarded the Ochsner Research Institute a $475,000 grant to study causes and cures for breast cancer.

Alton Ochsner is framed by the Clinic and Hospital bearing his name in the mid-1970s.

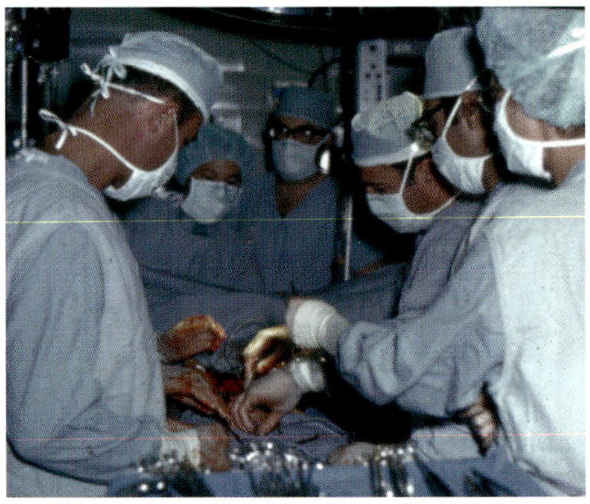

John Ochsner leads the team that performed the first heart transplant in the region in January 1970.

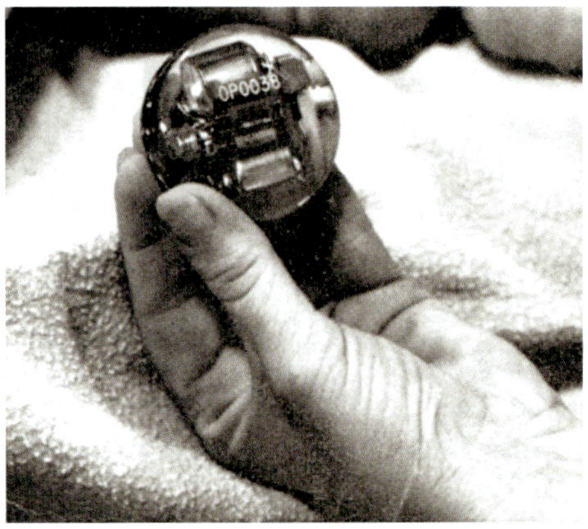

John Ochsner implanted a heart pacemaker in a nine pound, two ounce infant only 18 hours after birth.

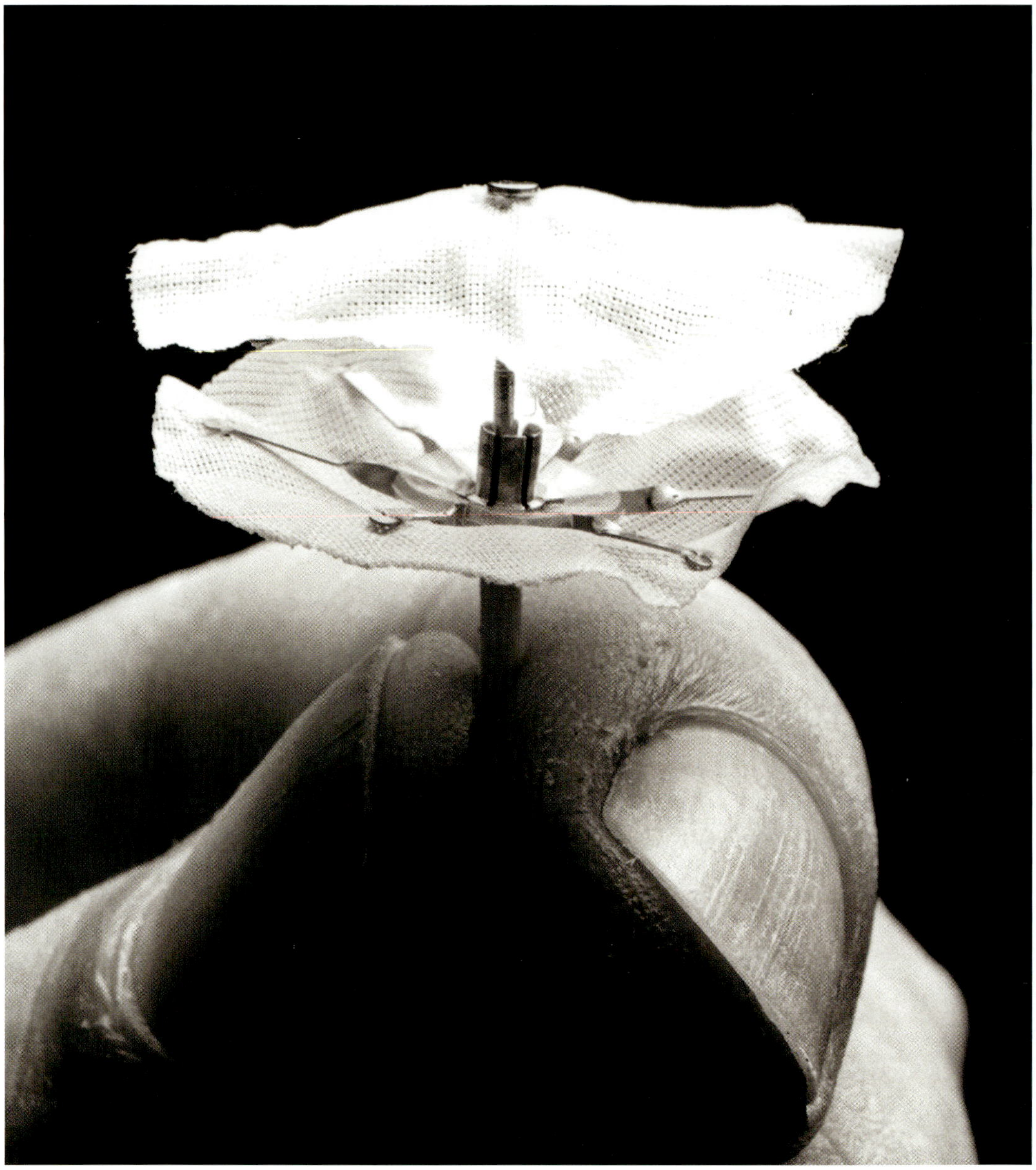

Terry D. King and Noel L. Mills closed the hole in the heart of a 17-year-old boy without surgery in 1973 with this umbrella catheter.

Dr. Jay Goldsmith coordinated airplane and ambulance transportation to make Ochsner Foundation Hospital the first in the region to utilize a two-way transport system in Pediatrics. The opening of Ochsner's Neonatal Intensive Care Unit (NICU) in 1972 made the Hospital a pioneer in NICU operation in the Gulf South region. It was a commitment on the part of Ochsner to treat its youngest and smallest patients with the same quality medical care available to their parents and grandparents. The transport team would stabilize newborns in the referring hospital before transporting them to the unit at Ochsner. This was an important first step in Ochsner's regionalization efforts.

Ochsner's Renal Laboratory, established in 1967, helped create the New Orleans Metropolitan Organ Procurement Program, making kidney transplantation a reality in the region in the late 1960s.

Ochsner physicians began performing kidney transplants in 1968, and by the early 1970s reported that patients were consistently living five years or more following transplant surgery with normal function and complete rehabilitation. By the late 1970s, Ochsner physicians were routinely performing liver transplants and transforming the lives of hepatitis victims who had previously been condemned to a slow, painful death.

Ochsner's growing reputation for surgical and medical advances was unmatched anywhere in the region. This fulfilled the five founders' vision for creation of a competitive clinic in the South.

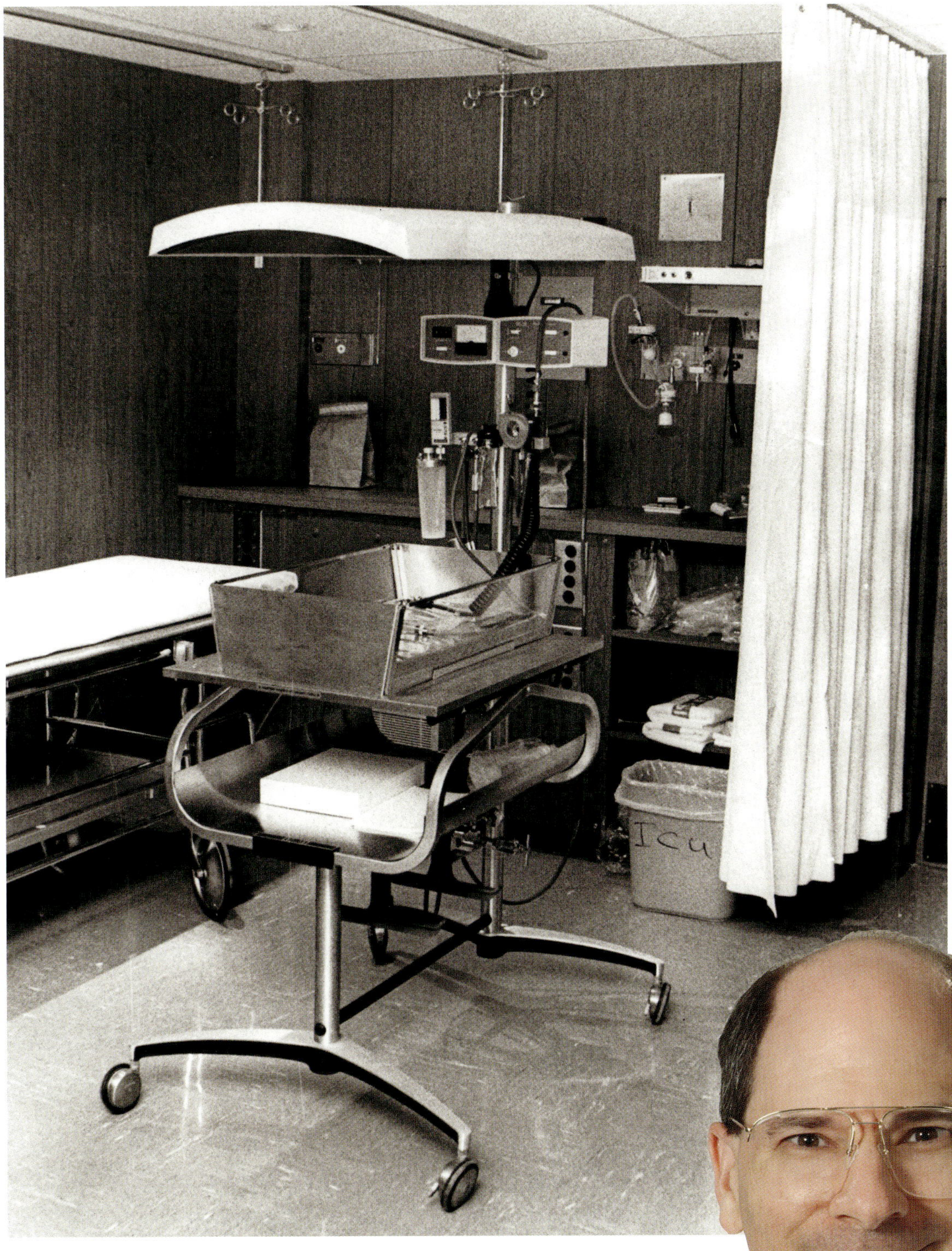

Ochsner's Neonatal Intensive Care Unit (NICU) revolutionized the care of at-risk newborns in the region.

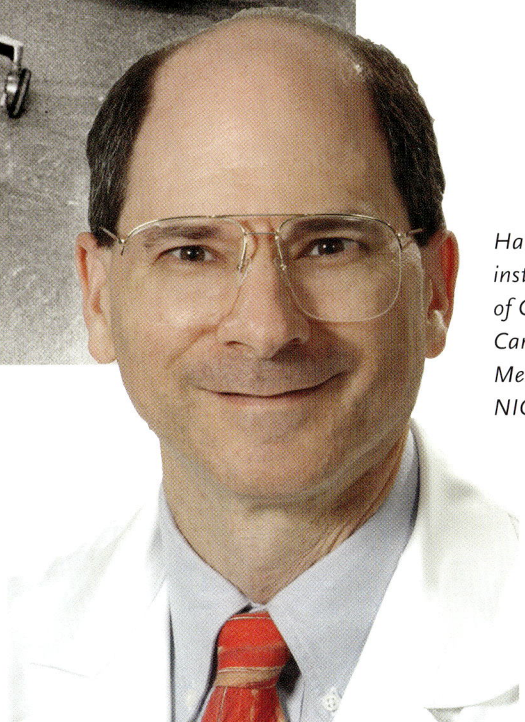

Harley Ginsberg, M.D., was instrumental in the expansion of Ochsner's Neonatal Intensive Care Unit (NICU) and is the Medical Director of Ochsner's NICU.

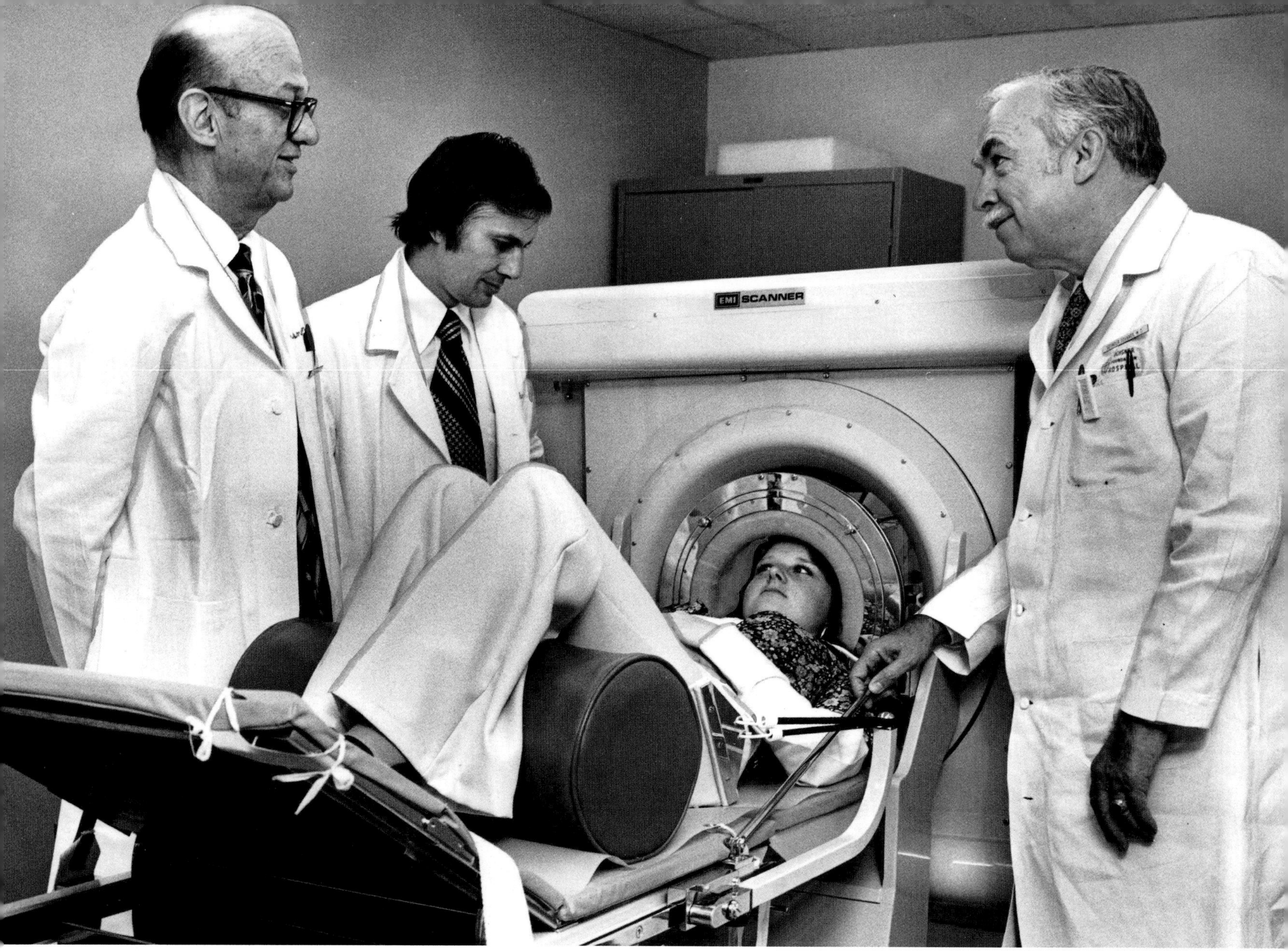

Ochsner was the first hospital in the region to use a computed tomography (CT) scanner to diagnose patients in 1974. Left to right are Merrill O. Hines, President of Alton Ochsner Medical Foundation and Director of Ochsner Clinic; Roger H. Tutton, Associate Head of the Department of Radiology; Jackie Berthelot and Seymour F. Ochsner, Chairman of the Department of Radiology.

PHASE I

Ochsner Clinic and Foundation Hospital administrators remained keenly aware that the contributions of John Ochsner, Albert Segaloff, Jay Goldsmith and many others would be impossible without the provision of first-rate medical facilities. To that end, the Foundation embarked upon a major building project that transformed the Jefferson Highway campus during the 1970s.

The first major expansion, early in the 1970s, resulted in the construction of an Intensive Care Unit, the new Monroe Hall, a Coronary Care Unit, as well as a new board room and administrative and business offices. In late 1970, the Foundation Trustees set a goal of $3.5 million for a fund-raising campaign, which would be used to pay for the extensive expansion.[1]

By the end of 1971, the campaign had raised $3.1 million, more than 90 percent of the original goal. Significantly, nearly half of the donations had come internally from the Foundation Board of Trustees, the Clinic partnership of physicians, and Clinic and Hospital personnel.[2] This expansion, which was complete by the end of the calendar year, was the last expansion funded entirely through a capital campaign.

The expansion of the business office allowed Ochsner to take a major step forward in automating the accounting and medical records function. Since 1968, the Hospital and Clinic had been working with the national accounting firm of Haskins and Sells to lay the groundwork for computerization of accounts. In July 1971, the Foundation took delivery of an IBM 30 Model 360 computer and entered the computer age.

The next expansion, later in the decade, would be financed by bonds issued by Alton Ochsner Medical Foundation and would be overseen by a new generation of Clinic and Foundation leadership.

EDGAR BURNS

As a new generation of leaders charted the future course of Ochsner Clinic and Ochsner Foundation Hospital, mortality inevitably began to lay its claims on the five men who had founded the Clinic more than 30 years before.

Dr. Edgar Burns came home from the office one day in late August 1973, laid down for his customary late afternoon nap and never woke up. Burns was 78 and was the first of the founders to pass away.[3]

Dr. W. E. Kittredge, one of Burns's longtime colleagues, described his friend in a eulogy as a consummate physician and an outstanding teacher. "He had the most powerful intellect of anyone I have ever known," Kittredge wrote. "He could see through the confusing aspects of a difficult diagnostic problem and get right to the heart of the matter in minutes. Graduates of his postgraduate training program are scattered the world over and have never lost their gratitude for his efforts on their behalf, nor their respect for his overall contribution to the teaching of Urology as a science."[4]

• WHAT OCHSNER MEANS TO ME •

"I'm excited that this journey doesn't just end with the clinical treatment we provide, but that we also strive to develop an even deeper, more profound RELATIONSHIP with a patient so that their experience here is more meaningful and rewarding."

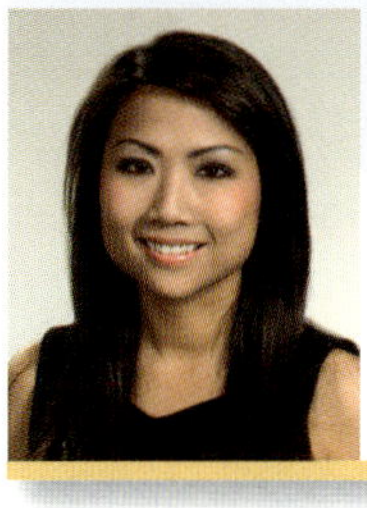

Nga Vu, Vice President, Operations, Ochsner Medical Center – West Bank Campus

To watch the full interview with Nga Vu, visit **ochsner.org/history**.

A NEW MEDICAL DIRECTOR

Two things happened to change Dr. Frank Riddick's life during the early 1970s. A Memphis native who arrived at Ochsner Clinic in 1961 by way of St. Louis, he had developed a successful Endocrinology practice by 1970. Then, colleagues in the practice got Riddick involved in the state chapter of the Society of Internal Medicine. He found he enjoyed society work and was soon elected to the Board of Trustees of the American Society of Internal Medicine.

The second and more lasting change came in 1972. Dr. Merrill Hines, who had succeeded Dr. Guy Caldwell as the Clinic Medical Director in 1959, was involved in a minor automobile accident and was unable to work for several weeks. Directors of the Alton Ochsner Medical Foundation decided it was time to groom a successor to Hines. They asked Riddick to take the position of Assistant Medical Director.[5]

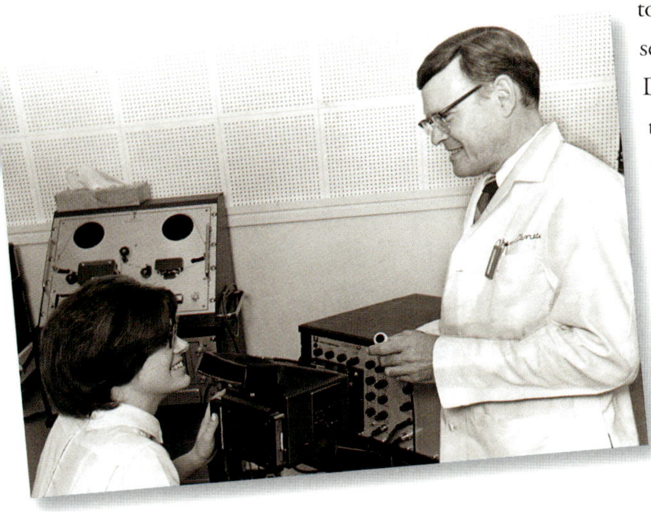

Cardiologist Charles B. Moore, M.D., and technician Cheryl Lawrence inspect a new echocardiograph machine in 1972, a time of transformative change in cardiac care.

Riddick assisted Hines with the major Hospital and Clinic expansions of the early to mid-1970s. Urged by the Ochsner Clinic Partnership, the Clinic's Board of Management directed him to undertake a major restructuring of the Clinic partnership agreement. "The agreement worked for an organization with a small number of founders/owners," said Riddick, "but didn't meet the needs of the 1970 partnership for management, governance and representation. The Board of Management was self-perpetuating and selection as a member was essentially a lifetime appointment."[6]

The rewritten partnership agreement made positions on the Board of Management elective, with six-year terms. The new agreement established the Medical Director as Chairman of the Board and Chief Executive Officer, selected by and serving at the pleasure of the Board. In 1975, Riddick replaced Hines as Medical Director, a position he would hold for the next quarter-century.

Hines, meanwhile, capped his career at Ochsner with election as Chairman of the Alton Ochsner Medical Foundation Board of Trustees.[7]

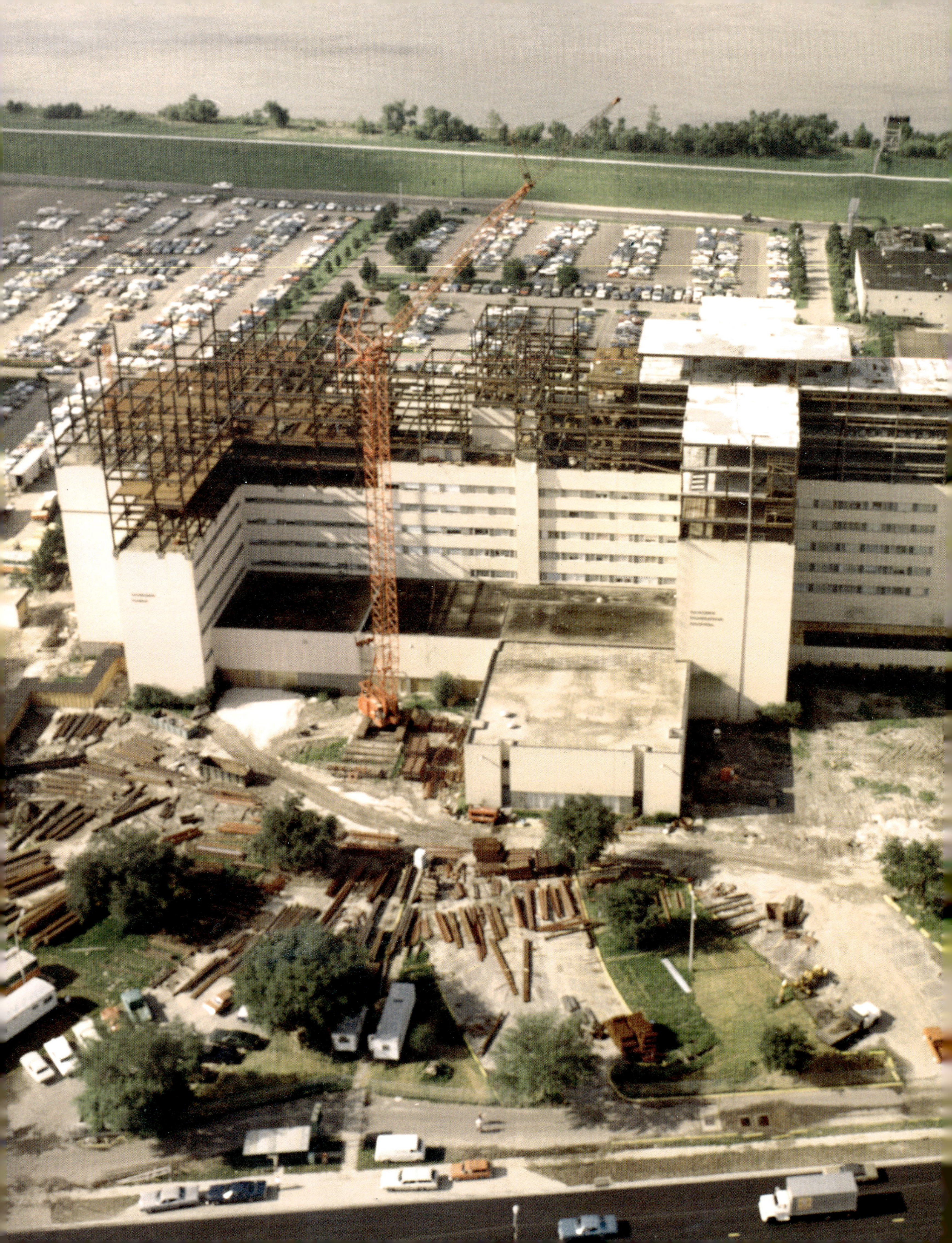

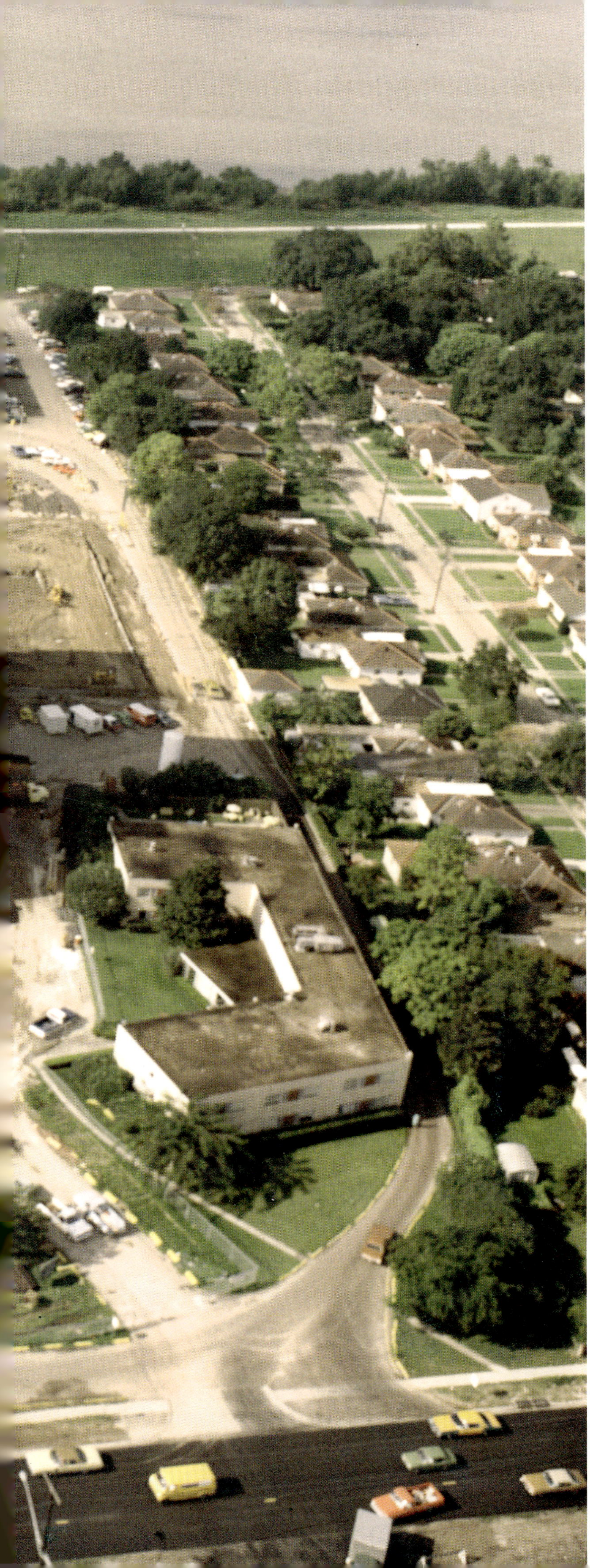

PHASE II

Riddick would be among the Clinic and Hospital leaders assigned the task of planning and overseeing the $60 million expansion program announced in the summer of 1975 and choreographing the successful presentation before the Health Planning Agency, whose sanction was required.

Since the completion of the Phase I expansion in late 1971, Ochsner Clinic and Foundation Hospital were bursting at the seams.

"At Ochsner we are now treating the third generation of patients and finding it extremely difficult to schedule appointments to meet their needs," Riddick said in June 1975. "We are now running about 430,000 patient visits a year in somewhat cramped quarters."[8]

The scope of the expansion was breathtaking. Trustees approved plans late in 1974 that called for major additions to literally every segment of the Jefferson Highway campus. The two-year program called for spending $60 million, most of which would be raised by issuing Health Education Authority of Louisiana (HEAL) bonds authorized by the State of Louisiana. Work began early in 1975, with construction scheduled for completion by the end of 1976.[9]

The bonds went to market in July 1975. Bobby C. Brannon, Financial Vice President and CFO of the Foundation, estimated the tax-free bonds would save Ochsner $18–20 million in interest compared to more traditional financing during the 25-year period in which the tax-free bonds were outstanding.[10] The Foundation was able to lock in all of its costs at the beginning of the construction project.[11]

The initial construction included a 102-room addition to the Brent House Hotel and the erection of a seven-level parking garage.[12] An air-conditioned mall connected the Brent House Hotel and garage with the Clinic and Hospital.

"At Ochsner we are now treating the third generation of patients and finding it extremely difficult to schedule appointments to meet their needs."

An aerial view of the ongoing construction work at the Jefferson Highway campus during the mid-1970s. The facility nearly doubled in size during the decade.

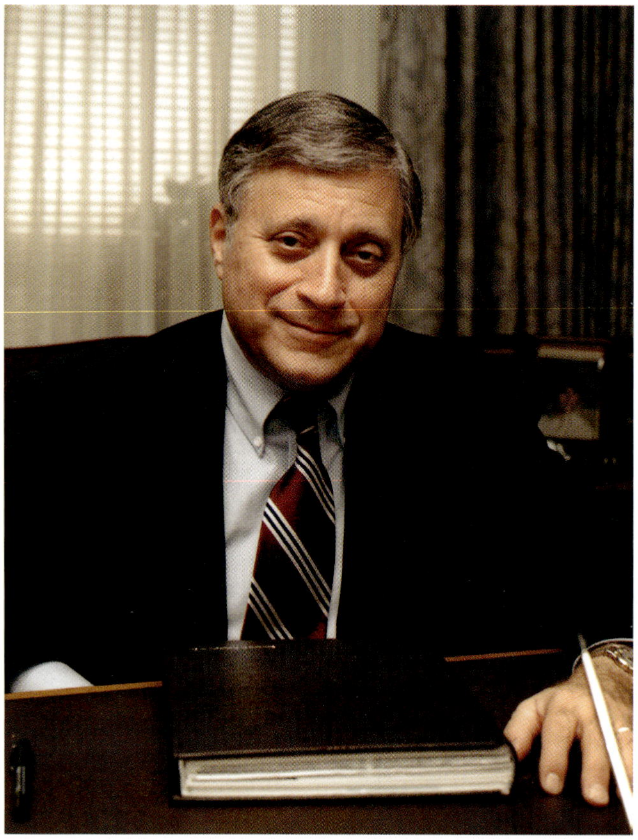

Edward Frohlich, M.D., published groundbreaking studies in hypertension research as director of Ochsner's research efforts during the 1970s.

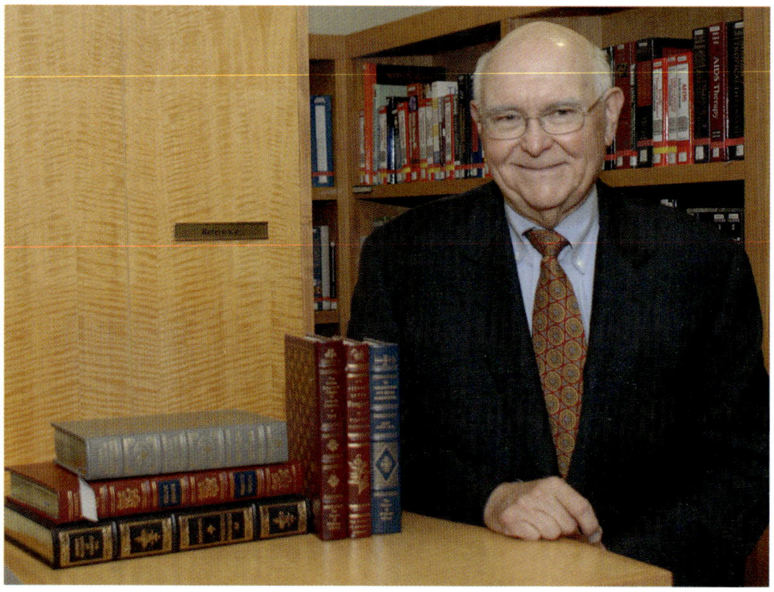

Carl G. Kardinal, M.D., was the Director of Clinical Cancer Research at Ochsner. In 2004, he received the Association of Community Cancer Centers' Annual Clinical Research Award for his extensive contributions to developing new cancer treatments, particularly for breast cancer.

RESEARCH

Research activities continued throughout construction. The reputation for excellence in Ochsner research efforts fostered by Dr. Albert Segaloff was further enhanced when Dr. Edward Frohlich came aboard as Director of Education and Research in 1976 to carry on what continued to be a primary founding principle of Ochsner. A New York City native and graduate of the School of Medicine at the University of Maryland, Frohlich came to Ochsner from the medical school at the University of Oklahoma, where he held an endowed chair. Prior to his tenure there, Frohlich spent five years conducting medical research and caring for patients at the Cleveland Clinic.

Frohlich helped pioneer the study of Cardiovascular Pathophysiology and is an internationally recognized expert in the field of hypertension and related research. "When I went to medical school," he said, "heart attack, stroke, malignant hypertension and kidney failure constituted the majority of hospital admissions."[13]

Frohlich worked with laboratory animals at the Cleveland Clinic and was firmly convinced that animal research was a critical part of any hypertension research project. When he arrived in New Orleans, he came with a colony of laboratory rats he purchased from the National Institute of Health (NIH) in Bethesda, Maryland. His rats joined the colonies of rats bred by Segaloff for breast cancer research. By the early 1980s, more than 7,000 rats occupied cages in the Richard Freeman Research Institute at the Jefferson Highway campus.[14]

"We bred all of our rats," Frohlich said. "We developed techniques with rats that helped the drugs work so much better. We took concepts to the lab and then back to the patient."[15]

Among those concepts was the use of beta-adrenergic blocking drugs in the treatment of hypertension. Frohlich made Ochsner a pioneer in therapy with what became known as "beta-blockers," a family of drugs that proved to be among the most effective in treating high blood pressure.

In 1985, Dr. Richard Ré led a major expansion of Ochsner's Division of Research that added to the laboratories of Cellular Immunology, Hepatology, Hypertension, Molecular Genetics, Molecular Immunogenetics and Molecular Oncology. The 1985 expansion was a recognition of the reality that the focus of medical research was getting ever smaller, moving from the

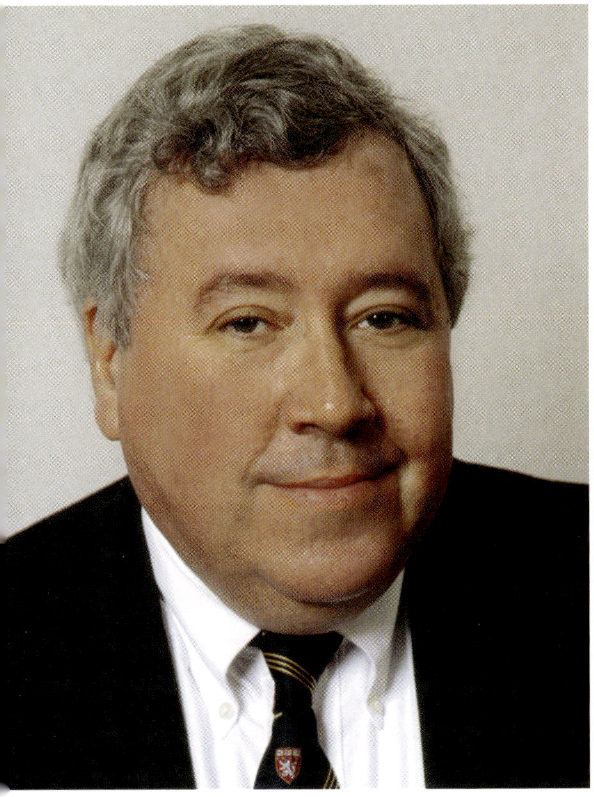

Richard Ré, M.D., carries on the tradition of Ochsner research pioneered by Albert Segaloff and Edward Frohlich.

organ to the cell to the molecule. He forged strong collaborative initiatives with the Biochemistry Department at LSU and with colleagues from Tulane. Ré also embarked on an internal campaign that laid the groundwork for the Division of Research's recruitment of top-grade scientists in the field of Molecular Biology.[16]

In 1986, Ochsner surgeons performed procedures that were the first of their kind in the region. Dr. John Ochsner led a team that performed the first pediatric heart transplant in the region, while another team accomplished the first pediatric liver transplant in Louisiana. Ochsner's growing reputation for surgical and medical innovations would continue to increase in the decades ahead.

Ochsner would make further research and medical advances during the 1980s and would focus its expansion efforts on the growing suburban and rural areas of southeastern Louisiana.

ALBERT SEGALOFF

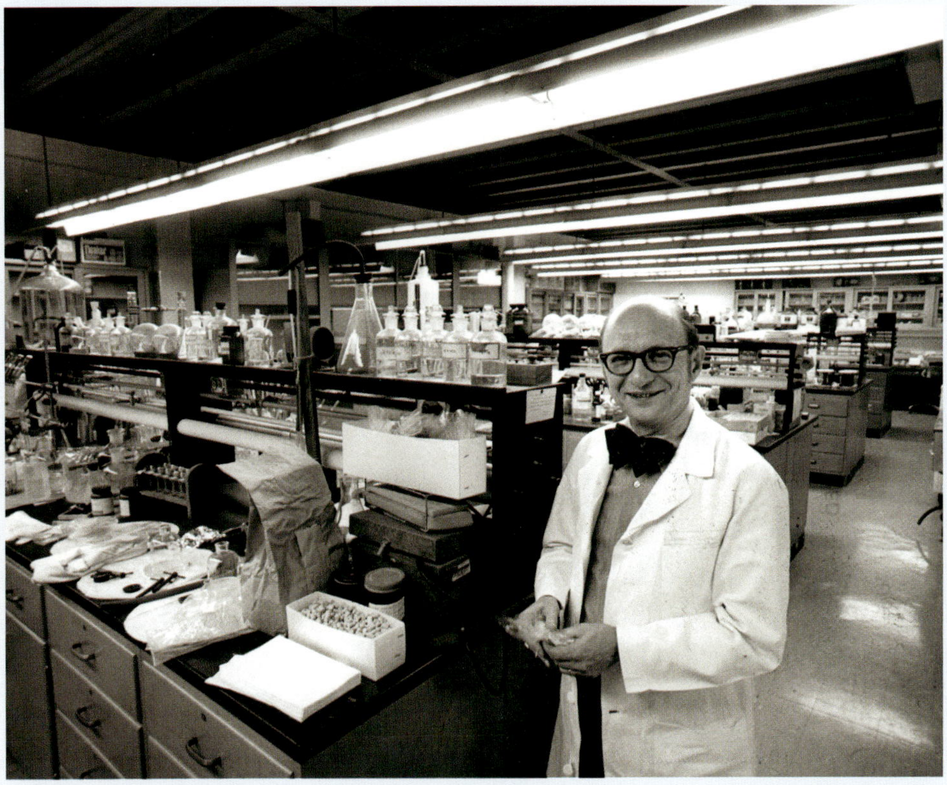

Dr. Albert Segaloff's research on breast cancer gave Ochsner a national reputation during the 1970s. Segaloff's laboratory rats were a key element in Ochsner research for decades.

For much of the 1960s and 1970s, Ochsner research created breakthroughs in the study of breast cancer. Dr. Albert Segaloff's work in the diagnosis and treatment of breast cancer gave Ochsner an international reputation.

Segaloff concentrated his work during the 1930s on the thymus gland, but by the time he arrived in New Orleans from Wayne State University in Detroit in 1945, Segaloff's work had shifted to how estrogen was metabolized in the human body. The work inevitably led to an investigation of the role that estrogen played in the development of breast cancer.[17]

Segaloff pioneered the use of rats for laboratory research in breast cancer. In his original laboratory facilities in the Martin Building, just down Prytania Street from the original Clinic building, Segaloff housed the rats in an enclosed second-story porch and used them in his research trials.[18]

Segaloff's research was invaluable in giving physicians around the world the tools to identify and treat breast tumors. He pioneered using testosterone to treat breast cancer and helped develop a standard for breast tumor measurement. Segaloff authored more than 100 journal articles in his specialty. Dr. Hector O. Ventura wrote that Segaloff played an important role, "not only in the basic understanding of breast cancer but in the multidisciplinary approach to the treatment of the disease."[19]

Segaloff died at his home in New Orleans at the age of 68 in February 1985.[20]

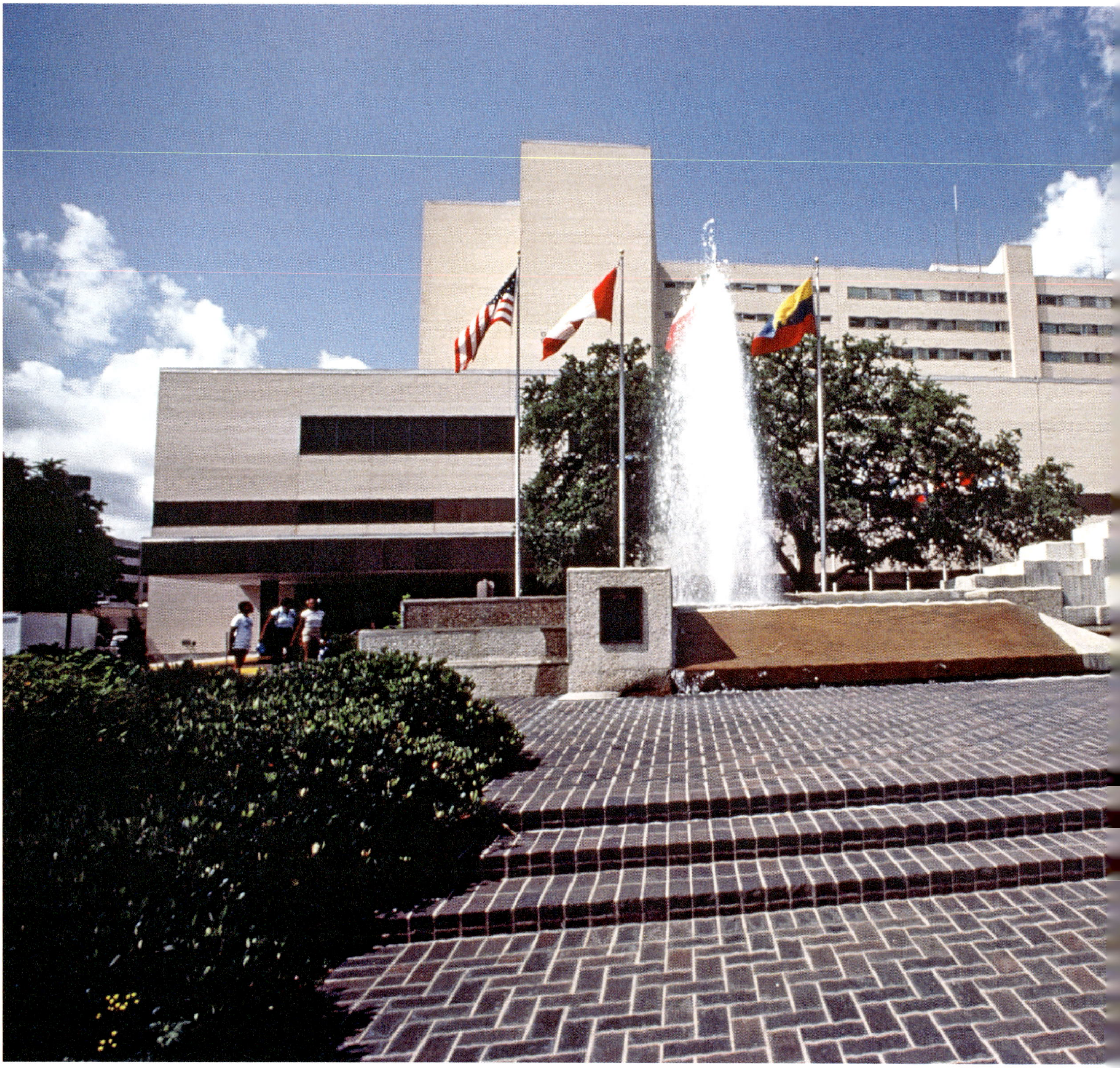

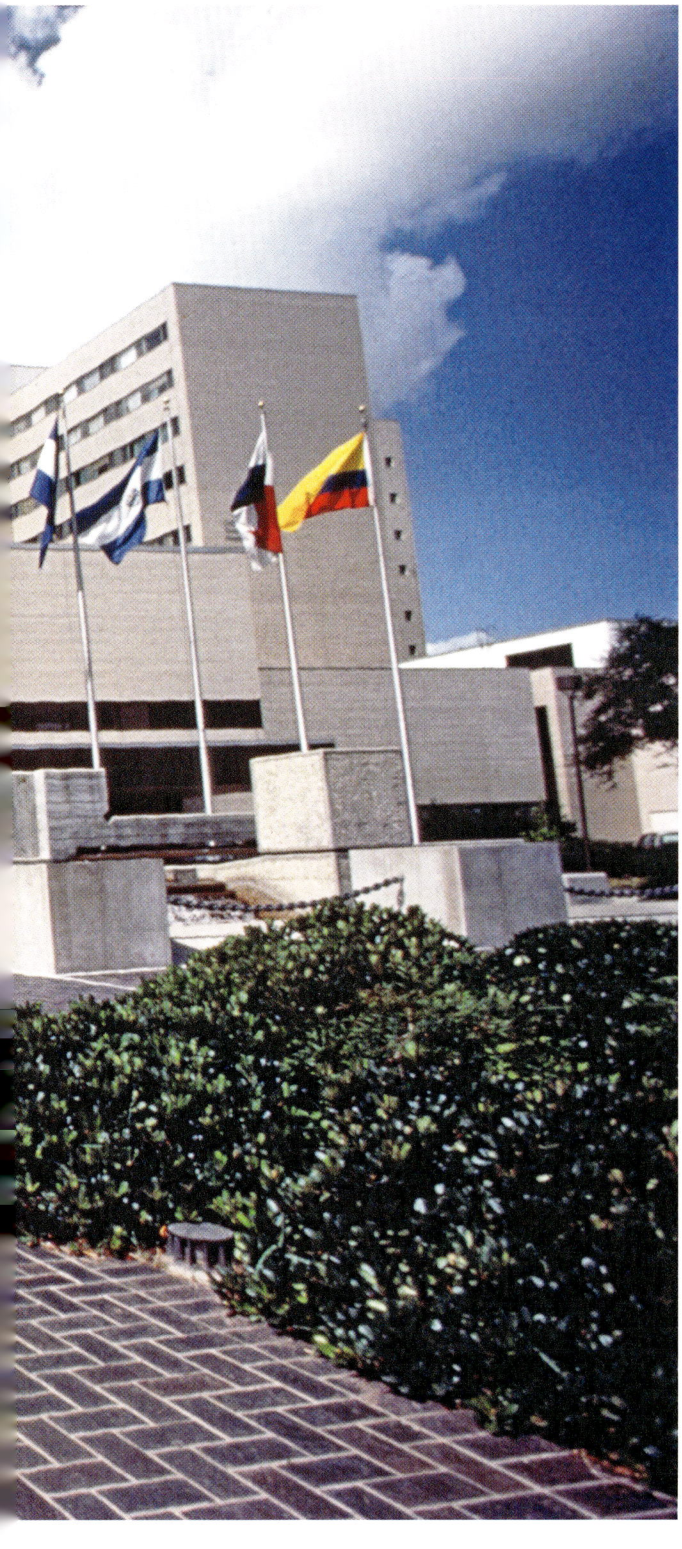

Alma and Russell Clark contributed to the construction of the Plaza of the Americas fronting Jefferson Highway in 1978, recognizing the institution's longtime international ties, especially for patients in Central and South America.

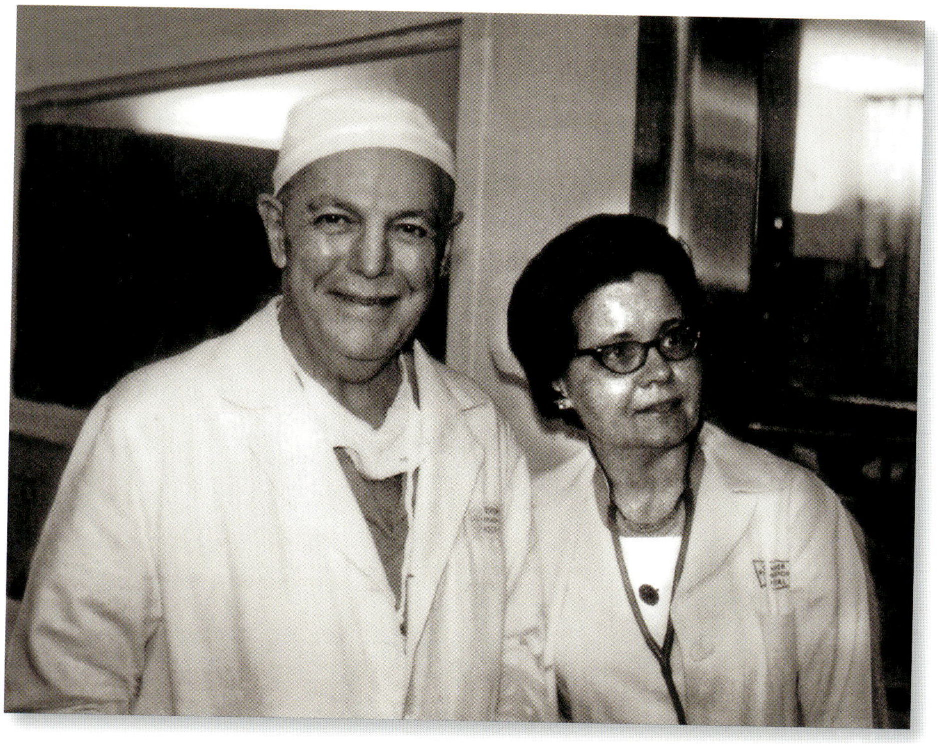

Among those who fondly remember working with Alton Ochsner is Julie Carnahan. Carnahan served Ochsner as a scrub nurse during the 1940s and 1950s.

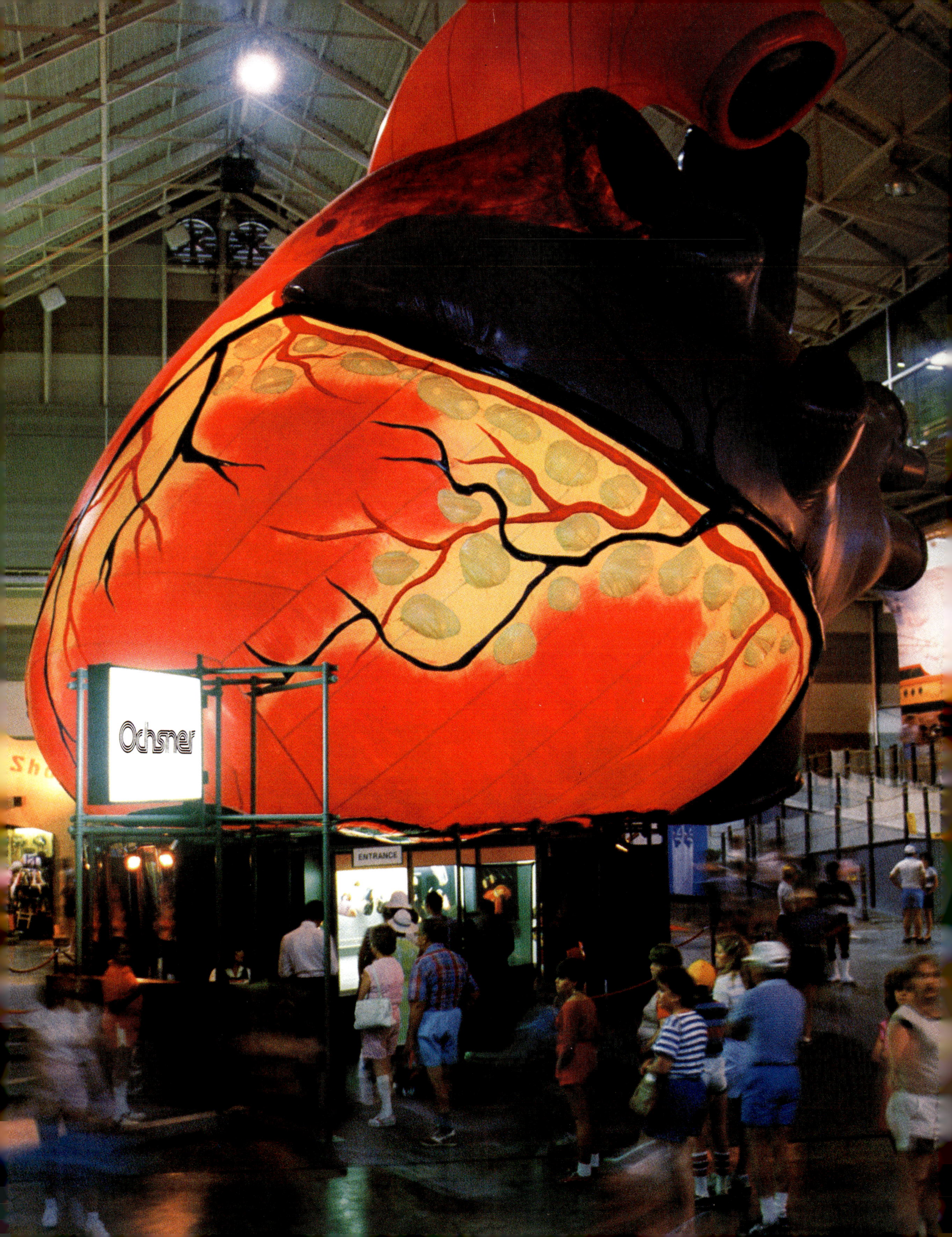
Ochsner
ENTRANCE

CHAPTER 6:

EXPANDING THE BASE

AT FIRST GLANCE, OCHSNER CLINIC AND OCHSNER FOUNDATION HOSPITAL experienced unrivaled prosperity during the 1980s. Admissions and revenues both steadily increased during the first half of the decade. However, inflation, a local and national recession and increasing government intervention in the healthcare segment of the economy all conspired to erode the traditional fee-for-service model of medicine by mid-decade.

These changing dynamics were complicated by the divergent views between the Ochsner Clinic Board of Management and the Foundation Board of Trustees. The sometimes passionate disagreement between the two entities would grow more intense during the 1990s but would lead inevitably to a formal unification and strengthening of the two organizations at the dawn of the twenty-first century.

Despite their differences, the Clinic and Hospital began an expansion outward from the Jefferson Highway campus in 1985 that would carry forward for the next quarter-century. Ochsner's growing community outreach initiative began a process of establishing neighborhood and regional clinics across southeastern Louisiana. The Clinic and the Foundation also established a Health Maintenance Organization (HMO), called the Ochsner Health Plan (OHP), to bring integrated healthcare to the people of the region.

Meanwhile, Ochsner's reputation for medical innovation strengthened during the 1980s with new advances in Diagnostic Radiology, Angioplasty, Pediatric Surgery and Neonatal Intensive Care. A decade of such promise and challenge, however, began on the saddest of notes.

Ochsner's 40-foot human heart was one of the big attractions of the 1984 New Orleans World's Fair.

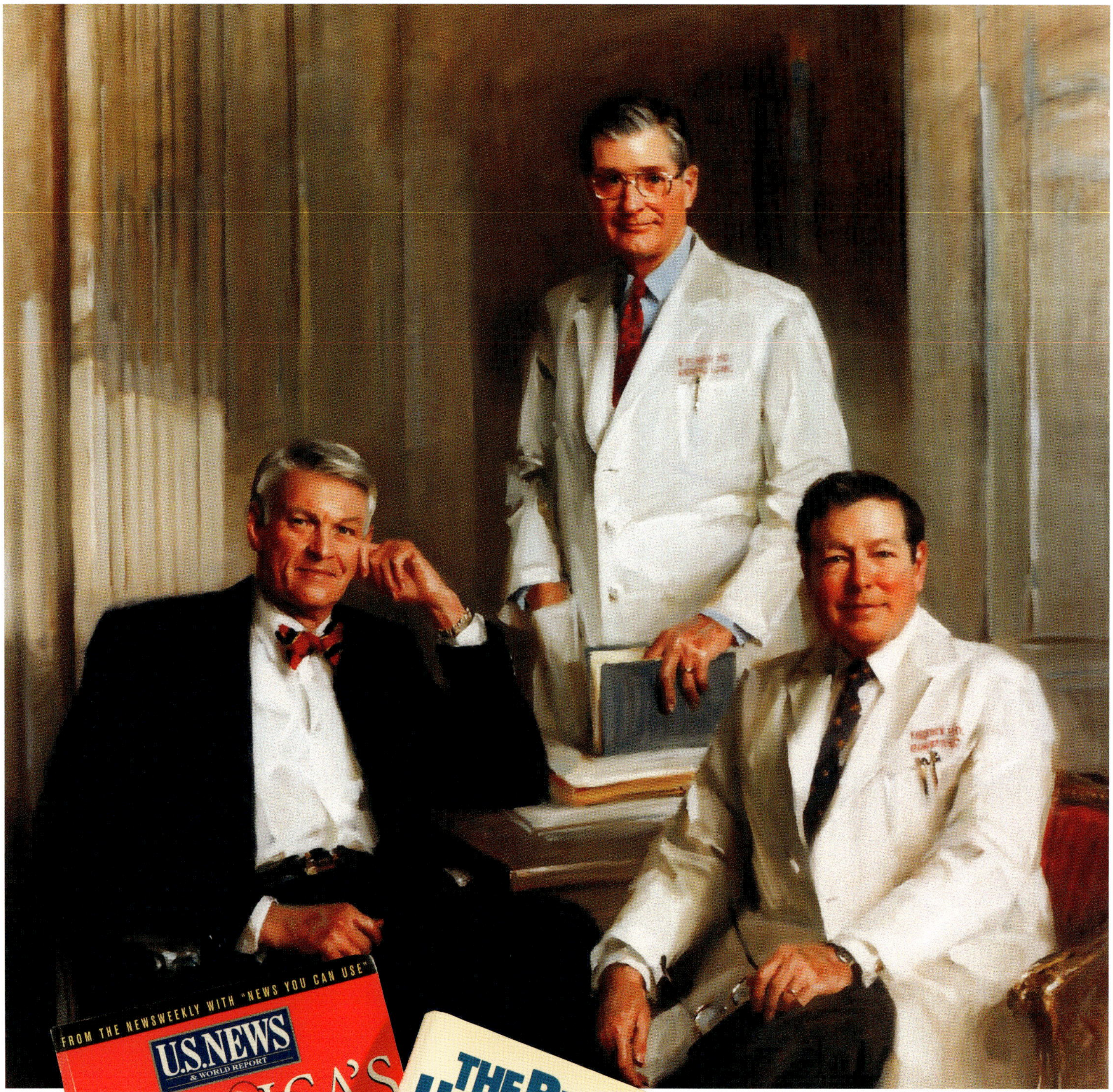

The leaders during the 1980s were J. Thomas Lewis, Chairman of the Board for the Foundation; George Porter, President of the Foundation; and Frank Riddick, Medical Director/CEO of Ochsner Clinic.

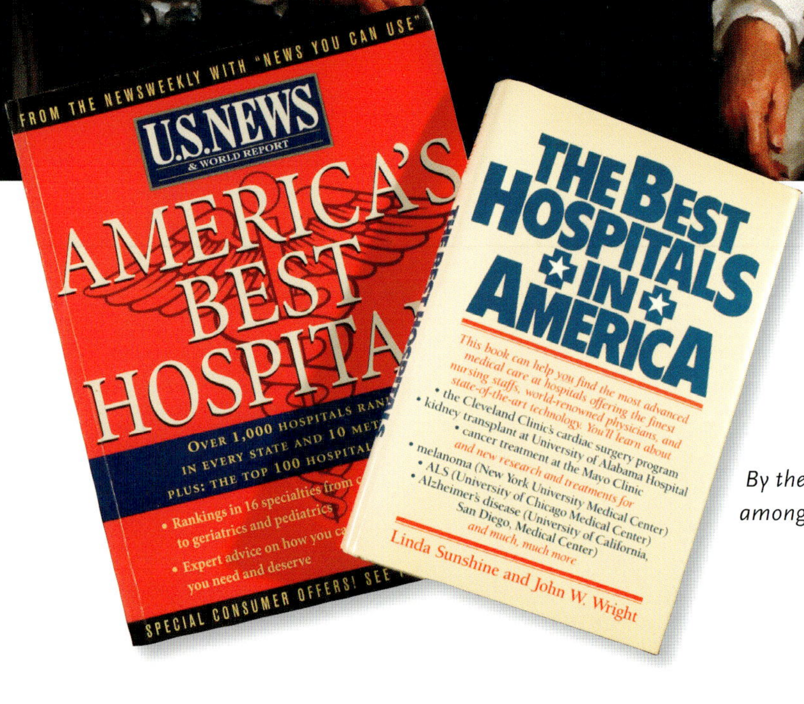

By the late 1980s, Ochsner was consistently ranked among the best hospitals in the United States.

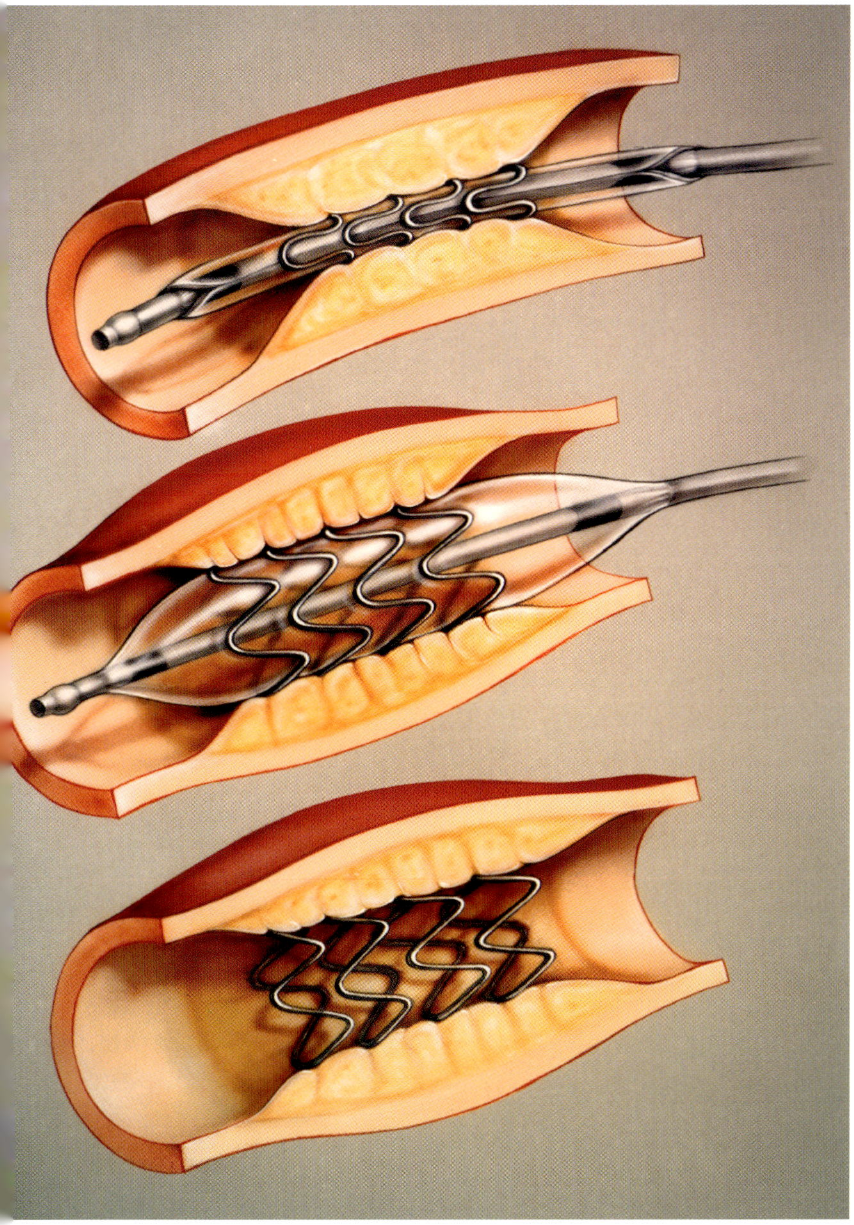

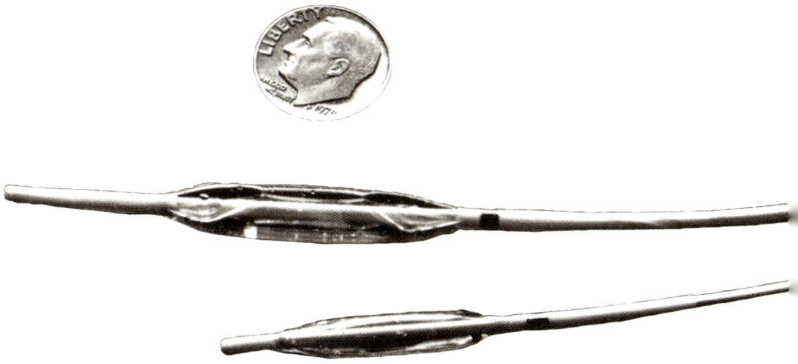

Device used by Cardiologist Lynn Skelton, who performed the first coronary angioplasty procedure at Ochsner in 1980.

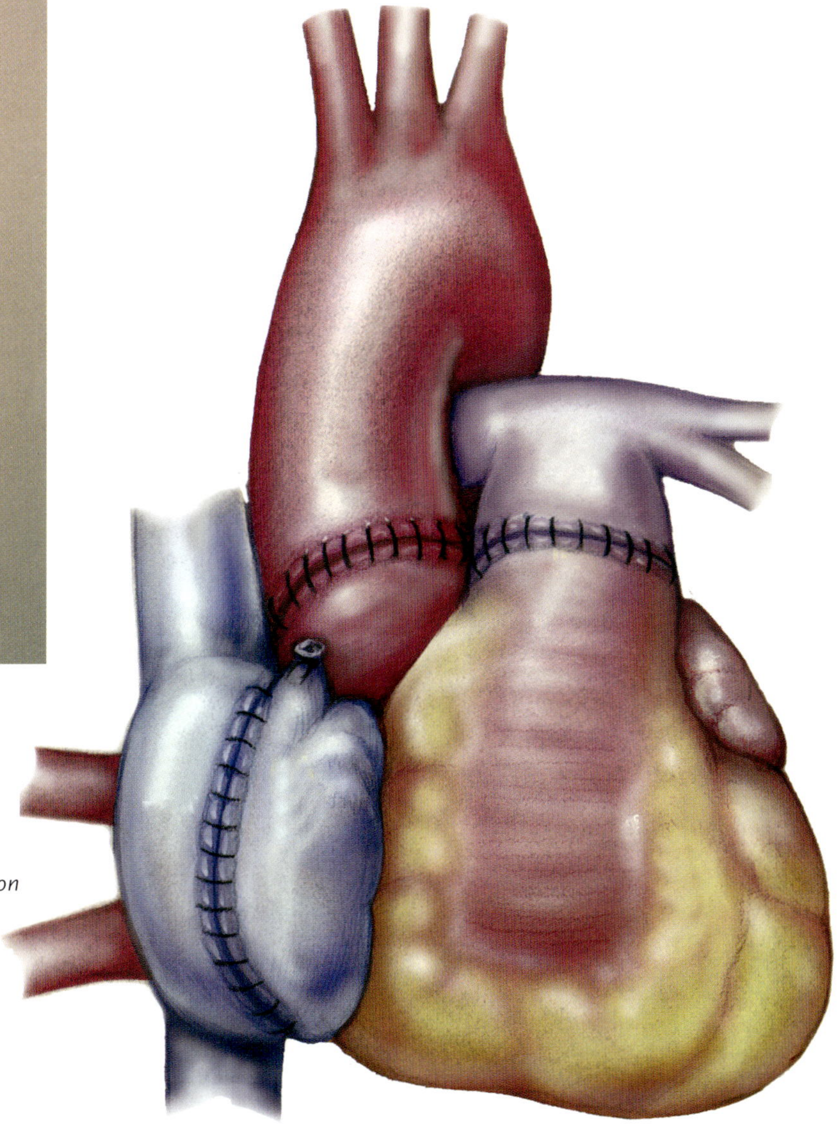

John Ochsner performed the first pediatric heart transplant in the region in 1986.

"We must get back to treating the individual," Ochsner told colleagues when he was in his eighties. "We must be doctors. We go off into one specialty or another, but we must continue to treat the individual. I feel we often treat only disease—we must treat people."

THE CHIEF PASSES

Dr. Alton Ochsner, who helped found the Clinic that bore his name just 40 years before, died at the age of 85 on September 24, 1981, at Ochsner Foundation Hospital.[1] Ochsner had suffered ill health for several years and had undergone heart surgery just three weeks before his death. He knew that the surgery might not correct the heart disease that was slowly killing him, but he told the surgical team to go ahead and give it their best effort. He, of all people, would understand if the surgery did not work.

During his career, Alton Ochsner had performed more than 20,000 operations, including 13 on his last official day at work, April 30, 1967. Even though he left the operating suite at the age of 70—according to the rule he and the other founders established when they started the Clinic—Ochsner continued seeing patients on a regular basis into his early eighties.

"My friends worry about me because they say I work too hard," Ochsner said on the occasion of his 80th birthday in 1976. "What they don't realize is that it is not work—it's fun. I love it."[2]

Alton Ochsner's later years were marked by both tragedy and happiness. His beloved wife of 45 years, Isabel, died during the spring of 1968 after fighting cancer for three years.[3] A year-and-a-half later, Ochsner met a Los Angeles widow at a California dinner party. Following a whirlwind courtship, Alton Ochsner married Jane Kellogg Sturdy in 1970, and the two enjoyed a very happy 10-year marriage.[4]

Alton Ochsner's death in 1981 was a reminder that an era was passing. Dr. Edgar Burns and Dr. Francis LeJeune Sr. preceded Ochsner in death. Dr. Guy Caldwell and Dr. Curtis Tyrone died within the 10 months following Ochsner's passing.

What the five founders left behind was a legacy of personal involvement with patients that typified Ochsner Clinic and Ochsner Foundation Hospital. "We must get back to treating the individual," Ochsner told colleagues when he was in his eighties. "We must be doctors. We go off into one specialty or another, but we must continue to treat the individual. I feel we often treat only disease—we must treat people."[5]

Alton Ochsner, May 4, 1896–September 24, 1981.

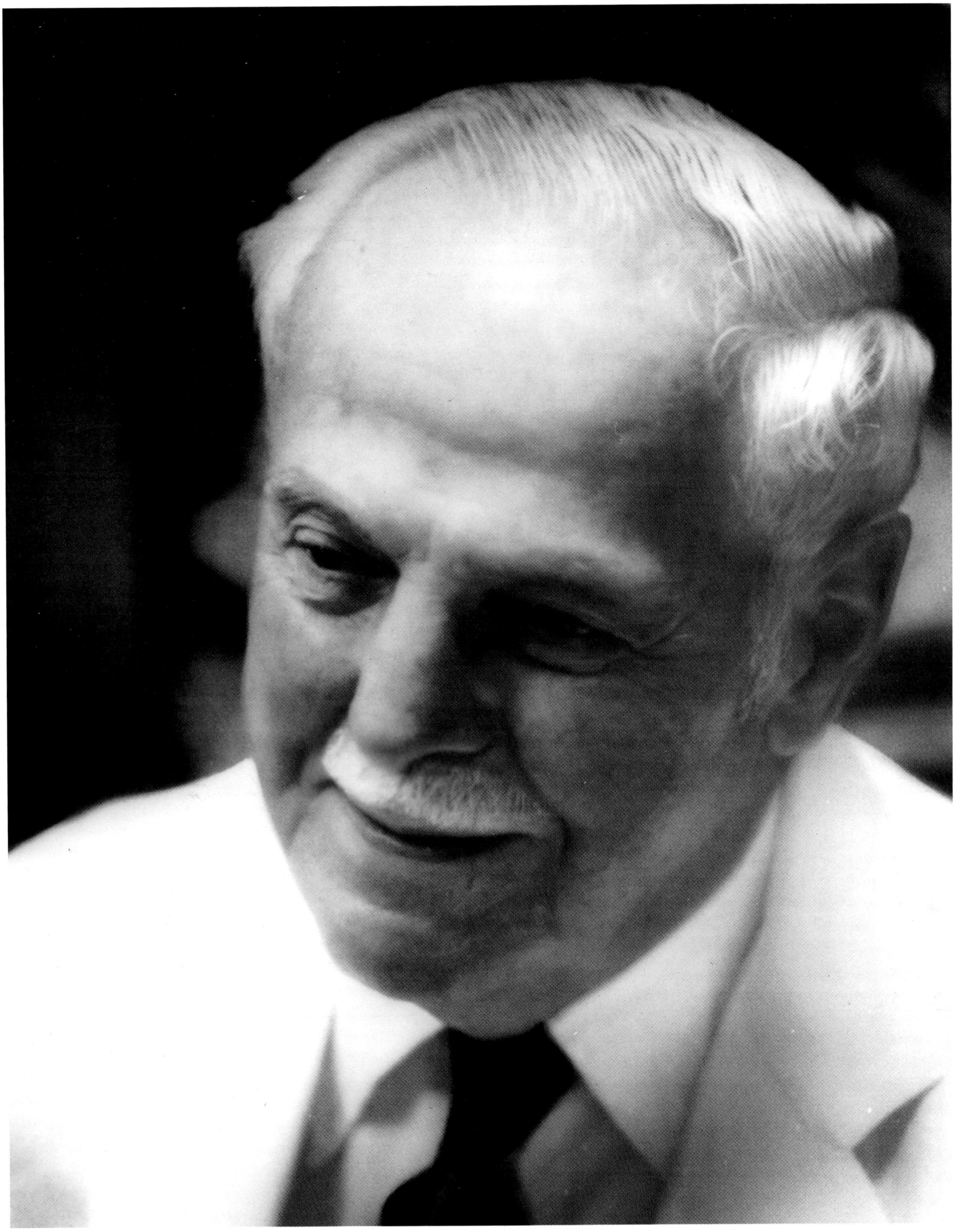

TREATING PEOPLE

Treating people with the latest advances in medical science and technology was something Ochsner as an institution did very well. Under the leadership of Dr. Carl Kardinal, Ochsner's Cancer Institute secured funding from the National Cancer Institute in 1983 to support Ochsner's Community Clinical Oncology Program (CCOP), which conducted clinical trials designed to speed cancer treatments to patients in southeastern Louisiana.

An Ochsner cardiologist conducted the first cardiac angioplasty procedure at the hospital in 1980, and surgeons re-attached a scrap metal yard worker's severed hand in a 10-hour operation that involved the reconnection of arteries, veins, nerves, tendons, bone and skin. In 1983, Ochsner's NICU became only the fourth hospital unit in the United States to utilize Extracorporeal Membrane Oxygenation (ECMO), introduced by Dr. Robert Arensman, for the treatment of "blue babies." ECMO helped stabilize a 13-ounce girl delivered in August 1987 by caesarean section at Ochsner Foundation Hospital and rushed to the NICU.

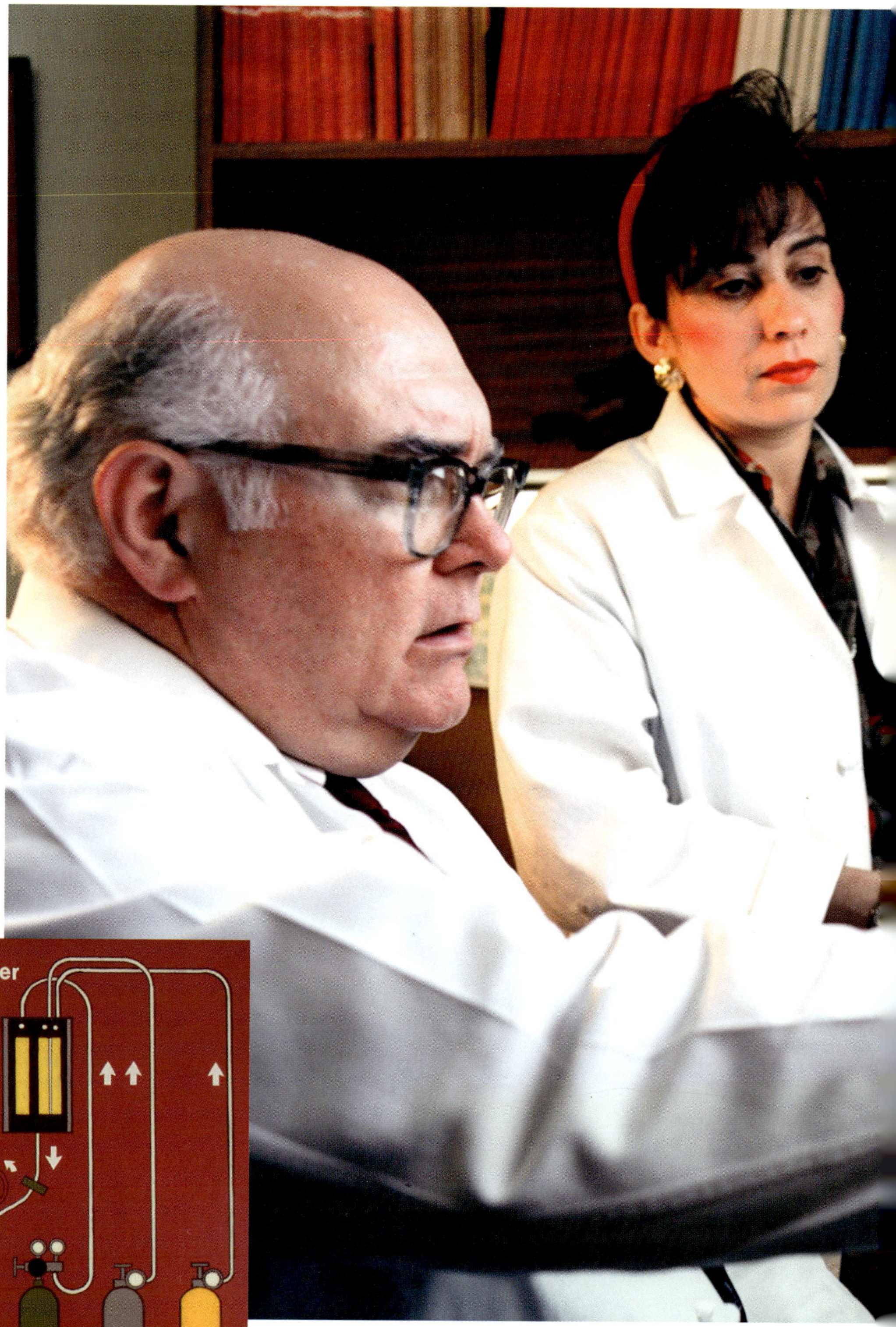

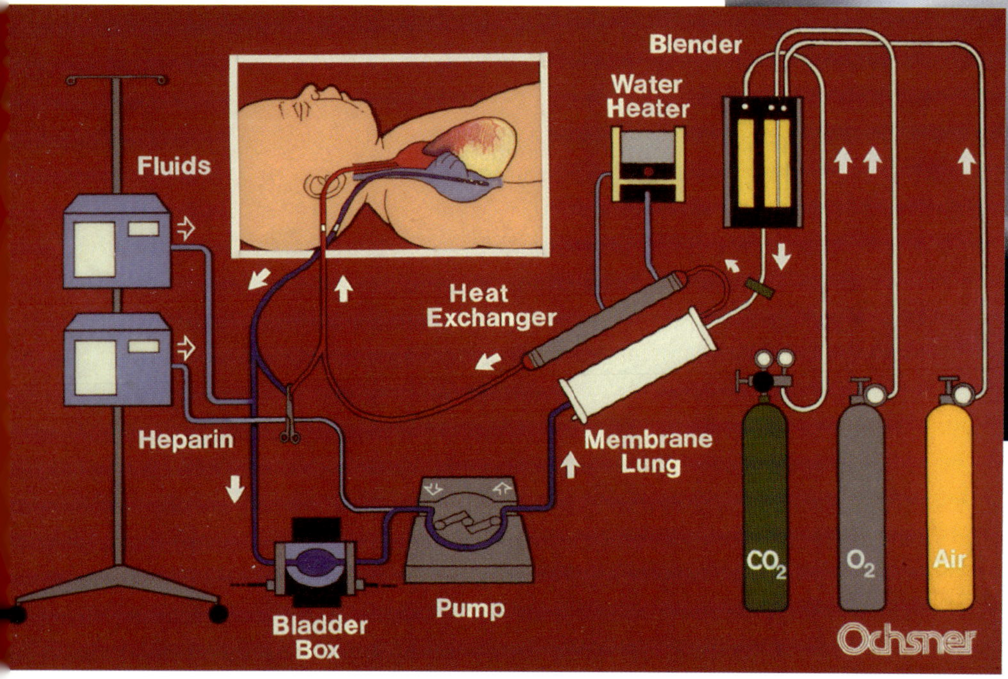

In 1983, Ochsner's Extracorporeal Membrane Oxygenation (ECMO) was the fourth such system in the United States and a godsend to local infants with congenital circulation problems.

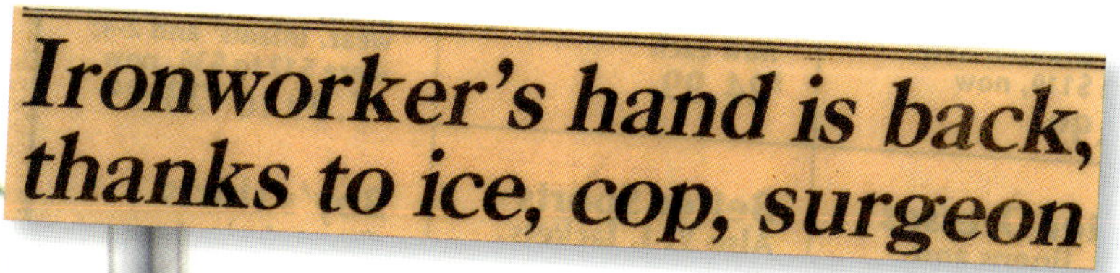

Ironworker's hand is back, thanks to ice, cop, surgeon

Ochsner Orthopedic Surgeon Jefferson Kaye led a team that re-attached a local ironworker's hand in a 10-hour operation in 1981.

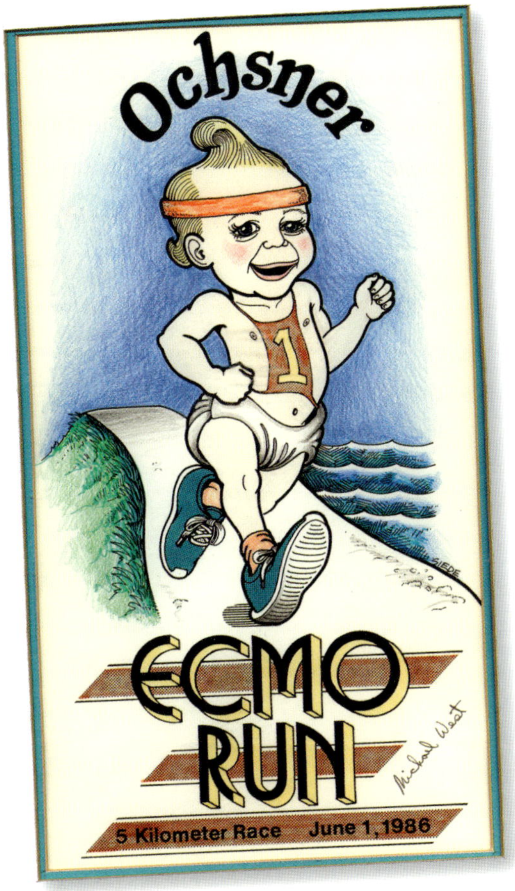

The Ochsner ECMO Run started in 1985 and was a way for staffers and the community to support children's healthcare at Ochsner.

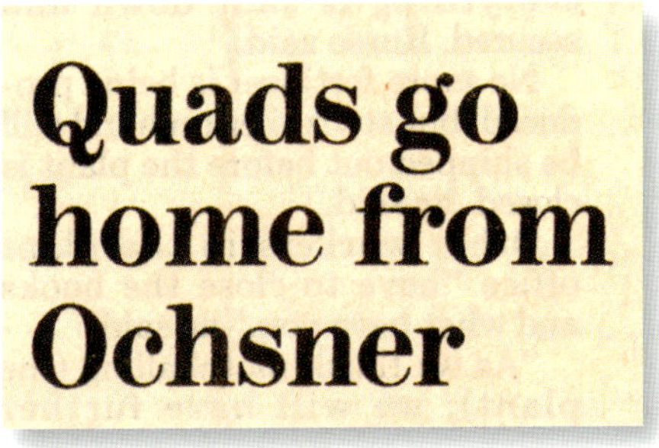

Quads go home from Ochsner

The first set of surviving quadruplets born in Louisiana went home from Ochsner in February 1987.

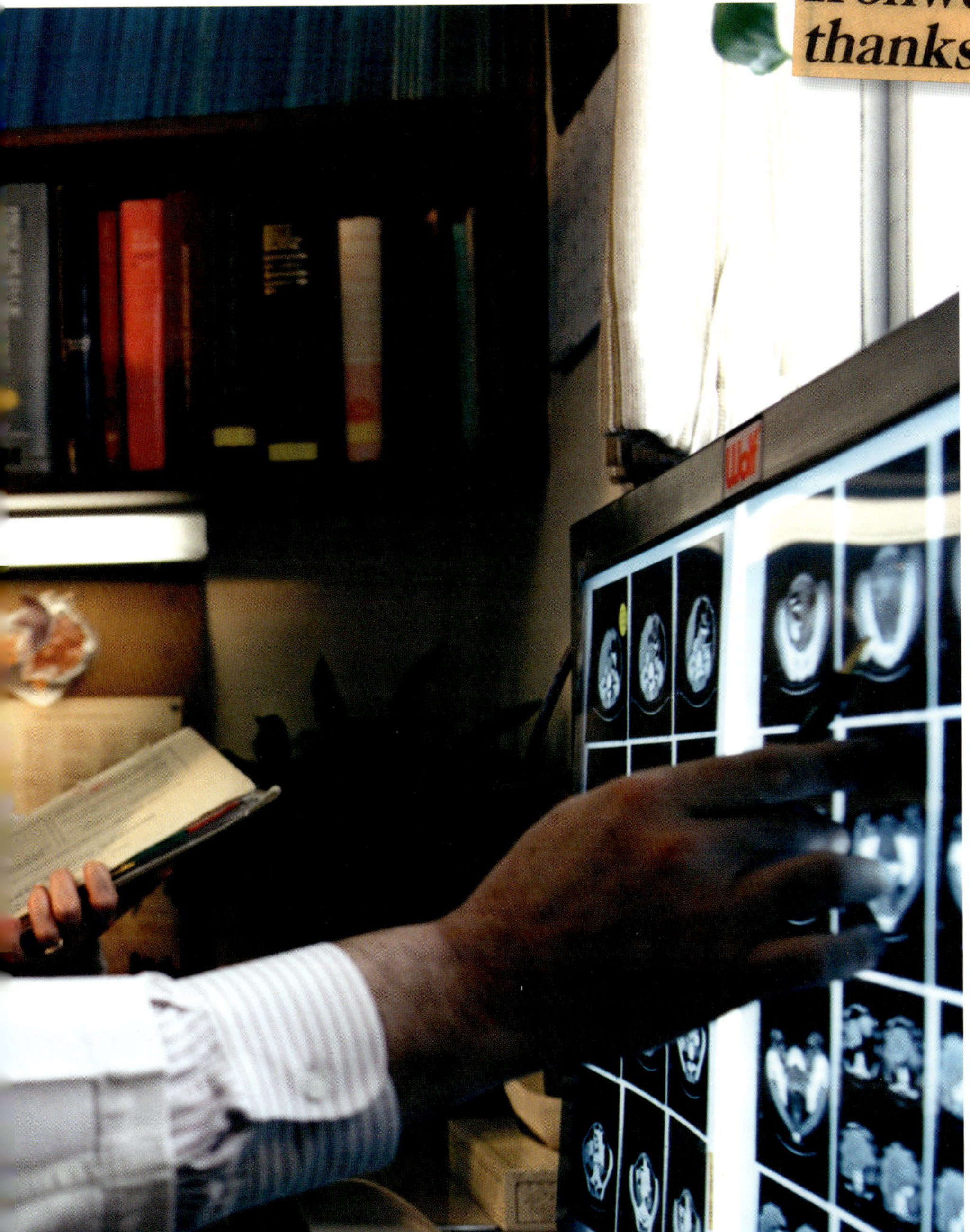

Carl Kardinal, M.D., Director of the Cancer Institute and Principal Investigator of the Ochsner Community Clinical Oncology Program, and Data Manager Nancy Rivera survey clinical trial x-rays in 1983.

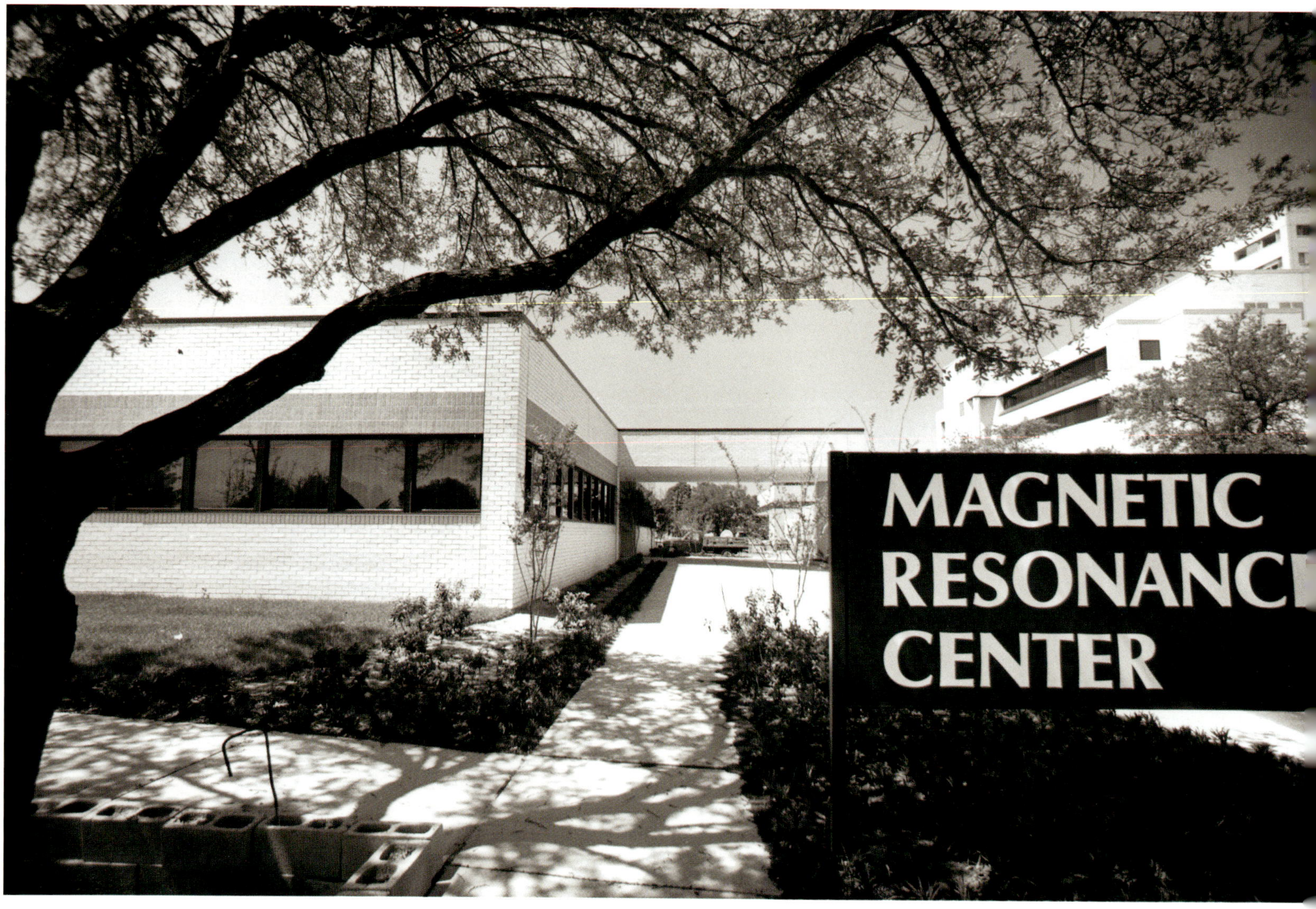

Magnetic Resonance Imaging (MRI), a new way for radiologists to peer inside the human body, required its own building in 1985.

MRI

Ochsner implemented one of the most potent diagnostic tools when it opened the area's first Center for Magnetic Resonance Imaging (MRI) during the spring of 1985 in a building separate from the Clinic and Hospital.

Radiology and Imaging made impressive strides during the 1980s, and Ochsner was an early adopter of the technology. The Department of Diagnostic Radiology conducted the first North American field test of a Computed Radiographic Imaging (CRI) system that promised better and cheaper images of the interior of the human body than conventional x-rays.[6] This advance would lead to digital radiography that became widely used during the 1990s.

Under the leadership of Dr. Christopher Merritt, Ochsner's Department of Diagnostic Radiology made quantum leaps in technology during the period. Dr. Michael A. Sullivan, whose father started the Gastroenterology Department at Splinter Village in 1945, joined the Ochsner Diagnostic Radiology staff in 1969. "When I started we could only examine the stomach and colon with barium during fluoroscopy," Sullivan said.[7] The relatively primitive radiological diagnostic abilities of the 1960s and 1970s gave way to much more sophisticated methods during the 1980s and 1990s.

Sullivan has experienced tremendous changes in Radiology during his career at Ochsner. The Department of Diagnostic Radiology obtained the 14th Computerized Axial Tomography (CT) scanner in the world in 1974. Two years later, Ochsner Radiologists, including Drs. Christopher Merritt, Edward Bluth and Michael Sullivan, began experimenting with Doppler and Color Doppler Ultrasound systems. In the mid-1980s, the department began working with digital radiographs.[8]

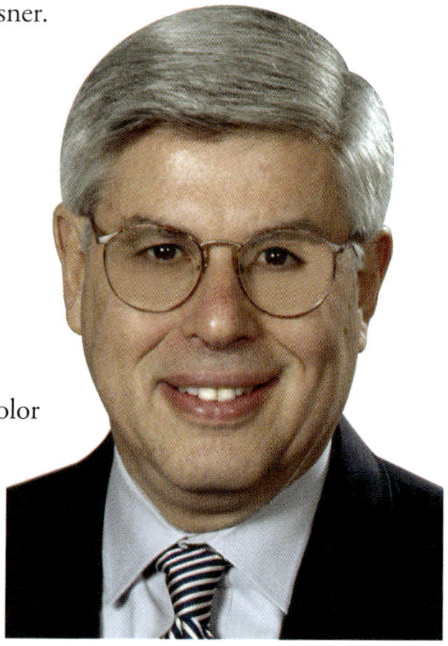

UNPARALLELED PROSPERITY

The period between 1974 and 1985 was one of unparalleled prosperity for Ochsner in particular and the medical community in general. Ochsner issued nearly $60 million in tax-exempt bonds to fund an expansion of the Hospital and Clinic during the mid-1970s. Ochsner Foundation Hospital added 131 beds at a cost of more than $29 million, and the Clinic staff grew to 140 physicians.[9]

Ochsner enjoyed steady growth during the 1970s and early 1980s. Admissions to Ochsner Foundation Hospital grew more than 26 percent in that era. Patient visits to Ochsner Clinic rose 11 percent between 1980 and 1985 and operating revenues for the Foundation jumped from $80 million in 1981 to $123 million in 1985.[10]

Dr. George Porter, a courtly Tarheel and Duke University Medical School graduate, came to Ochsner in 1964 to specialize in Hematology and Oncology. During 1980, he became President and CEO of the Alton Ochsner Medical Foundation. As such, Porter presided over much of the Foundation's growth during the early 1980s and witnessed the growing rift between the Clinic and the Foundation. Some of the discord stemmed from the 1975 financial restructuring mandated by the IRS.

"The Clinic was a cash-based partnership," Porter said. "The Foundation's main job was to generate capital to put into the institution. Part of the tension was that the Clinic's board felt we weren't putting the money back in."[11]

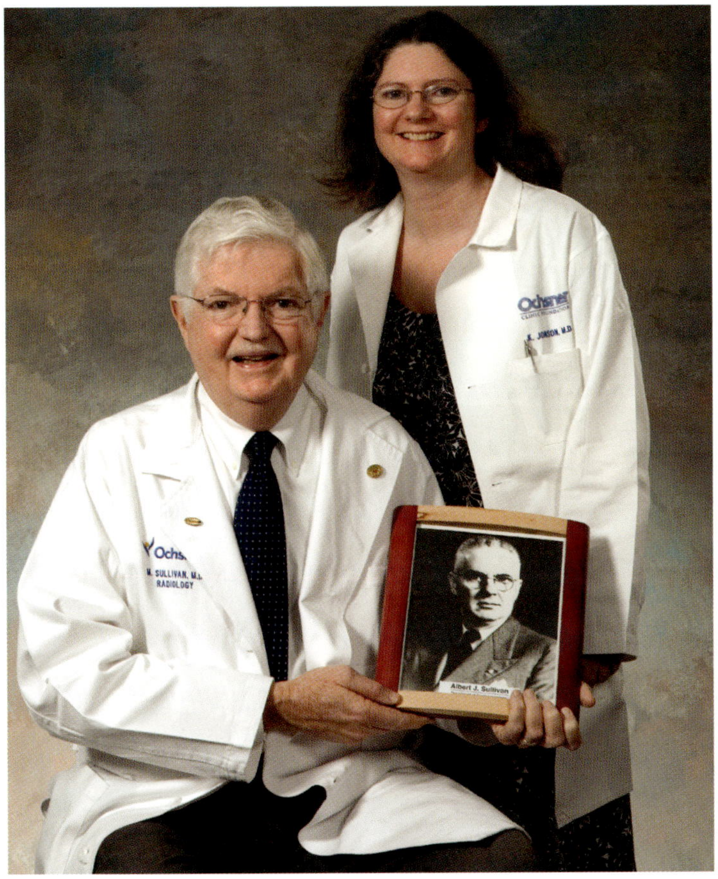

Ochsner has been caring for generations of Louisiana families for over 60 years. In that time, Ochsner has also employed generations of families. One of the most recent members of "Ochsner Generations" is Internist Kristin Johnson, M.D., the daughter of Ochsner Radiologist Michael A. Sullivan, M.D., who has been with Ochsner since 1969. Michael Sullivan, in turn, is the son of Albert J. Sullivan, M.D., who founded the Section of Gastroenterology at Ochsner and was on staff from 1945 to 1951.

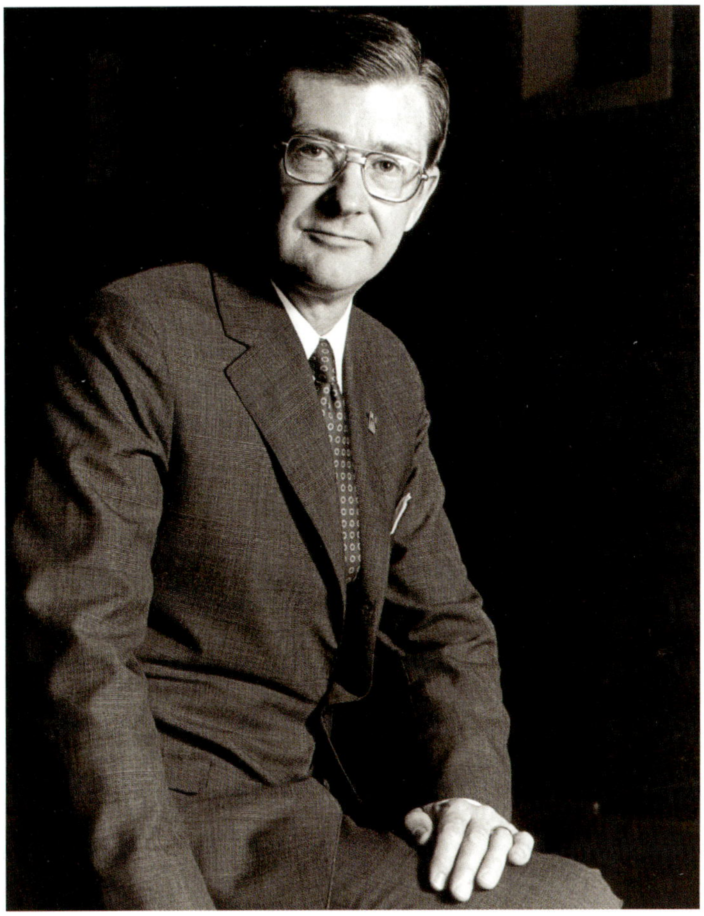

George Porter, M.D., guided the fortunes of the Foundation through the tremendous changes of the 1980s while safeguarding the institution's reputation for providing the best patient care in the region.

Edward Bluth, M.D., is the Chairman Emeritus of the Department of Radiology and heads the Section of Ultrasonography.

CHANGING DYNAMICS

Increasing scrutiny of the interactions between for-profit and not-for-profit entities highlighted problems intrinsic to the relationships between Ochsner Clinic and the Foundation. The organizations were mutually dependent and the sharing of resources became progressively more difficult. Regulatory constraints greatly slowed decision making and undermined teamwork.

The early 1980s, in the words of a 1985 Ochsner study, were "the last years of the golden age of fee-for-service, cost-plus medicine."[12] Healthcare administrators began to learn to live with the advent of HMOs, Preferred Provider Organizations (PPOs) and new Medicare reimbursement formulas, such as the Diagnostic Related Groups (DRGs). For New Orleans and the adjacent Gulf Coast region, the economy went from bad to worse in 1984 when the oil boom collapsed in the wake of the national recession.

"Everything worked until 1984–1985 when the money got tight," said George Porter. "We were spending money on expensive equipment. And we were facing unprecedented changes in medicine and medical finances."[13]

Something had to be done. The Clinic and Foundation boards came to the conclusion that the perilous times presented opportunities for Ochsner to expand beyond its Jefferson Highway base. Getting to that point, however, required changing attitudes that had evolved over nearly 40 years.

THE RISE OF SPECIALTIES

The roots of these challenges went back to the emergence of an era of medical specialization after World War II. During the 1950s and 1960s—an era of tremendous growth at Ochsner—patients tended to equate specialist care with high quality. The rapidly growing health insurance industry provided increased income to specialists, and society's respect accompanied the specialist role in American healthcare. Ochsner Clinic created a Section of General Internal Medicine during the 1970s but still found it difficult to recruit and retain physicians for primary care services.

Meanwhile, the administration of President Richard M. Nixon began pushing the concept of the HMO—essentially a closed-panel, prepaid group practice—as a vehicle to improve quality and hold down costs of medical care. Dr. Frank Riddick represented Ochsner at an early 1970s California conference on the topic of managed care. He reported back to the Clinic partnership that Ochsner was a specialized referral center in which virtually none of the physicians were devoting the bulk of their professional time to primary care. Furthermore, the attitudes of many of the Clinic partners were not fully supportive of embracing primary care. He concluded that if Ochsner Clinic were to become involved in managed care, it would require commitment to recruiting, nurturing and retaining primary care physicians who would provide services at sites away from the high technology teaching site on Jefferson Highway.

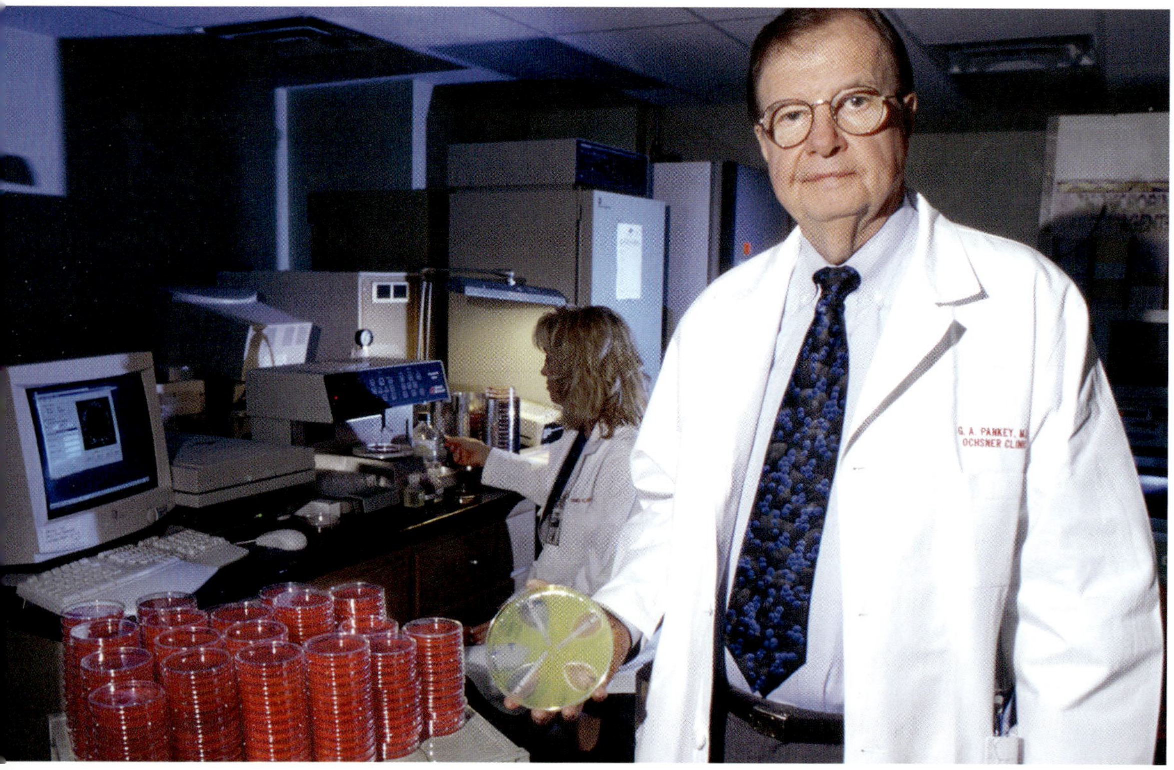

George Pankey, M.D., is Ochsner's Director of Infectious Diseases Research and is an internationally recognized and honored expert in the field of infectious diseases.

KICKING THE HABIT

In 1985 and 1986, Ochsner honored its namesake founder with two actions, one tangible and visible to the community-at-large and the second a policy decision that Dr. Alton Ochsner would have endorsed wholeheartedly.

The first action was the erection of a larger-than-life-sized bronze statue of Alton Ochsner in a brick courtyard adjacent to the fountain in the Plaza of the Americas at the front of the Jefferson Highway campus. The eight-foot-tall, half-ton statue captured Ochsner in a typical pose, his feet apart and his hands thrust into the pockets of a lab coat. The gift of New Orleans financier Louis J. Roussel Jr. and his son, Louis J. Roussel III, the statue was completed by New York sculptor Marc Richard Mellon.[14]

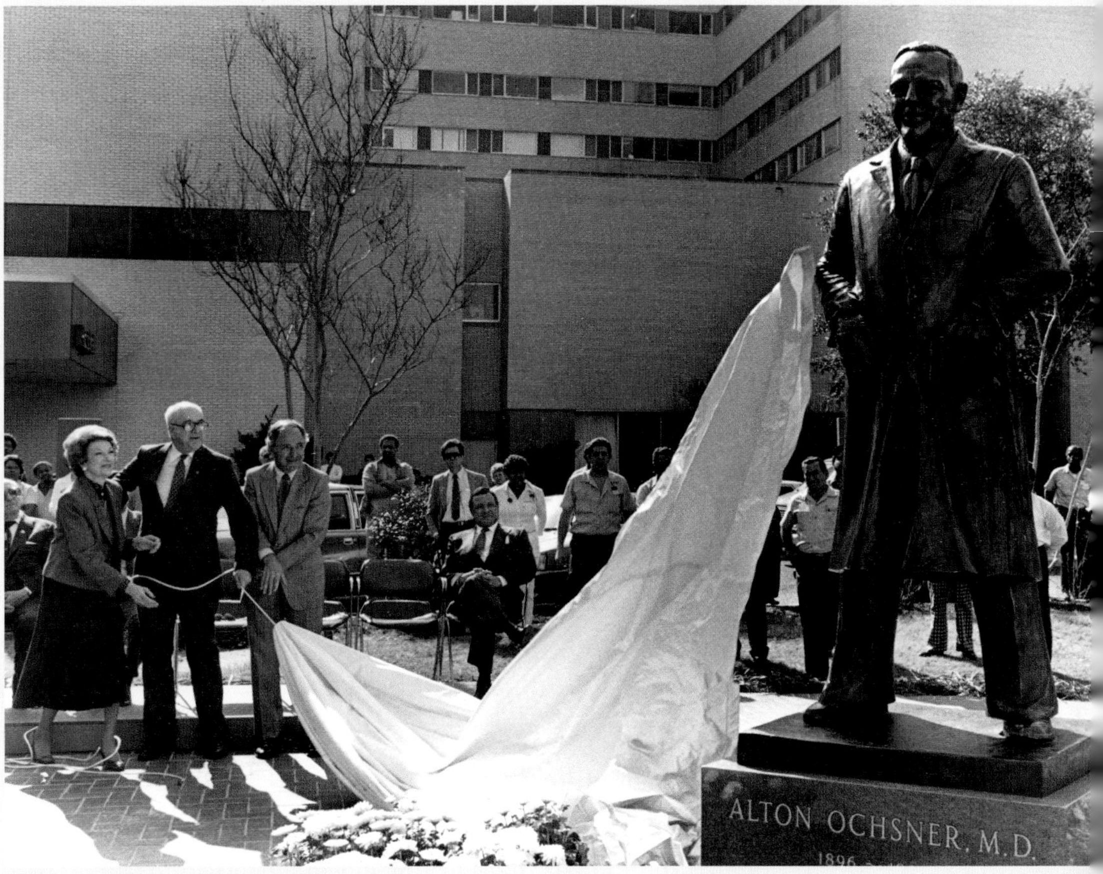

Five years after his death, Alton Ochsner was captured in bronze by sculptor Marc Mellon. Three of Alton Ochsner's children, including Sis Ochsner Mann, Alton (Akky) Ochsner Jr. and John Ochsner, unveiled the statue.

"I was trying to get a sense of Dr. Ochsner's great strength and character," Mellon said, explaining the statue's bold pose. "I wanted the quality to be there in the sculpture, so that people who knew him would feel his presence."[15]

The second action occurred on January 1, 1986, when all of the Ochsner facilities, including the Jefferson Highway campus and the neighborhood health centers, officially became smoke-free. Since initially publishing his pioneering research linking cigarette smoking to lung cancer, Alton Ochsner spent the remainder of his life warning against the dangers of smoking. Later in 1986, Ochsner presented the first Alton Ochsner Award Relating Smoking and Health to Dr. Oscar Auerbach at the annual convocation of the American College of Chest Physicians.[16]

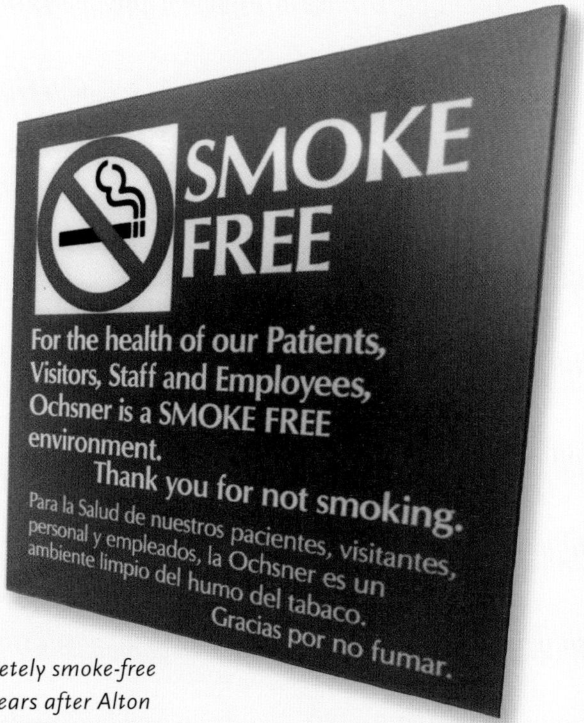

Ochsner went completely smoke-free in 1986, almost 50 years after Alton Ochsner first identified a link between cigarette smoking and lung cancer.

EXPANSION

By the early 1980s, Ochsner's traditional role as a tertiary care referral center was under siege from several threats. There was significant competition from local and regional institutions and specialists. Services traditionally restricted to referral centers such as Ochsner entered the healthcare mainstream and were no longer reimbursed at premium rates by insurance carriers. Patients' ability to choose care at Ochsner was limited by the steering mechanisms imposed by employer-based managed care plans.

Management's strategic planning considered several options to assure continued access to Ochsner's services. Not everyone agreed that steps for change were necessary, let alone the scope and direction of that change. Potential costs were a universal concern.

Some on the Clinic Board of Management insisted that the concerns were overblown and that patients would continue to seek quality care at Ochsner. Others on the Foundation Board of Trustees worried that the changes would convert Ochsner from high quality specialized care to something more diluted. Some Clinic partners resisted the idea of practicing at regional sites.

The shrinking number of primary care physicians at the Jefferson Highway campus could not generate the volume of referrals necessary to support the number of specialized physicians at Ochsner. Local initiatives had been tried, including strengthening staffing in the Emergency Department, establishing helicopter transport services and signing industrial medicine contracts to manage on-site services to maritime and industrial plants up the Mississippi River corridor.

Further complicating matters during the early 1980s was the prospect of competition from HMOs and PPOs. Managed care plans, typically directed by health insurance firms, enrolled entire populations of employees and steered them to a provider network of individual physicians, group practices and medical institutions that had agreed to provide services to the covered population at a pre-negotiated, usually highly discounted rate. At the same time, the federal government continued to sharply discount Medicare and Medicaid rates to participating physicians and medical institutions.

Ochsner was faced with three choices regarding managed care plans. The organization could simply avoid participation in any and all HMOs and hope that they would quickly fade from the scene. It could participate in another's plan and bank on being large enough that it could have a dominant voice in the plan, or it could create its own managed care plan and forge ahead into the brave new world of HMOs.

Ochsner chose to create its own managed care plan. Participation in an Ochsner prepaid managed care plan would mandate the ability to provide services close to where patients lived as a prerequisite for attracting Ochsner Health Plan subscribers. Creation of neighborhood and regional clinics became a key component of developing the Ochsner Health Plan.

TRUE SATELLITES

By the mid-1980s, the Clinic and Hospital were undergoing a metamorphosis from what Laura L. Etchen, then Vice President and Director of Planning, described as "a large, single-location tertiary care center into a much larger, fully diversified, multi-location system."[17]

In 1985, the strategy underlying Ochsner's transformation from a single campus on Jefferson Highway to a regional system that served patients across southeastern Louisiana became much clearer. With the competition for the healthcare dollar

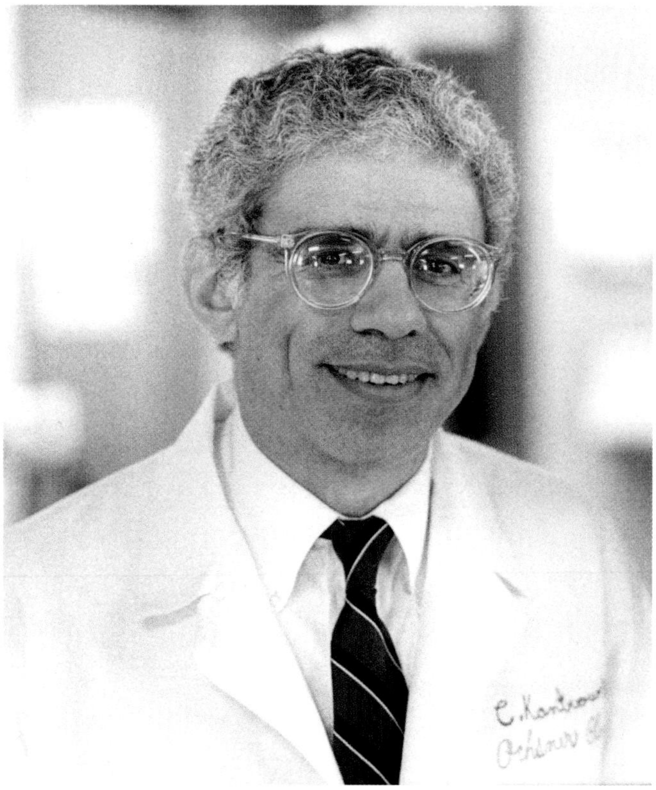

Charles M. Kantrow Jr., M.D., was the first Medical Director of Ochsner Clinic of Baton Rouge. He was instrumental in the development of the Clinic and the recruitment of its initial professional staff.

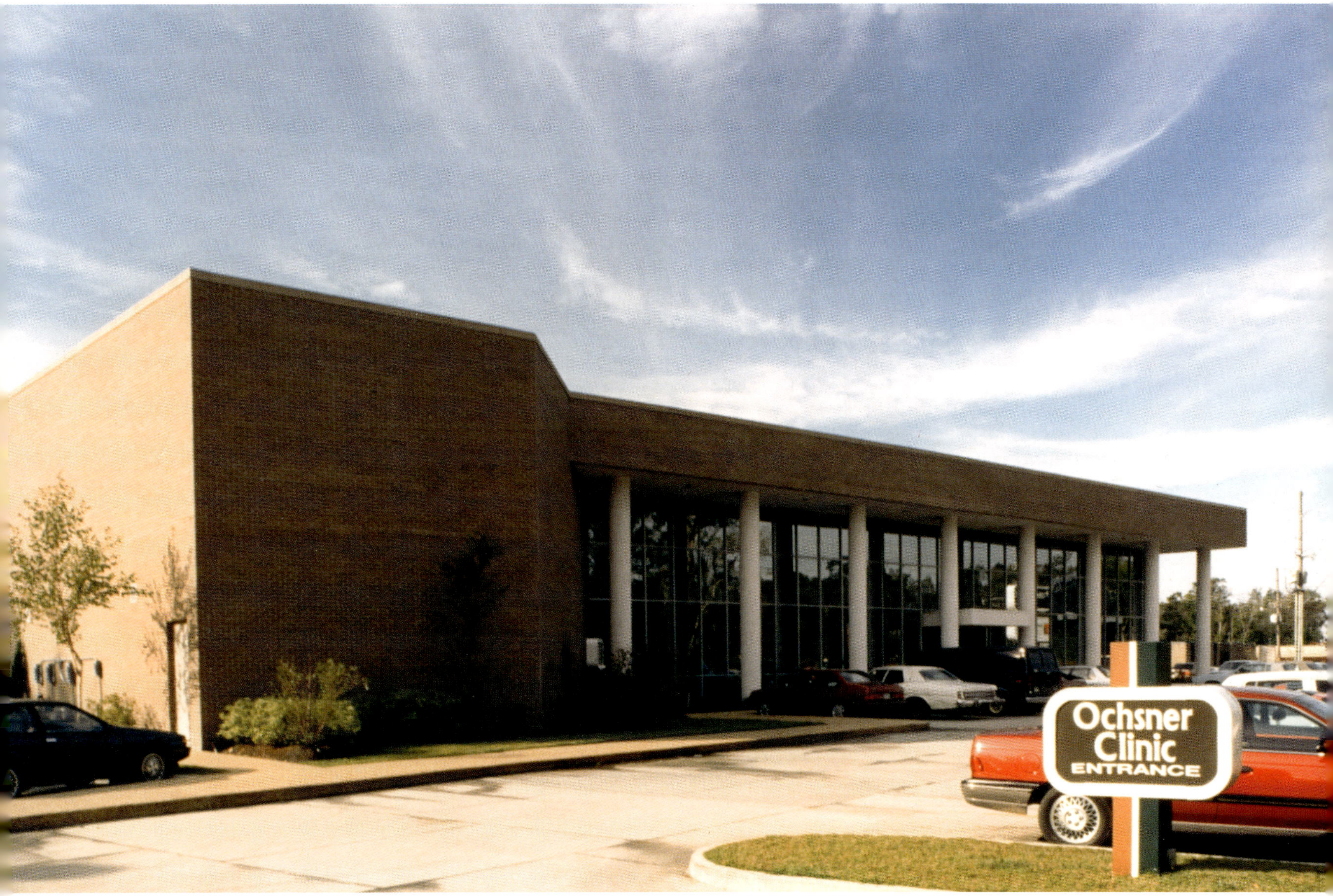

Ochsner Clinic–Lapalco on the West Bank of New Orleans was one of the institution's first neighborhood health centers in 1985.

growing ever more fierce, Ochsner resolved to bring its internationally renowned, patient-focused medical care closer to the patients it was already serving. Ochsner's move into satellite healthcare was motivated by the twin goals of adding value for patients and improving community health. Just as the founders had taken a huge risk in 1942 to open a specialty Clinic on Prytania Street, Ochsner took a similar risk during the mid-1980s, one that helped make a difference to the community in the years to come.

Between 1985 and 1987, Ochsner opened satellite clinics in New Orleans East, Kenner, the West Bank, Slidell, Metairie and St. Tammany Parish. Ochsner Clinic–Mandeville was based on the highly regarded and successful family practice of Drs. Jerry Keller and Roy Gregory. Nephrologist Charles Kantrow Jr., a member of Ochsner Clinic's Board of Management and a native of Baton Rouge, pioneered the first true regional facility, Ochsner Clinic of Baton Rouge, and guided recruitment of its staff and establishment in the community during its first decade.[18]

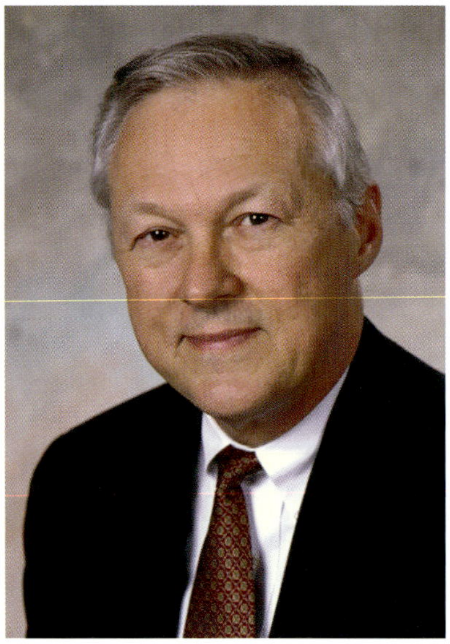

Rudolph "Rudy" Ehrensing, M.D., served as Chair of the Department of Psychiatry and Associate Medical Director for Personnel Affairs.

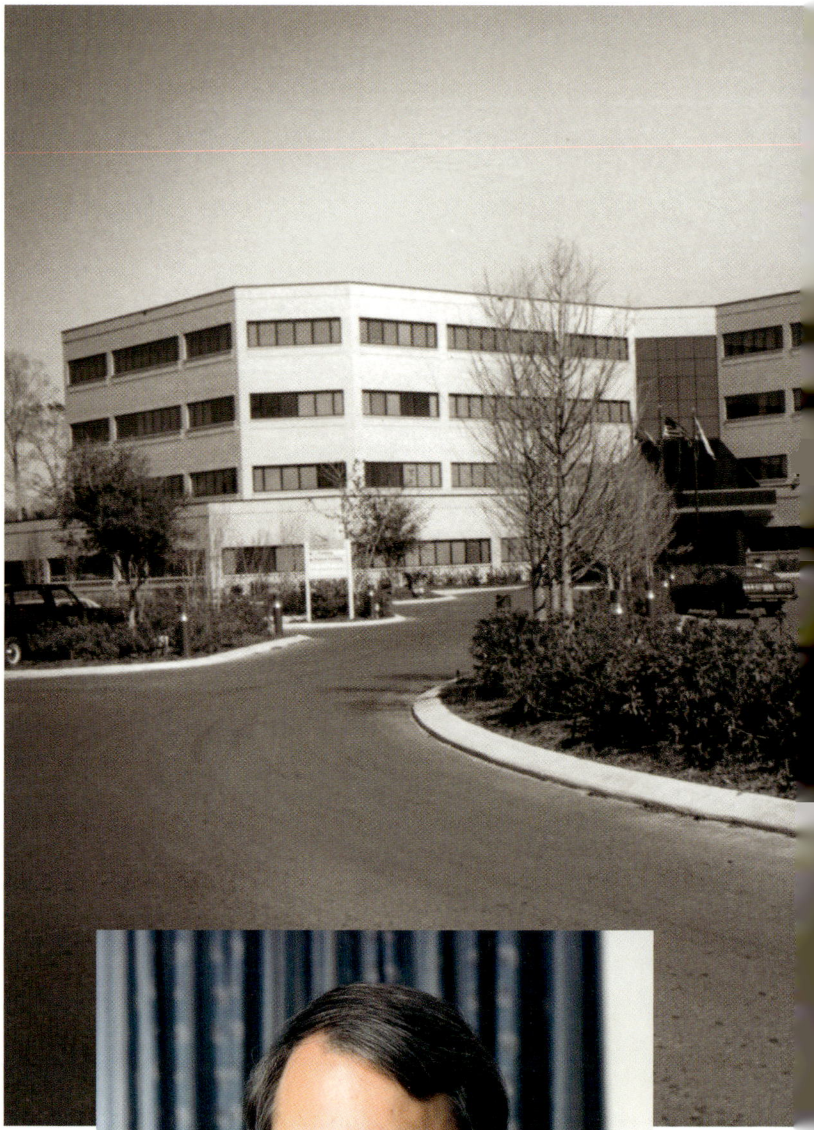

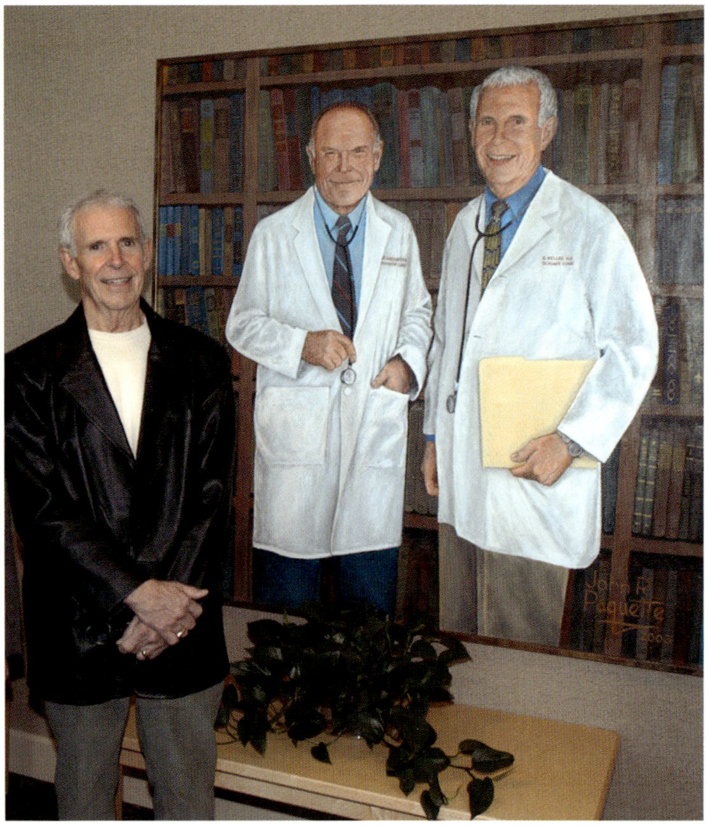

Gerald Keller, M.D (left in the portrait) and Roy Gregory, M.D. (standing to the left and right in the portrait) incorporated their family practice on the North Shore with Ochsner to become Ochsner Clinic - Mandeville.

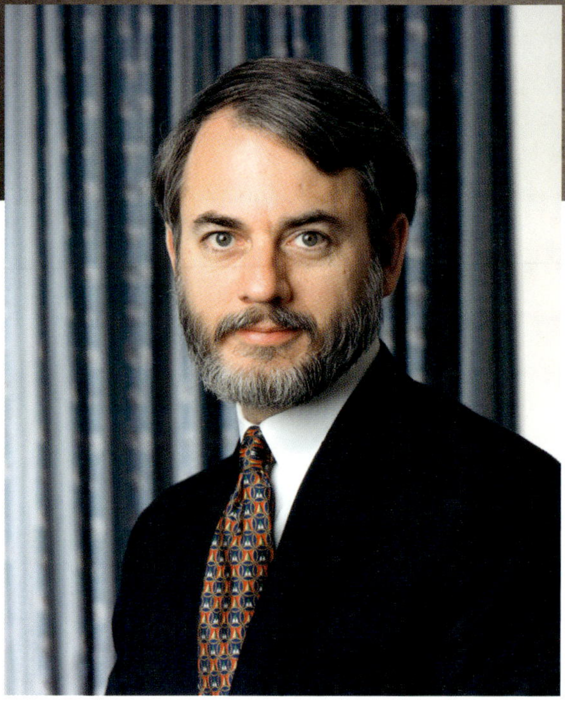

Michael Tooke, M.D., former Associate Medical Director of Ochsner Clinic from 1992 to 1994, played a role in developing the neighborhood health centers and establishing primary care services at Ochsner.

'A PROFOUND EFFECT'

In the decade ahead, Ochsner would continue its mission of bringing exceptional patient care, research and education to the people of southeastern Louisiana. It would also offer residents of the region the option of joining the Ochsner Health Plan to enjoy some of the best medical care available in the region.

In the process, however, lay the seeds of discord between the Clinic and the Foundation that would sow dissension between the two entities for the next 20 years. Creation of the neighborhood and regional satellite network had a profound effect on the components of the Ochsner System, and the burden fell unequally on the Clinic. The recruitment of professional staff was the responsibility and prerogative of Ochsner Clinic. In other settings, it was often a hospital that undertook the development of a referral network by purchasing physician practices, hiring physicians and running primary care practices in order to secure or retain a referral base. This typically proved to be a money-losing proposition requiring subsidies from the hospital. Healthcare planners estimated conducting each physician practice cost a hospital $100,000 annually, which the hospital hoped to make up by increased volume of admissions and provision of ancillary services in the acquired practices.

At Ochsner, the Clinic group practice bore the expense of the regionalization effort, while many of the benefits accrued to the Hospital. For a variety of reasons, the Clinic group did not wish to cede the right to hire the physicians.

Although the satellite network was essential to the success of the Ochsner Health Plan, the Plan was in no position to subsidize Ochsner Clinic's expenses incurred in the establishment and maintenance of the network.

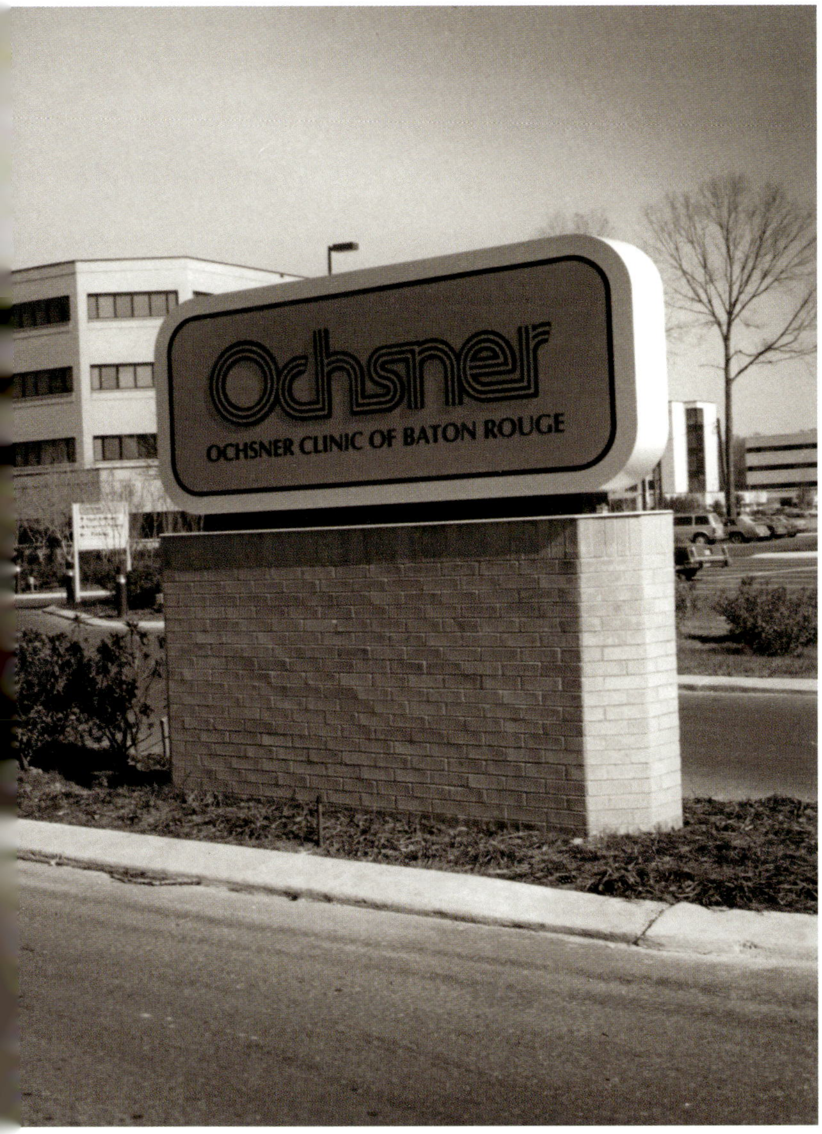

Ochsner Clinic of Baton Rouge opened in 1985 as Ochsner's first truly regional clinic. Nephrologist Charles Kantrow, Jr. shepherded the Clinic through its first decade of growth.

• WHAT OCHSNER MEANS TO ME •

"To me, Ochsner means being able to provide services to the COMMUNITY close to home, but also having access to the resources of a much larger community of hospitals."

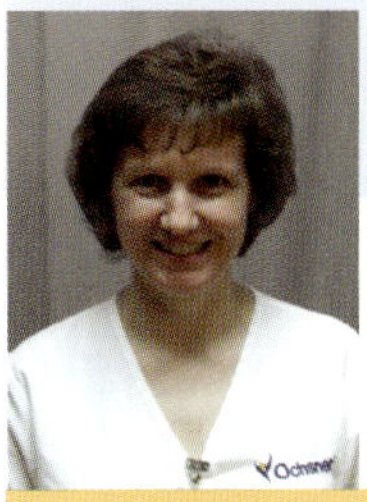

Ann Savoie, Outpatient Infusion Nurse,
Ochsner St. Anne General Hospital

To watch the full interview with Ann Savoie, visit **ochsner.org/history**.

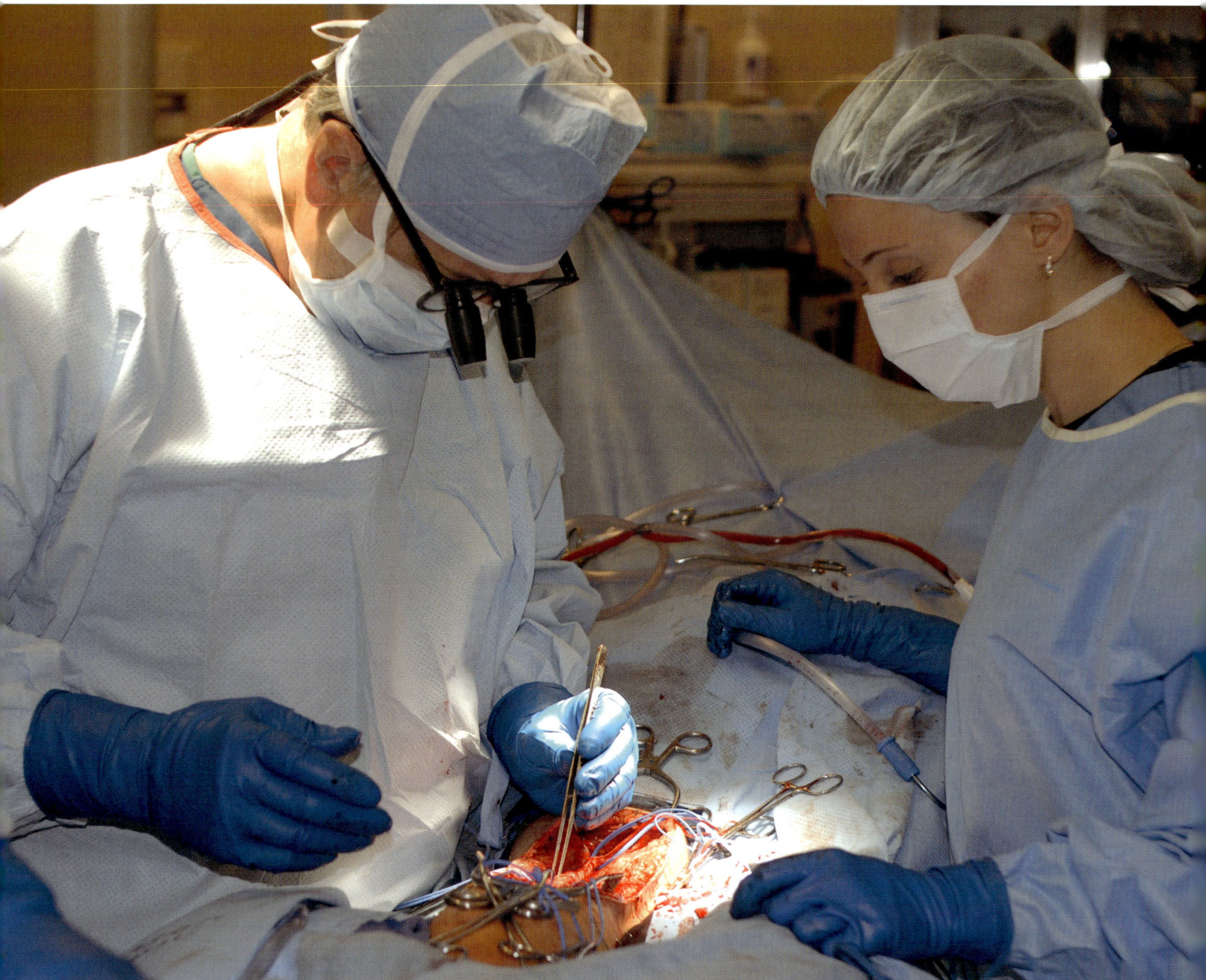

CHAPTER 7:

IMPROVING THE COMMUNITY'S HEALTH

THE 1990s WERE PERHAPS THE MOST DIFFICULT DECADE in the history of Ochsner; the organization, however, achieved major accomplishments during the period. It emerged as a multi-disciplinary, integrated healthcare system with expansion of the neighborhood and regional clinics and growth of the Ochsner Health Plan, the organization's HMO. Ochsner medicine, education and research also continued to advance during the 1990s. Ochsner surgeons performed the first successful heart-lung transplant in Louisiana in 1990, enhancing its reputation for cutting-edge patient care. Ochsner consolidated the research facilities into a new Ochsner Biomedical Research Building on the Jefferson Highway campus in 1993.

External and internal pressures, however, threatened the ties that held Ochsner together. A Clinic/Foundation unification initiative early in the decade never gained traction and led to continued dissension. A failed merger with a Catholic health group created management turnover, and Clinton administration initiatives to rein in healthcare costs further eroded the fee-for-service medical model that had been the pillar of the Ochsner financial structure since the early 1940s.

Ochsner surgery teams have been contributing to Ochsner's surgical legacy for two-thirds of a century.

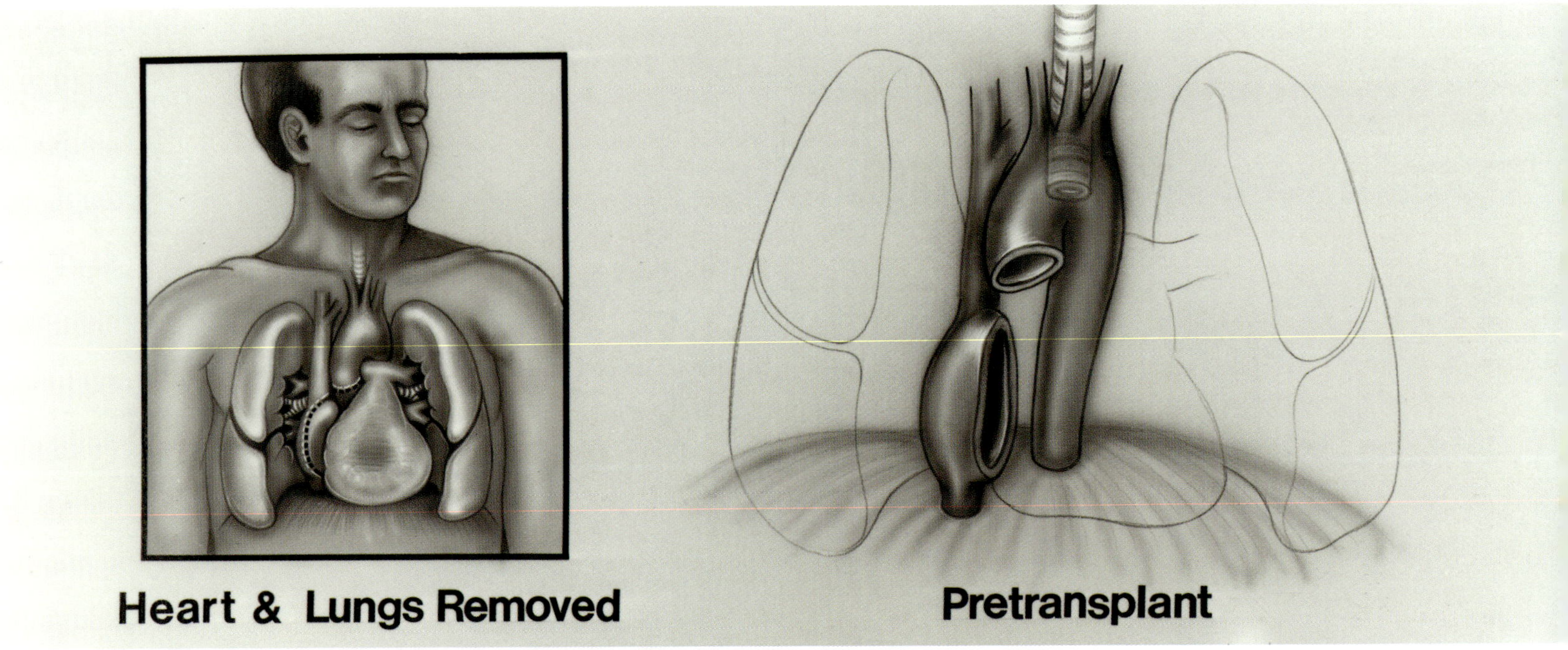

THE OCHSNER HEALTH PLAN

Ochsner's emergence as a fully integrated healthcare provider during the 1990s was attributed in part to the growth of the Ochsner Health Plan.

HMOs began entering the New Orleans marketplace in 1985. Prior to that time, a combination of private individual and group insurance and Medicare/Medicaid was the traditional method of health insurance in the nation at large; the addition of Louisiana's system of charity hospitals to the mix made the state unique. HMOs, however, were clearly the wave of the future in 1985, and some estimates predicted that 85 percent of Americans would be covered by HMOs or PPOs by the turn of the twenty-first century.[1]

"They decided that healthcare costs needed to be restrained," explained George Porter, who was President of the Alton Ochsner Medical Foundation in 1985. "The HMO is basically an insurance company. It had to be capitalized. Ochsner Clinic drew up plans to develop an Ochsner HMO. I agreed wholeheartedly and told the somewhat skeptical Chair of the Foundation's Finance Committee that the Foundation and the Foundation Hospital needed to participate in the project."[2] Ochsner had moved beyond a focus on specialty care and into an independent model with a very large and geographically diverse primary care presence.

Ochsner was a multi-disciplinary practice, and the decision to start an HMO generated some internal conflict. Bobby Brannon, Vice President and Director of Finance, recalled participating in discussions about forming an HMO in 1984 and early 1985. "There was a bit of a philosophical question for the physicians," Brannon said. "The question involved specialty care versus primary care. There was a concern we would dilute ourselves under the HMO framework."[3]

The Ochsner Health Plan was thinly capitalized with only $100,000, permitted by the Louisiana Insurance Commission because the owners would be at risk for providing professional and hospital services. The Ochsner Health Plan began operations in 1985, with 70 percent owned by Ochsner Clinic and 30 percent owned by the Foundation. Through the late 1980s, the health plan experienced rapid growth in membership. There were 11,000 members in 1986 and 41,000 in 1987, after a little over one year of operation.[4] By 1990, the number of HMO members had doubled to 80,000.[5]

By the mid-1990s, the Ochsner Health Plan was developing provider network relationships with physician groups and hospitals across the Gulf Coast of Louisiana. More than 600 Ochsner and affiliated physicians were offering services through the Ochsner Health Plan.[6]

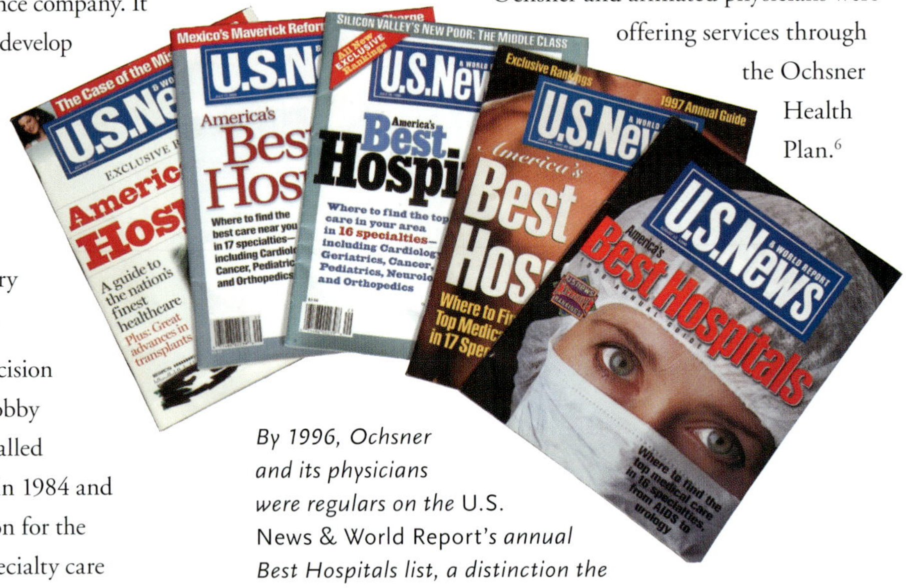

By 1996, Ochsner and its physicians were regulars on the U.S. News & World Report's *annual Best Hospitals list, a distinction the Hospital would enjoy over the next 15 years.*

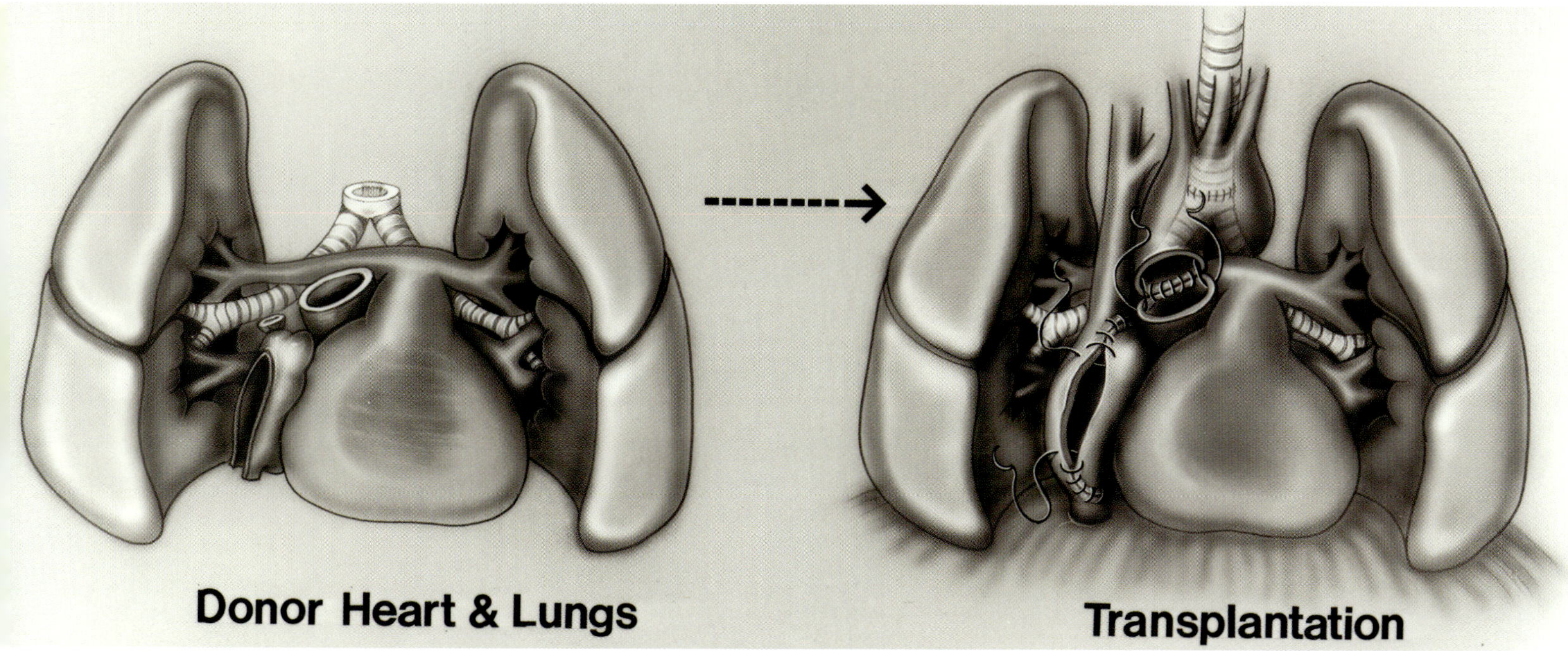

Ochsner surgeons performed the first heart-lung transplant in Louisiana in 1990, another first for the Hospital.

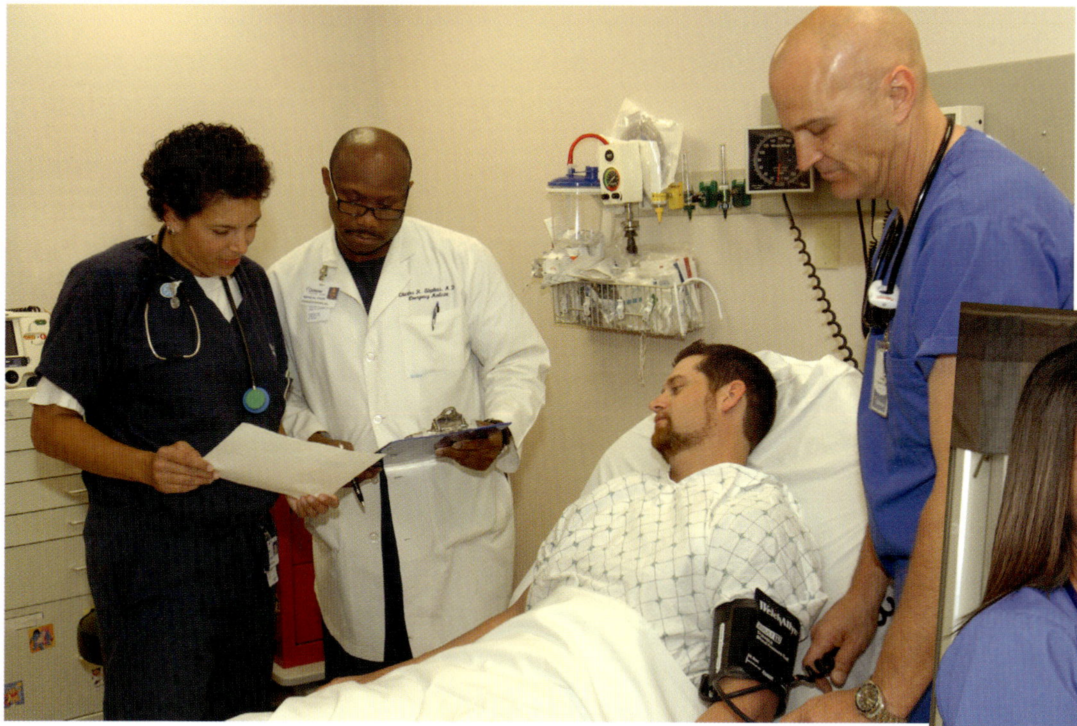

Since 1942, Ochsner has prided itself on the quality of its physicians and staff.

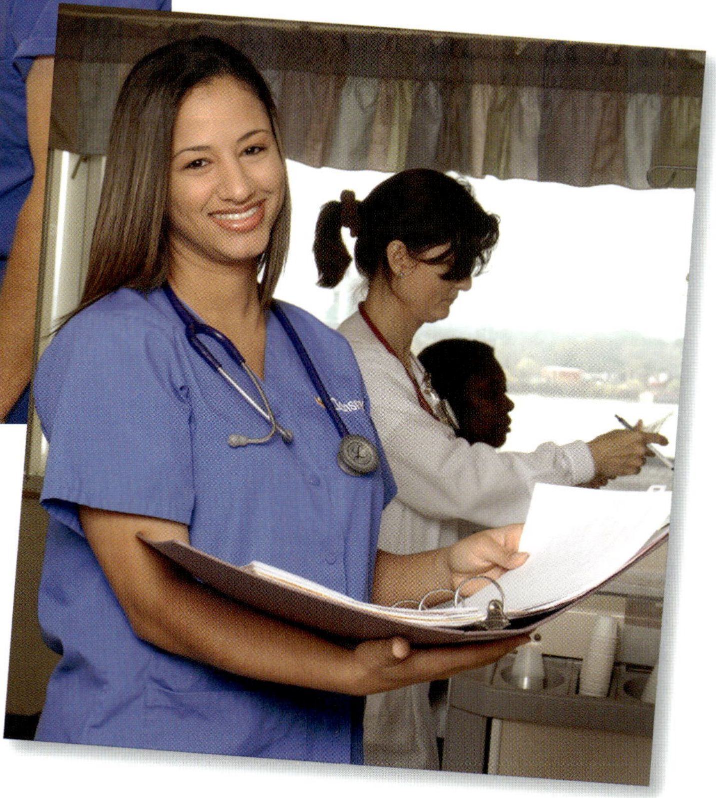

Ochsner nurses are part of the human face of medicine that characterizes Ochsner's focus on treating the patient, not just the disease.

THE NEIGHBORHOOD HEALTH CENTERS EXPAND

Rapid growth of the Ochsner Health Plan placed great demands on Ochsner Clinic to expand the neighborhood health centers significantly to handle the expanded enrollment. "The plans allow us to enhance our service to the communities near each clinic's location," explained Dr. Michael Tooke, Assistant Medical Director of Ochsner Clinic and Medical Director of Ochsner Health Plan. "The neighborhood clinics are an integral part of the community."[7]

The ambitious expansion plan called for doubling the size of the clinic in Slidell and construction of a brand new building for the clinic in Kenner. The clinic in New Orleans East doubled its size during the spring of 1990, and architects were drawing up plans to add four stories to the Metairie clinic building on Veterans Memorial Boulevard. A major expansion for one of the West Bank clinics was planned for mid-1991.[8]

Following the expansion of the original five neighborhood health centers, Ochsner embarked on a program of adding new clinics during the late 1980s. By 1994, the neighborhood health center system included Covington, Uptown New Orleans, Metairie, Destrehan, Hammond and three in Baton Rouge.[9] Ochsner's expansion into the community has continued to make a difference in the healthcare opportunities offered to residents of the region.

In 1991, the Foundation acquired Elmwood Fitness Center at the Elmwood Shopping Center on South Clearview Parkway in Harahan. Located just three miles from the Jefferson Highway campus, the acquisition of Elmwood Fitness Center emphasized Ochsner's emergence as a total healthcare organization. Dr. George Porter, Foundation President, called the acquisition "a very natural fit" and pointed out the preventive medicine benefits available to Ochsner patients.[10]

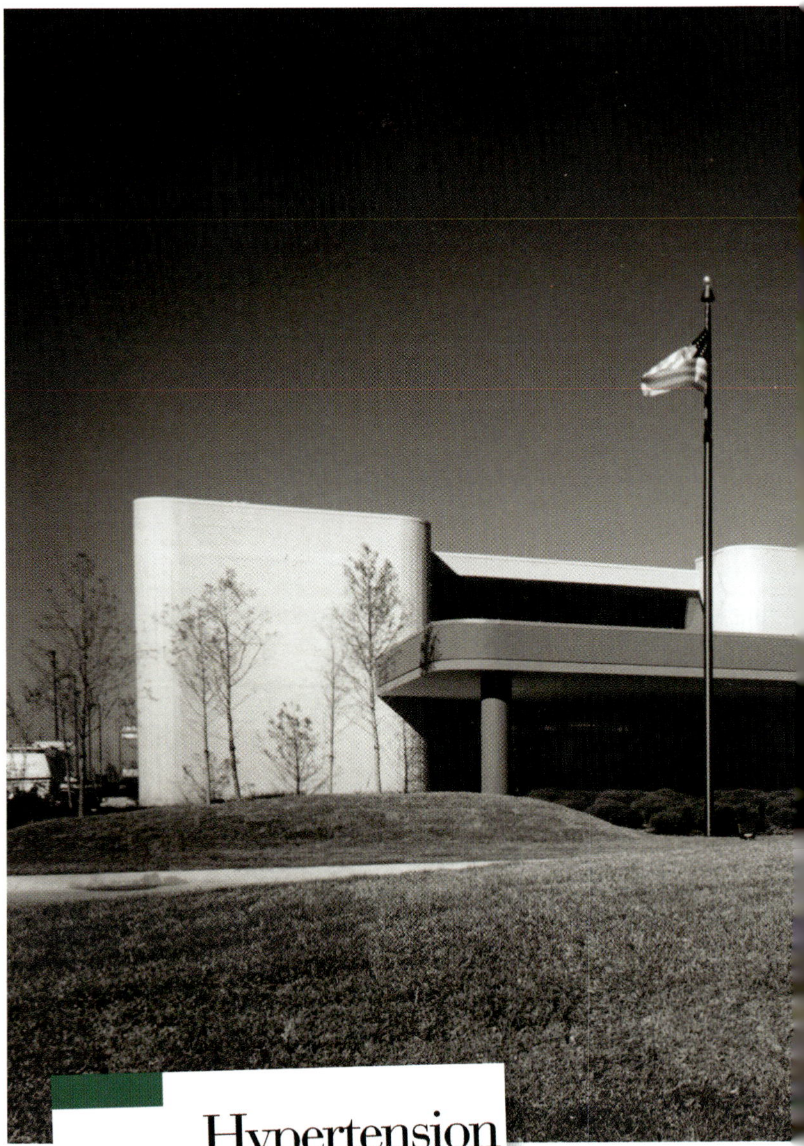

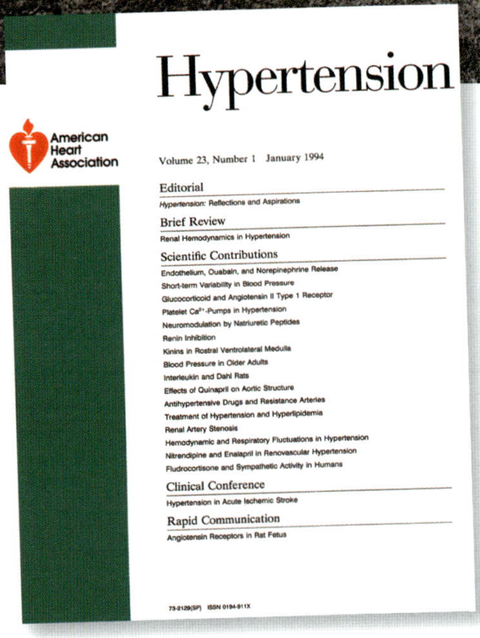

Hypertension

American Heart Association

Volume 23, Number 1 January 1994

Editorial

Hypertension: Reflections and Aspirations

Brief Review

Renal Hemodynamics in Hypertension

Scientific Contributions

Endothelium, Ouabain, and Norepinephrine Release
Short-term Variability in Blood Pressure
Glucocorticoid and Angiotensin II Type 1 Receptor
Platelet Ca^{2+}-Pumps in Hypertension
Neuromodulation by Natriuretic Peptides
Renin Inhibition
Kinins in Rostral Ventrolateral Medulla
Blood Pressure in Older Adults
Interleukin and Dahl Rats
Effects of Quinapril on Aortic Structure
Antihypertensive Drugs and Resistance Arteries
Treatment of Hypertension and Hyperlipidemia
Renal Artery Stenosis
Hemodynamic and Respiratory Fluctuations in Hypertension
Nitrendipine and Enalapril in Renovascular Hypertension
Fludrocortisone and Sympathetic Activity in Humans

Clinical Conference

Hypertension in Acute Ischemic Stroke

Rapid Communication

Angiotensin Receptors in Rat Fetus

73-2129(SP) ISSN 0194-911X

The American Heart Association named Ochsner's Edward D. Frohlich Editor-in-Chief of the prestigious journal Hypertension.

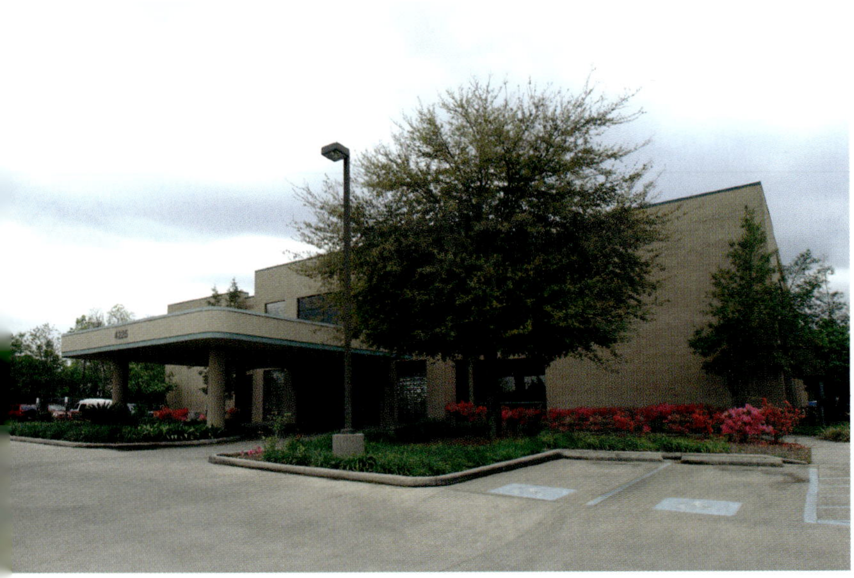

Ochsner Clinic–Lapalco moved into a new 54,000 square-foot building in 1992.

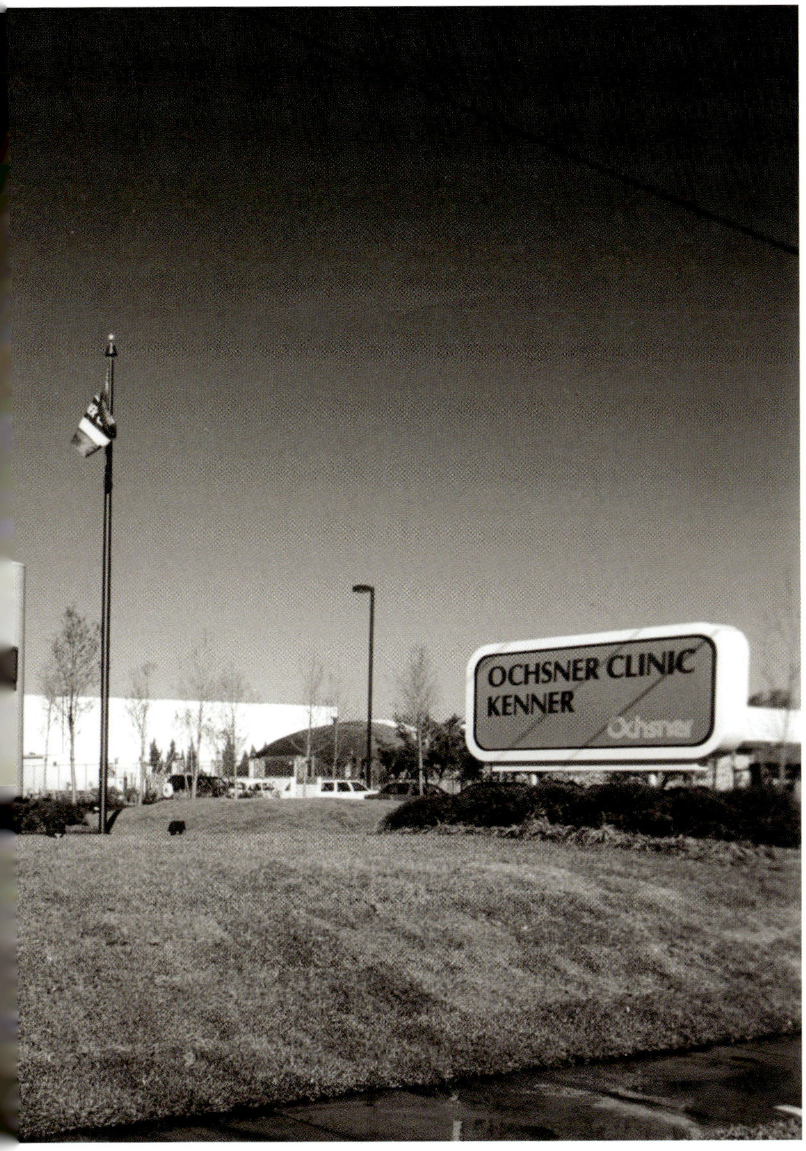

In 1992, Ochsner replaced the original Ochsner Clinic–Kenner with a new facility.

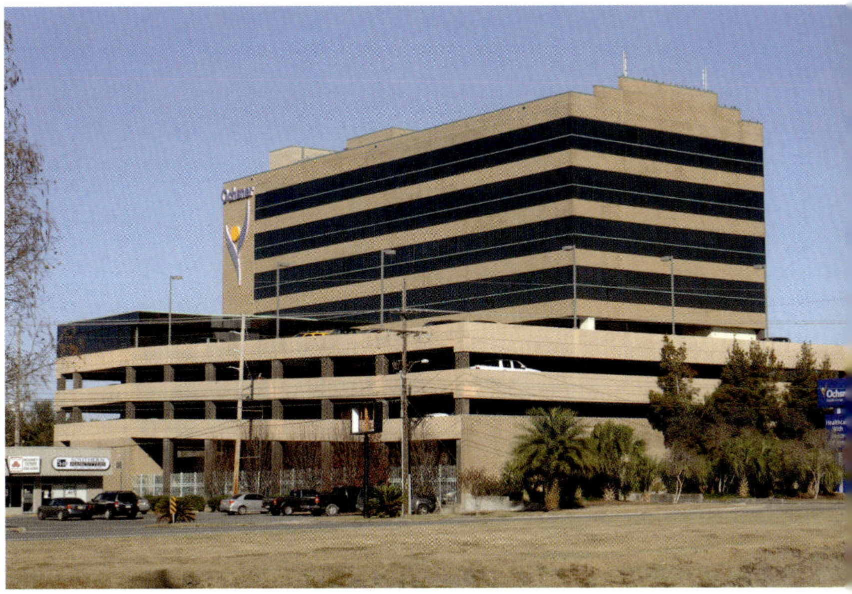

A full seven stories, Ochsner Health Center in Metairie is the most visible neighborhood heath center outreach effort, along with Ochsner Health Center in Baton Rouge and Ochsner Health Center in Covington.

• WHAT OCHSNER MEANS TO ME •

"I think of Ochsner as being a big family. Over the years I've made a lot of friends and associates and we've experienced a lot together. Anytime anyone was in need, people were there to help. We were always CONNECTED."

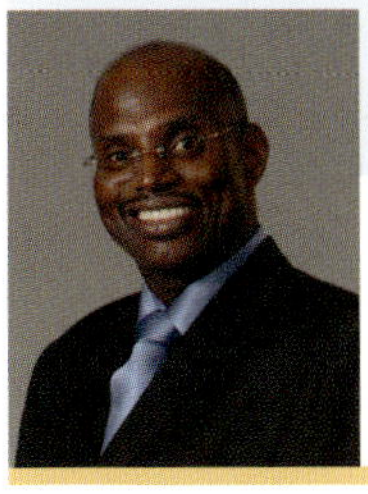

Floyd Grayson, A/V Technician,
Ochsner Medical Center

To watch the full interview with Floyd Grayson, visit **ochsner.org/history**.

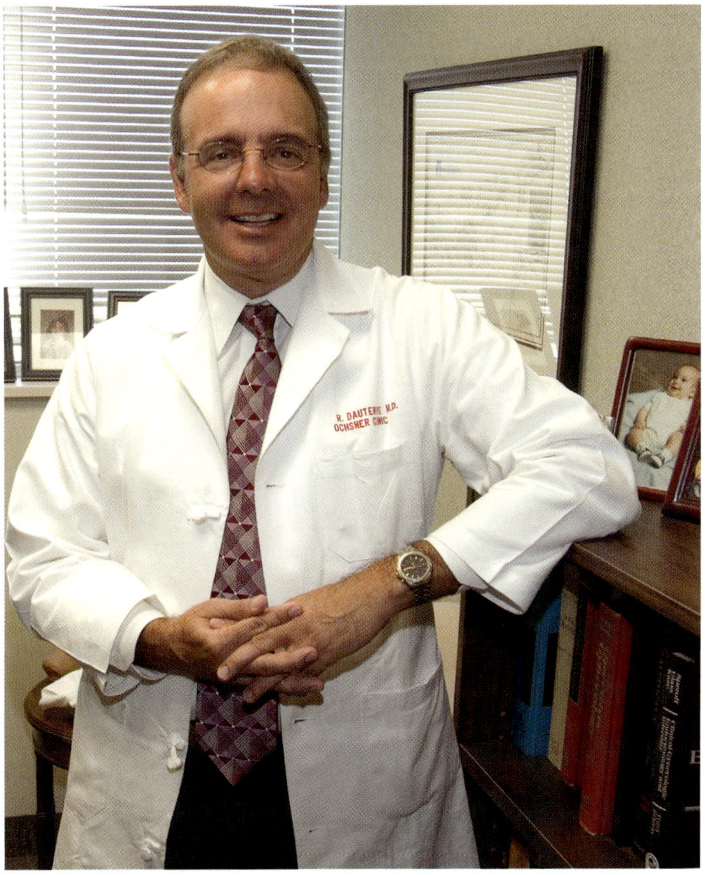

Ralph F. Dauterive Jr., M.D., is the Vice President of Medical Affairs – Ochsner Medical Clinic – Baton Rouge and Associate Medical Director of Surgical Services – Ochsner Baton Rouge Region.

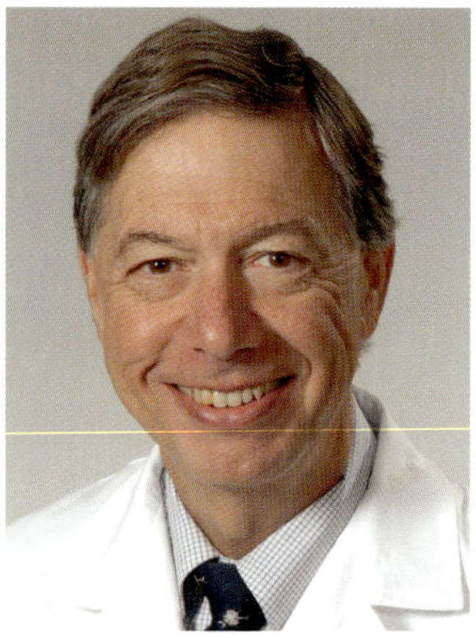

Ochsner's Chair of Medicine and board member Joseph Dalovisio, M.D., served as the Associate Director for Medical Specialties.

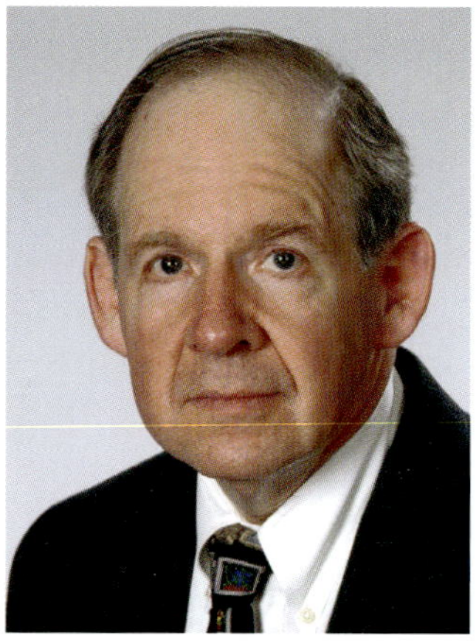

Lawrence Blonde, M.D., serves as Director, Ochsner Diabetes Clinical Research Unit, Department of Endocrinology, Diabetes and Metabolic Diseases, Ochsner Clinic Foundation and Associate Internal Medicine Residency Program Director, Ochsner Medical Center, New Orleans. He directed a number of clinical trials and research during his more than 30 years at Ochsner. Blonde is a nationally known clinical investigator in diabetes.

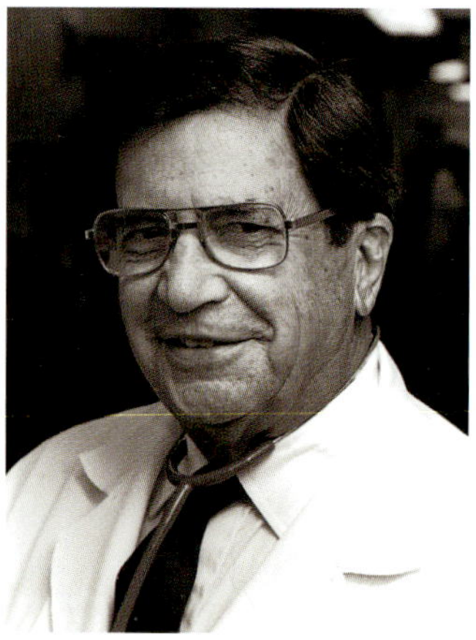

Thomas E. Weiss, M.D., was the founder and Chair of Ochsner's Section of Rheumatology and a board member of Ochsner Clinic and the Alton Ochsner Medical Foundation. A revered teacher and practitioner who garnered international acclaim, Weiss lends his name to the annual Thomas E. Weiss, M.D. Outstanding Alumnus Award.

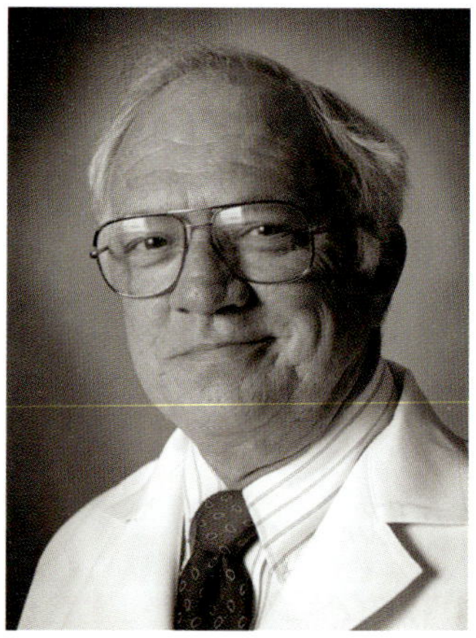

Gordon B. McFarland, M.D., was a major force in the Department of Orthopaedic Surgery for more than 30 years. A hand surgeon, he was involved in research on tendon repair and prostheses for replacement of damaged joints. McFarland directed the Mary Sherman Bone Pathology Laboratory.

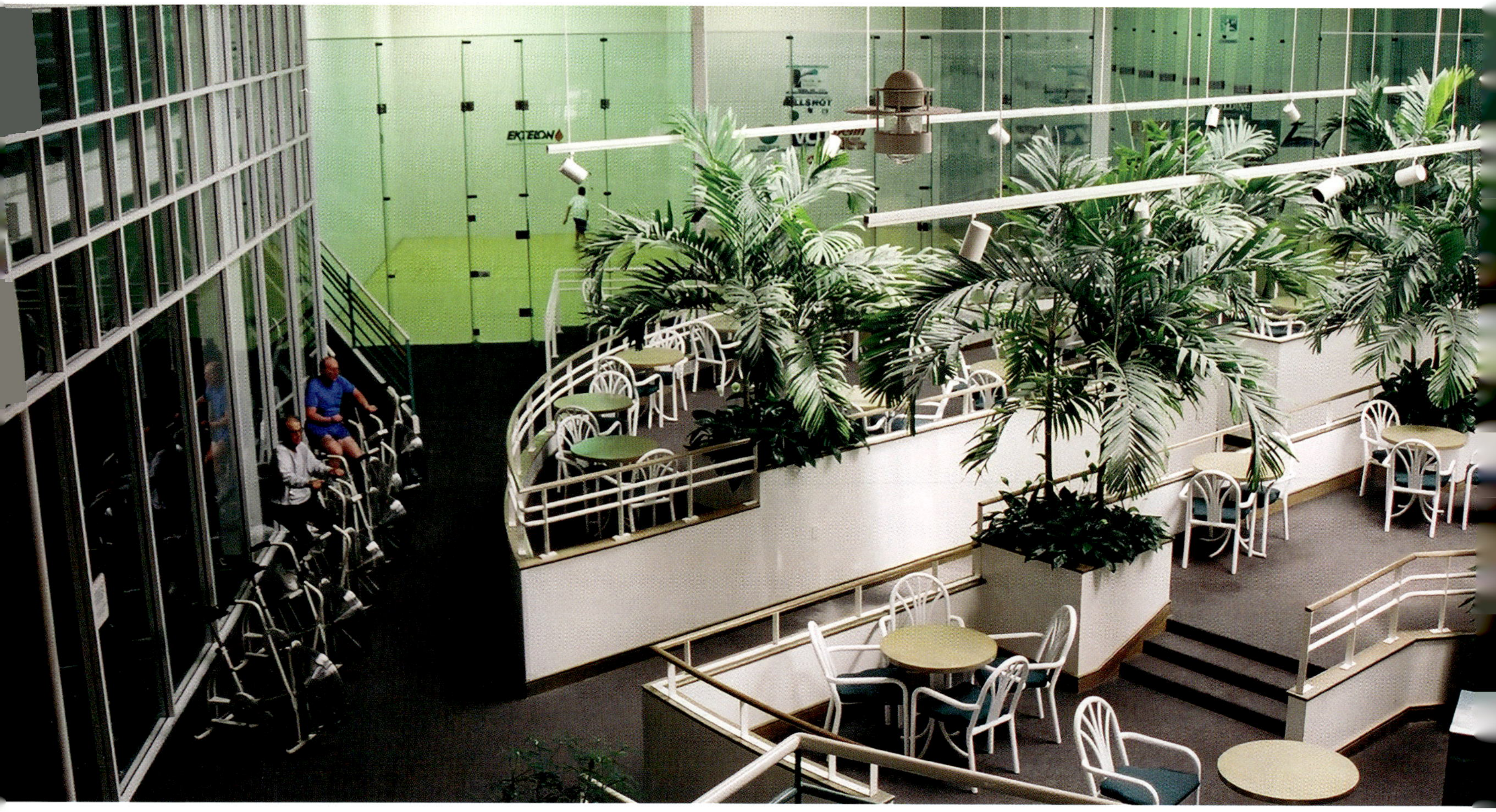

Ochsner acquired Elmwood Fitness Center in 1991 because of Ochsner's commitment to the total health of its patients.

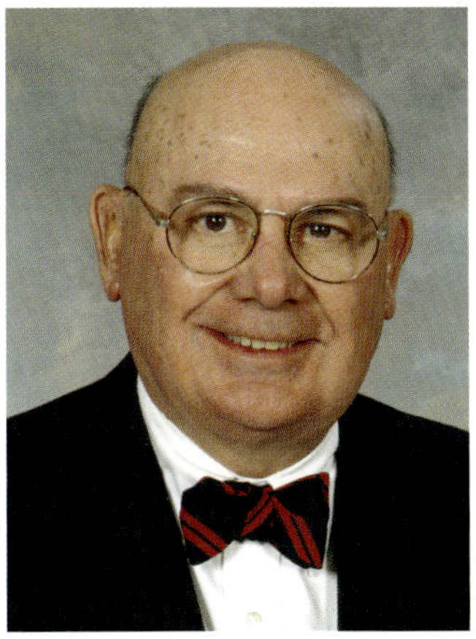

Edward Connolly, M.D., was Chair of Ochsner's Department of Neurosurgery. A respected leader in the New Orleans medical community, Connolly served in a variety of professional leadership roles at Ochsner.

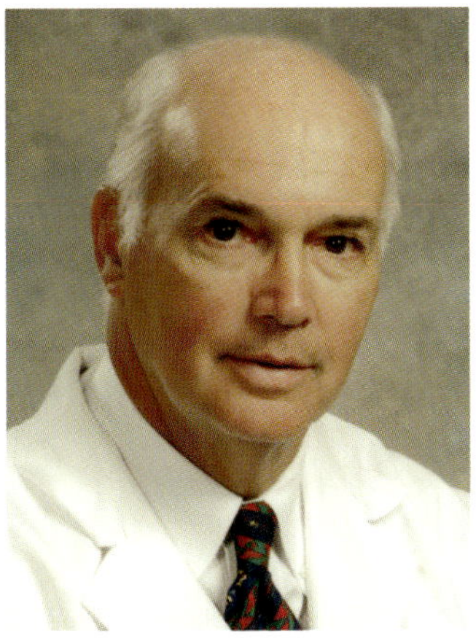

A longtime member of the professional staff at Ochsner and former Department Head of Pulmonary Diseases, W. Brooks Emory, M.D., has always been very popular with his patients.

MORE CHANGES AHEAD

The early 1990s were a time of intense ferment for the nation's healthcare industry. The election of Bill Clinton to the United States Presidency in 1992 opened a passionate debate about reforming the delivery of medicine and the way society paid for healthcare. Inside Ochsner, a fierce debate was taking place over the direction the Clinic and the Foundation Hospital would follow in the fast approaching twenty-first century.

The crux of the problem, as it had been for 15 years or more, was the difference in financial structure between the Clinic and the Foundation. The Foundation was a tax-exempt corporation. Its major financial goal was to invest money back into the Hospital and other Foundation facilities. The Clinic was a taxable partnership that employed physicians in addition to the partners and by 1991 had more than 1,700 total employees.[11] Each partner owned a capital account plus a proportionate share of the accounts receivable. The shift from traditional fee-for-service medicine to prepayment for over half the professional services required a change in the technique for valuation of partnership shares to prevent wild swings in the accounts.[12]

"There were 200-plus partners," said Dr. Richard Guthrie, who served on the Clinic's Board of Management during the mid-1990s. "It was very unwieldy."[13]

THE OCHSNER JOURNAL

In the 1950s Dr. Alton Ochsner published a journal dedicated to national and international medical practices informing the medical community about current research and innovation at Ochsner. Nearly 50 years later, the journal was revived to support Ochsner's commitment to patient care, research and education.

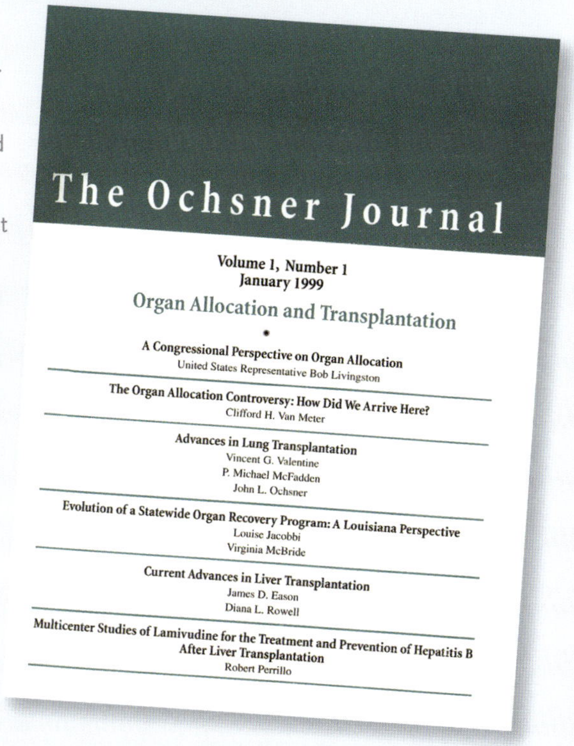

The Ochsner Journal

Volume 1, Number 1
January 1999

Organ Allocation and Transplantation

A Congressional Perspective on Organ Allocation
United States Representative Bob Livingston

The Organ Allocation Controversy: How Did We Arrive Here?
Clifford H. Van Meter

Advances in Lung Transplantation
Vincent G. Valentine
P. Michael McFadden
John L. Ochsner

Evolution of a Statewide Organ Recovery Program: A Louisiana Perspective
Louise Jacobbi
Virginia McBride

Current Advances in Liver Transplantation
James D. Eason
Diana L. Rowell

Multicenter Studies of Lamivudine for the Treatment and Prevention of Hepatitis B After Liver Transplantation
Robert Perrillo

The Ochsner Journal, *which began publishing in 1999, gives the Clinic's physicians and research scientists another vehicle to report on their clinical trials and research findings.*

Befitting Ochsner's reputation for quality research dating back to the earliest days of Ochsner Clinic, Editor-in-Chief Dr. Robert Perrillo continued Dr. Alton Ochsner's legacy with the unveiling of *The Ochsner Journal* in 1998. This quarterly publication was started to support Ochsner's Mission to improve the health of the community and from the beginning has provided an active dialogue on practice standards in healthcare.

Following Hurricane Katrina, Dr. David E. Beck, Chairman, Department of Colon and Rectal Surgery, was appointed the new Editor-in-Chief of *The Ochsner Journal* and instilled renewed interest in this publication. *The Ochsner Journal* today continues to present applicable scientific information on a wide range of medical topics. Submitted manuscripts are subjected to peer review by the editors and other experts in the field. Appropriate articles published in the journal offer Continuing Medical Education credit through the Ochsner Clinic Foundation Department of Continuing Medical Education. Popular sections include a basic science section and a review section that provides concise commentary about controversial and timely topics of interest or relevance to physicians, scientists, nurses, administrators and others associated with the medical community.

FIRST ATTEMPT AT UNIFICATION

The Clinic and the Foundation had begun to move further apart during the mid- to late-1980s. When interest rates dropped mid-decade, the Clinic secured bank financing and ownership interest for some of its construction projects, rather than just leasing space from the Foundation. Both organizations benefited from the outreach initiative embodied by Ochsner neighborhood health center growth. The Foundation Hospital was able to sustain occupancy rates, and both organizations were able to spread overhead costs over a larger base than just the Jefferson Highway campus.[14]

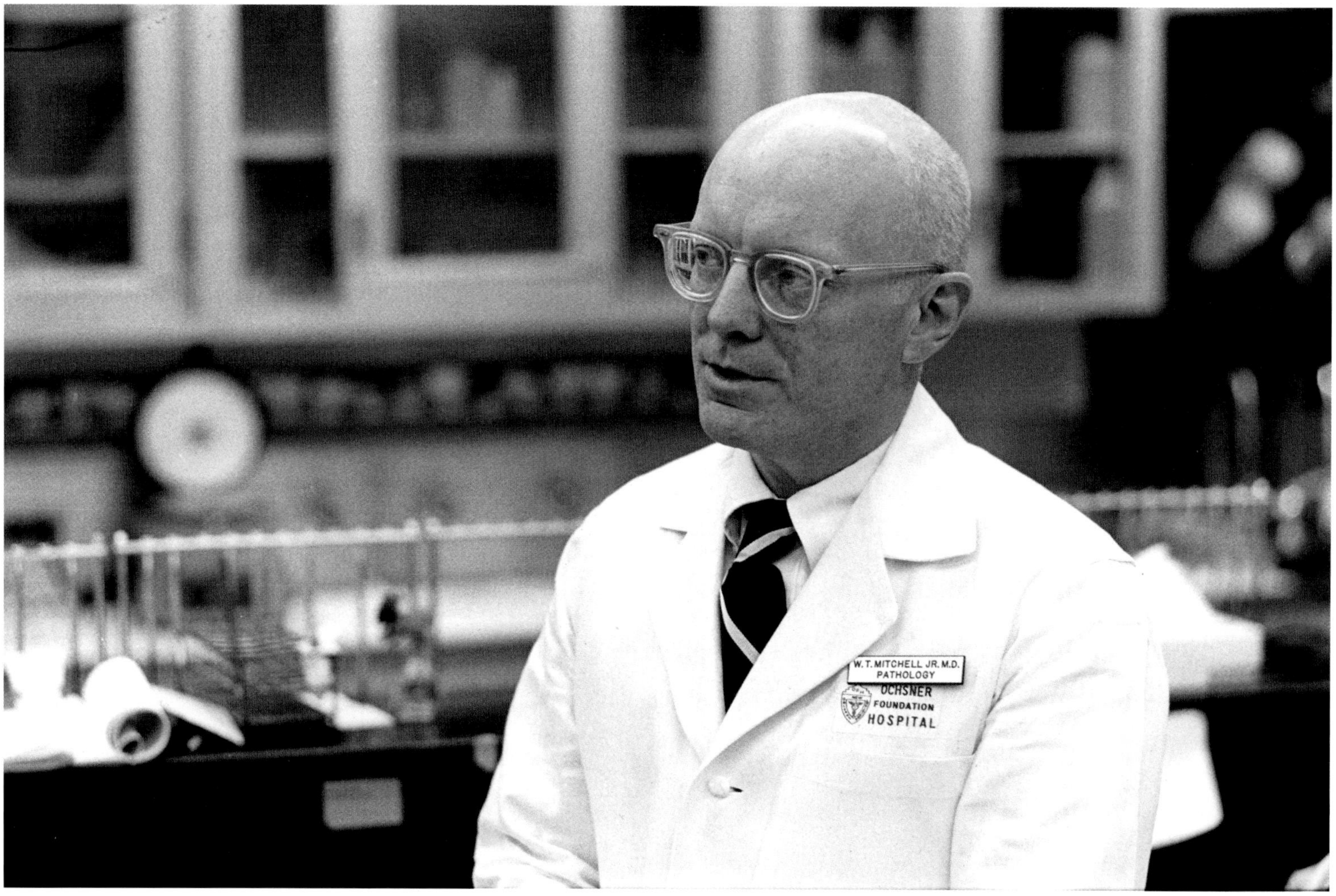

William T. "Billy" Mitchell Jr., M.D., headed Ochsner's Department of Pathology and the Division of Anatomic Pathology for many years. Mitchell had a well-deserved local and national reputation in the area of Surgical Pathology.

In 1988, Ochsner hired the Hay Group to review the organizational ties between the Clinic and the Foundation. The consultant recommended the two groups unify.

"The Clinic group was thinking about a merger with the Foundation," Guthrie explained. "At the time—1988–1989—there were two separate management groups. They had to get everybody on the same page."[15]

Negotiations dragged on for nearly a year and floundered on how to value the financial assets of the Clinic. "Using asset valuation techniques, the debt incurred by the Clinic for expansion of the Ochsner patient base in New Orleans and Baton Rouge decreased the monetary value of the Clinic from the perspective of the Foundation," a 1991 report concluded.[16] Unable to agree on an equitable financial model for unification, the Clinic Board of Management and the Foundation Board of Trustees agreed to abandon the effort. During the next 11 years, there would be other unsuccessful attempts to unify the two organizations.

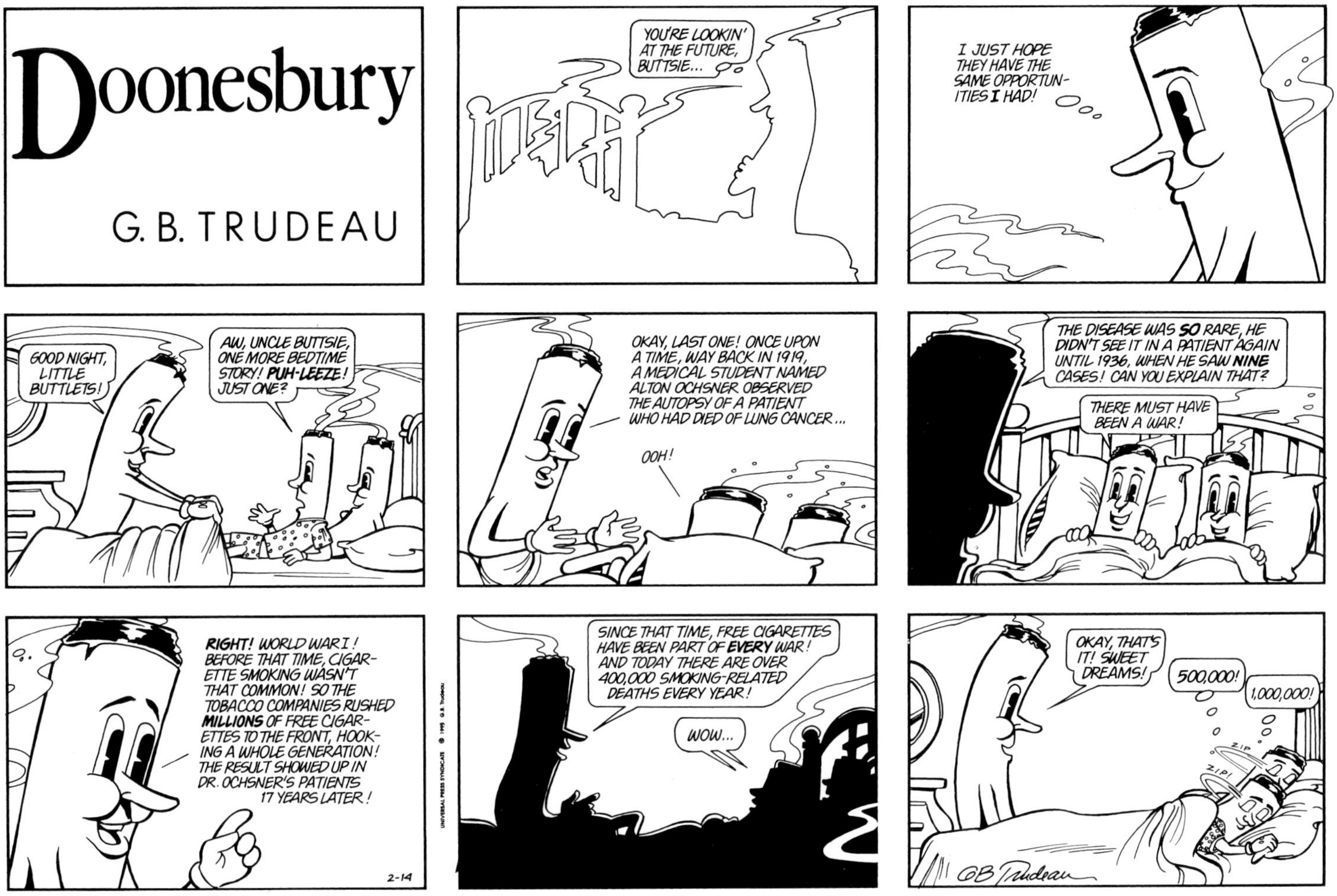

Garry Trudeau's Doonesbury *comic strip featured a 1993 character, Mr. Butts, who informed Americans about Alton Ochsner's pioneering work in uncovering the link between smoking cigarettes and lung cancer.* DOONESBURY © 1993 G. B. Trudeau. Reprinted with permission of UNIVERSAL PRESS SYNDICATE. All rights reserved.

CHANGES AT THE TOP

Ochsner Clinic emerged from the failed negotiations at the end of the 1980s sobered by the experience and mindful of the need to change. Clinic leadership demanded that the Foundation invest money in some much needed facility maintenance and expansion, and held out the threat of moving the group practice away from the Foundation Hospital. The Foundation took the threat seriously, and in 1991 abandoned 17 years of separate leadership when it agreed to name Dr. Frank Riddick, Medical Director of the Clinic, as CEO of the Foundation.[17]

Riddick came into office with a set of goals and clearly defined powers—and one huge disadvantage. He had to give up the job in three years.

"The partnership agreement required that I step down at the end of 1994 because I would be 65 years old and no longer a partner. I was eligible to continue serving as CEO of the Foundation, however, until a suitable successor was named," Riddick said. "We spent almost the whole year of 1992 in a search process with the idea that if we did have an external candidate selected, that would provide two years of tutelage before I had to step down. And we had a broadly constituted search committee."[18]

The search committee's choice was an insider with a long medical pedigree. Dr. Michael Tooke, a longtime physician at Ochsner, succeeded Riddick as the Medical Director of Ochsner Clinic and Managing Partner of the Clinic Partnership late in 1992. The son and grandson of doctors, Tooke pledged Ochsner would focus on "attentive, compassionate service" to patients.[19] When Riddick retired as Medical Director of the Clinic at the end of 1994, Tooke was to replace him as CEO of the Foundation.

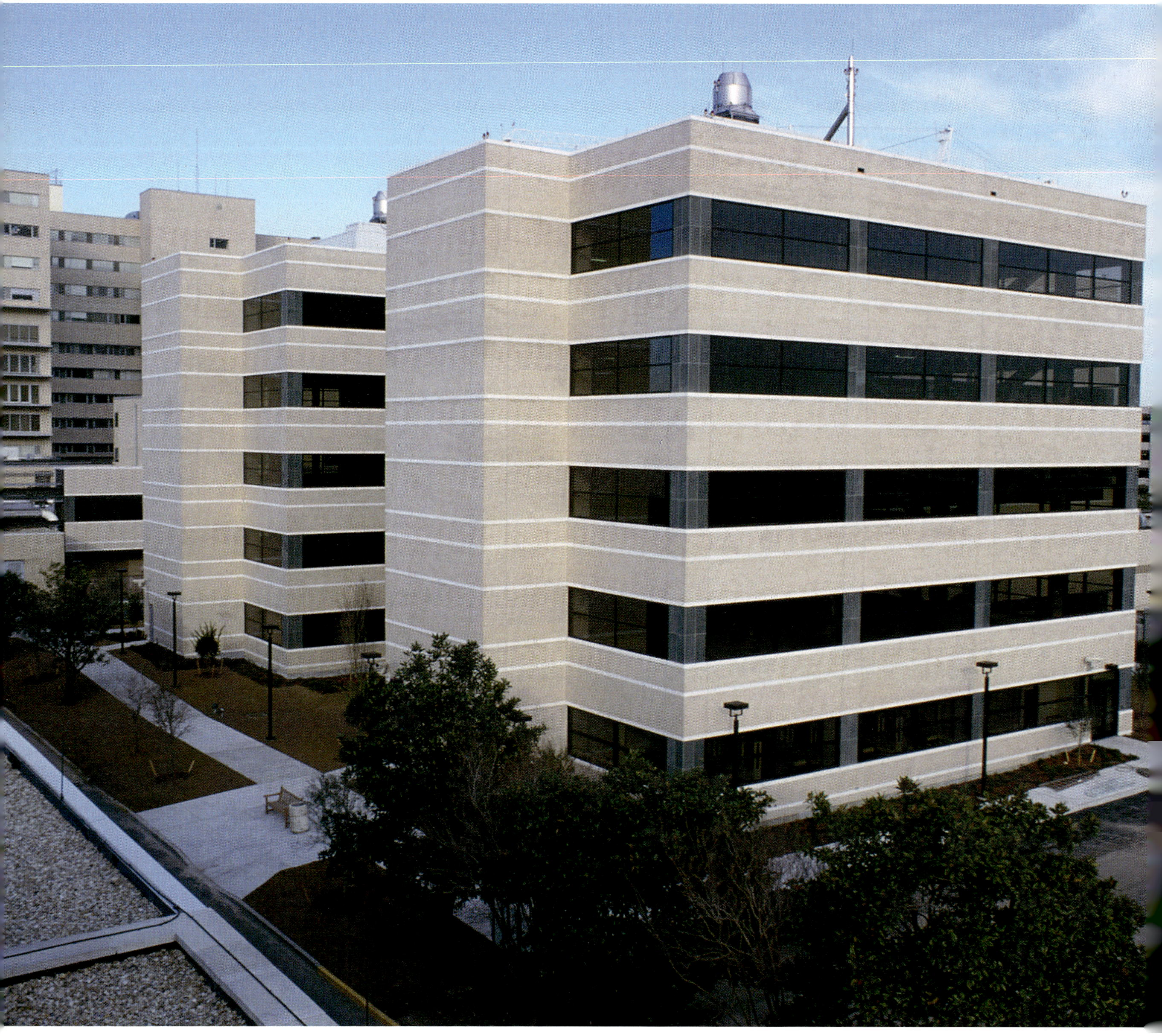

The new Ochsner Biomedical Research Building on the Jefferson Highway campus opened in 1993 and fulfilled the vision of the founders for a facility that combined clinical practice, medical education and research.

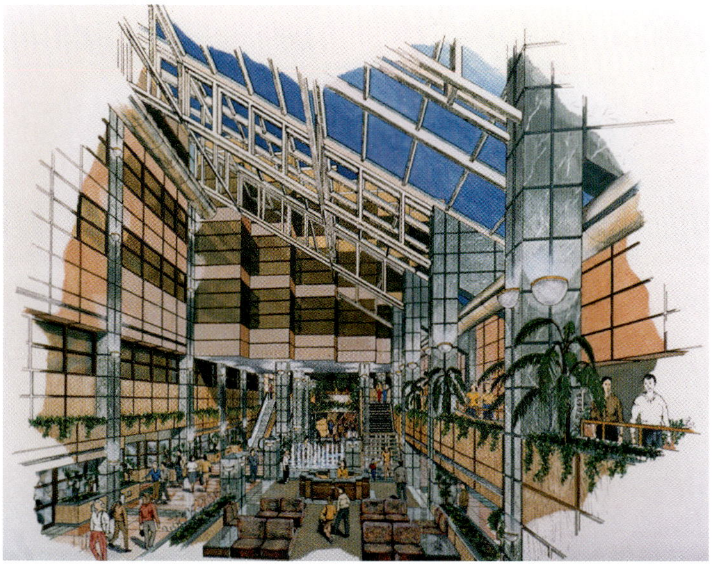

The 1993 opening of the Atrium Tower connected the garage with the Clinic and gave visitors the feeling of passing through an enclosed mall.

TAKING CARE OF THE SICKEST PATIENTS

Michael Tooke only spent a little over two years as Clinic Managing Partner. There were accomplishments of which he was intensely proud. "We created a true integrated health system," Tooke said. "It was the whole ball of wax. In the state of Louisiana, we had the highest severity case mix index, and we had the lowest per case charge. We took care of the sickest patients with incredible efficiency. We had very little duplication, and that's the bottom line."[20]

During 1993, the Foundation strengthened Ochsner's reputation for research when it completed the new Ochsner Biomedical Research Building on the Jefferson Highway campus. The 16,000-square-foot Molecular Genetics Research Facility included the laboratories of the Richard Freeman Research Institute. The Research Division also opened facilities for cardiovascular, transplant and surgical research, continuing the emphasis on medical research the founders had established a half-century before.[21]

Tooke represented the Clinic in 1993 in yet again another round of discussions with Tulane about a closer relationship between the two institutions.[22] "We had a series of very serious negotiations," Tooke said. "We were looking at a joint operating agreement that would have created quite a medical system. I think we got very close. It was a fascinating negotiation, and there were elements of it that would have been neat."[23]

'THE SISTERS PROMISED MORE THAN THEY COULD DELIVER'

The end of discussions with Tulane was followed in short order by the termination of a health plan merger with an order of Catholic nuns who operated a number of hospitals in Louisiana. Ochsner announced the agreement to form a statewide health network with the Sisters of Charity of the Incarnate Word Health System of Houston, Texas. The Sisters operated hospitals in Shreveport, Alexandria and Lake Charles, complementing Ochsner's presence in New Orleans, Baton Rouge and Houma.[24]

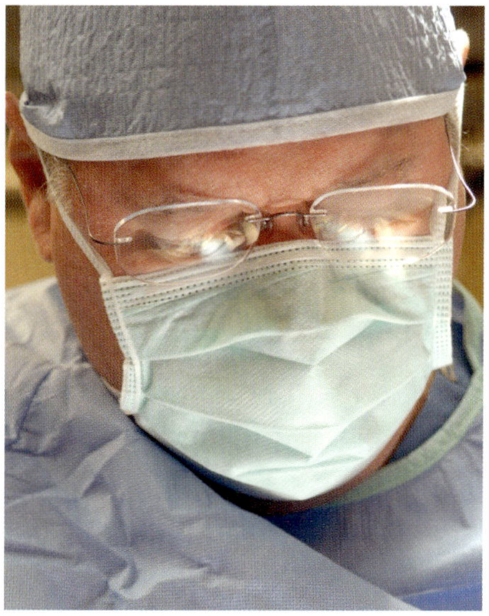

Masked and gowned for surgery, John Bowen III is the Chairman Emeritus of Ochsner's Department of Surgery and is a Vascular and General Surgeon.

Tooke became a champion of the merger agreement with the Sisters of Charity, primarily because he felt a statewide presence was necessary to deal with the healthcare changes advocated by the Clinton administration. By the time Ochsner and the Sisters of Charity started negotiating seriously, however, a national coalition of physicians and insurance companies had blunted the proposed Clinton health plan.

The Sisters of Charity did not have effective group practices at their Louisiana hospitals, and problems quickly arose over the procedure for joining the Ochsner Health Plan with the HMO operated by the Sisters. "Although the Sisters claimed expertise in providing cost-effective prepaid services in their institutions, the Sisters promised more than they were able to deliver," Frank Riddick said.[25] Since the Clinic owned 70 percent of the Ochsner Health Plan, Tooke found himself at odds with the Clinic Board of Management. When the merger agreements fell apart in early 1995, Tooke resigned his position with Ochsner Clinic and took an executive position with a Baltimore, Maryland, healthcare system.

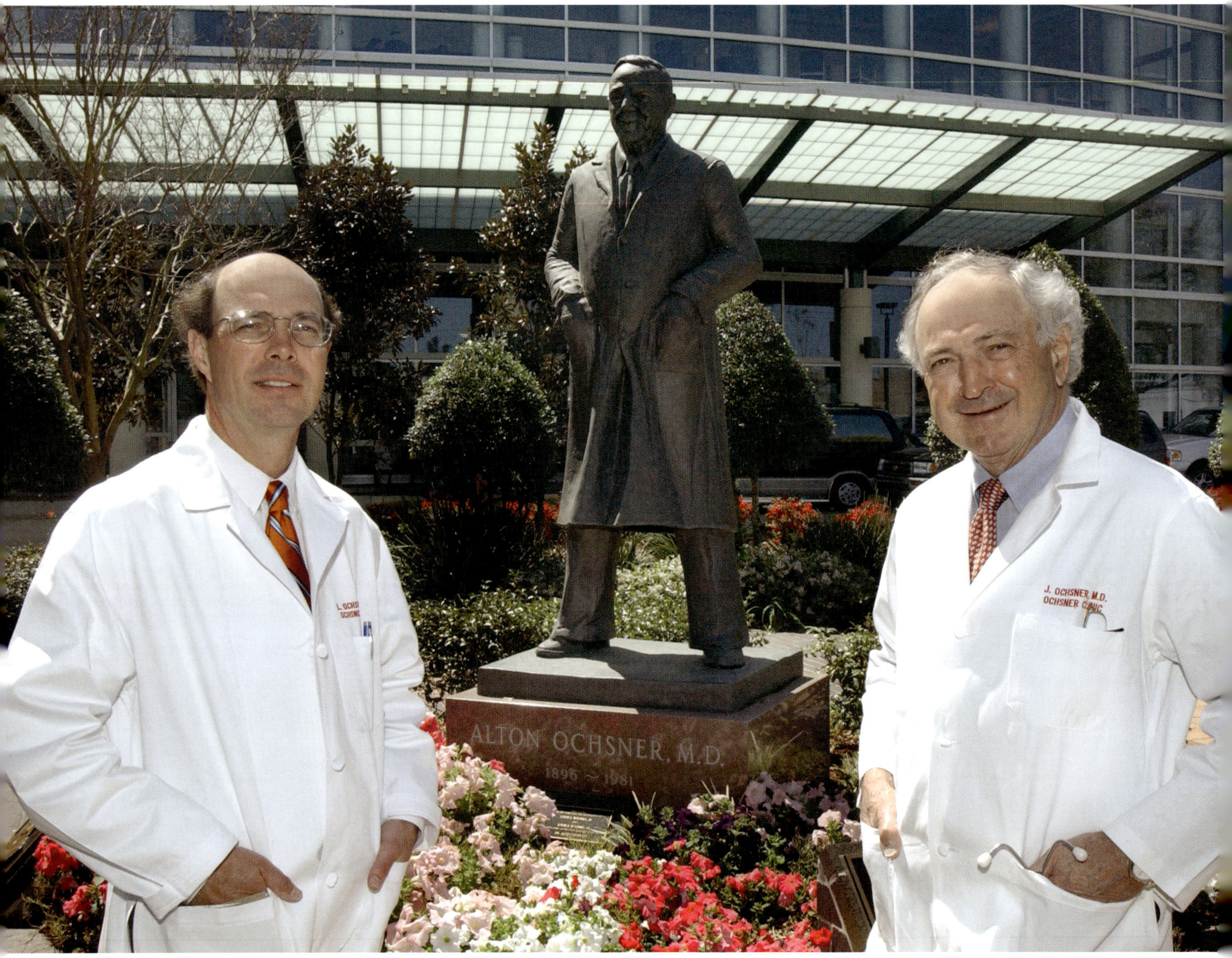

John Lockwood Ochsner, left, and his father, John Ochsner, pose with the statue of Alton Ochsner, three generations of Ochsner surgeons.

CHAPTER 8:

THE CHALLENGE OF 21ST-CENTURY CHANGE

AS OCHSNER APPROACHED THE 21st-CENTURY, the medical complex that Alton Ochsner and the four other founders had established nearly 60 years before was both taking advantage of external opportunities and facing internal pressures.

The flagship Ochsner Clinic and Ochsner Foundation Hospital were enjoying a reputation for quality healthcare unmatched anywhere in the region. Lay magazines and peer-reviewed journals considered Ochsner a model for what a truly integrated healthcare system could be. In 2000, the Hospital expanded the Emergency Room and moved it to an entrance off Jefferson Highway. At the same time, the expanded Critical Care Tower added 10 new operating rooms to the complex.

Ochsner's system of regional and neighborhood health centers delivered quality care to the growing number of patients living in the New Orleans suburbs and along the highly populated Mississippi River corridor connecting New Orleans with Baton Rouge. The Ochsner Health Plan gave the Clinic and Hospital a managed care brand that set Ochsner apart in the increasingly competitive Louisiana healthcare marketplace.

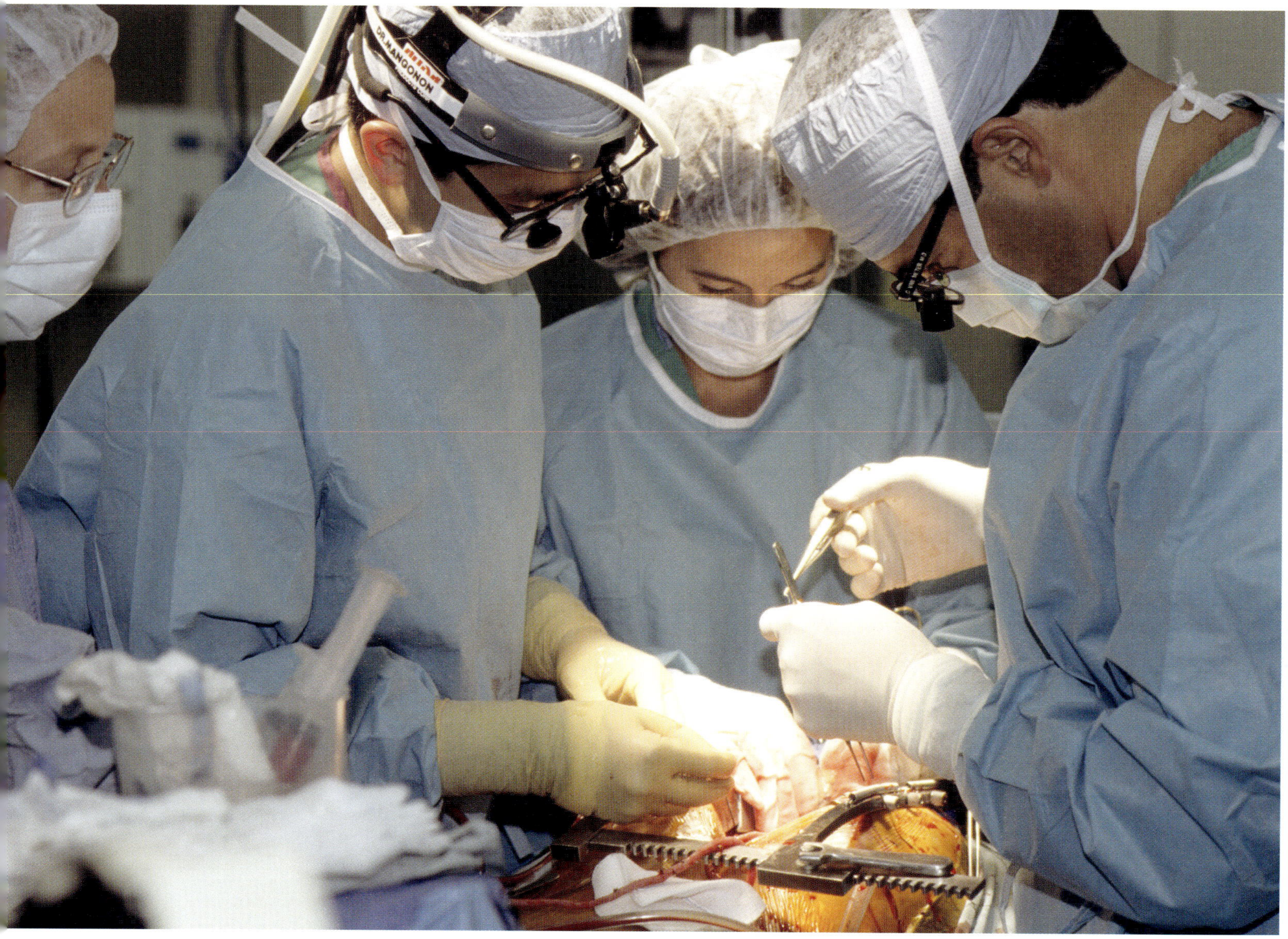

Clifford Van Meter Jr., M.D., (right) and team performing open heart surgery, a specialty at Ochsner since the 1970s.

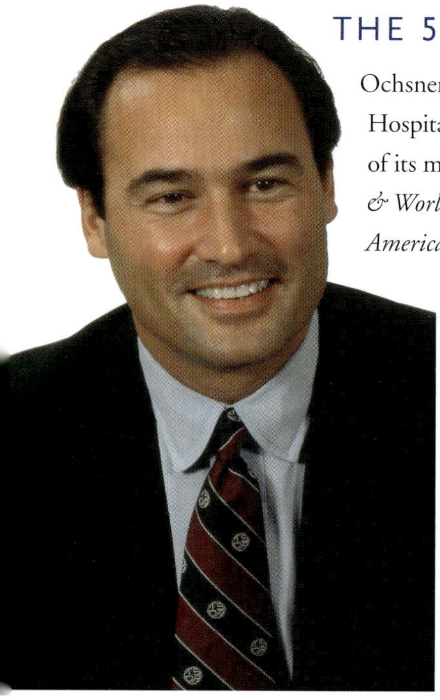

THE 500TH TRANSPLANT

Ochsner Clinic and Ochsner Foundation Hospital maintained and improved the quality of its medical care. In August 2000, *U.S. News & World Report* recognized Ochsner as one of *America's Best Hospitals* for the fourth straight year. The magazine singled out the Hospital as one of the nation's 50 best in the areas of Heart, Urology, Rheumatology and Gynecology. Ochsner was the only hospital in the region to receive the magazine's coveted "50 best" designation.[1]

Clifford Van Meter Jr., M.D., led the surgical team that performed the 500th heart transplant at Ochsner, just 30 years after John Ochsner performed the first.

Ochsner confirmed its reputation for quality medicine in January 2000 when a surgical team led by Dr. Clifford Van Meter Jr., in conjunction with the medical team led by Dr. Mandreep R. Mehra, performed its 500th heart transplant.[2] It had been only 30 years since Dr. John Ochsner had performed the Hospital's first heart transplant in 1970.

The 500th transplant placed Ochsner in elite company. Of the 282 U.S. transplant centers, Ochsner was one of only six centers to have achieved the surgical milestone. Ochsner joined transplant centers at the Cleveland Clinic Foundation, University of California Los Angeles, Presbyterian Hospital in New York, Temple University Hospital in Philadelphia and the Texas Heart Institute at St. Luke's Hospital in Houston in reaching the 500-transplant level.[3] Ochsner was in distinguished company, indeed.

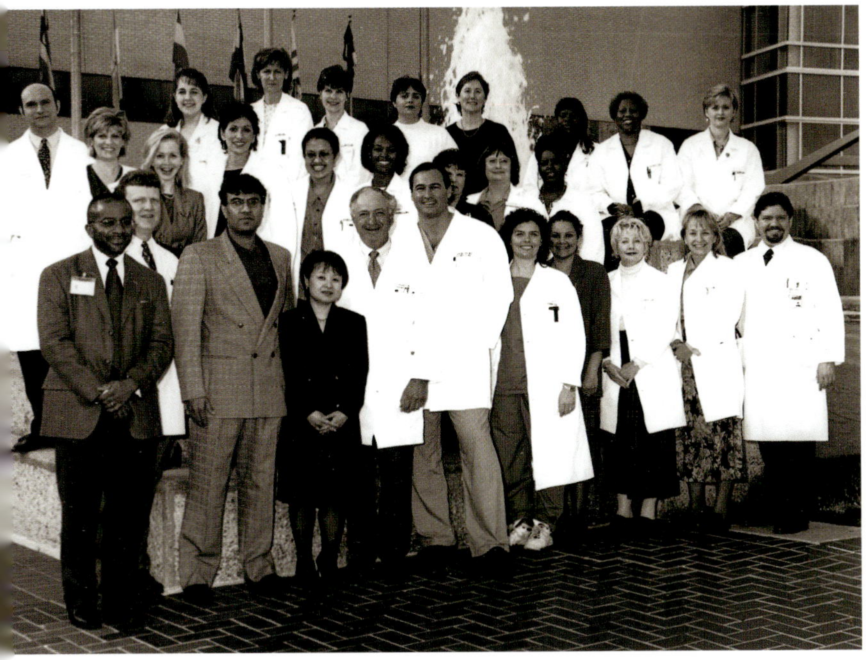

The Ochsner transplant team achieved its 500th heart transplant in 2000, one of only six U.S. transplant centers to pass that mark.

Ochsner surgeons performed 114 transplants in the period between 1997 and 1999 alone. Survival rates of 85 percent after one year and 70 percent after five years were well above the national averages.[4]

"In contrast to early days," said John Ochsner, "we now have hundreds of people involved in the transplant program. In the early days we only had three or four people on the entire team. It has gone from a very scary and unpredictable procedure, because of a lack of knowledge and equipment, to a procedure that is very safe and effective."[5]

Ochsner's growing expertise in transplant surgery required expansion of Ochsner Foundation Hospital's surgical and intensive care facilities. In September 2000, Ochsner opened its new three-story Critical Care Tower on the Jefferson Highway campus. Designed to be expandable up to 14 stories, the $47 million Critical Care Tower centralized and improved patient access to the new Emergency, Surgery and Intensive Care Departments. The facility featured a 34-bed Intensive Care Unit and added 10 new operating rooms for Ochsner Foundation Hospital.[6]

INITIATIVE FOR THE NEW CENTURY

Often overlooked in the story of healthcare financing is the role that generous contributions play at organizations such as Ochsner. Since logging the first contribution of $21,500 to Ochsner Clinic in 1944, Ochsner has been the recipient of millions of dollars in gifts, donations and endowments.

For nearly 30 years, Charles Heim was the face of Ochsner giving. Hired in 1981 as the Director of Development, Heim oversaw capital campaigns and planned giving that funded everything from the first MRI machines, to the Atrium Tower in 1993, to the Initiative for the New Century in 2000.

Heim's travels in search of contributions for Ochsner took him across a broad swath of the Gulf Coast, from Texas to Florida. "New Orleans was very strong in petroleum and petrochemicals for years," Heim said of his travels. "A lot of executives and professionals whose careers took them to New Orleans came to Ochsner for healthcare. A lot of those people wound up in Tampa and Houston."[7]

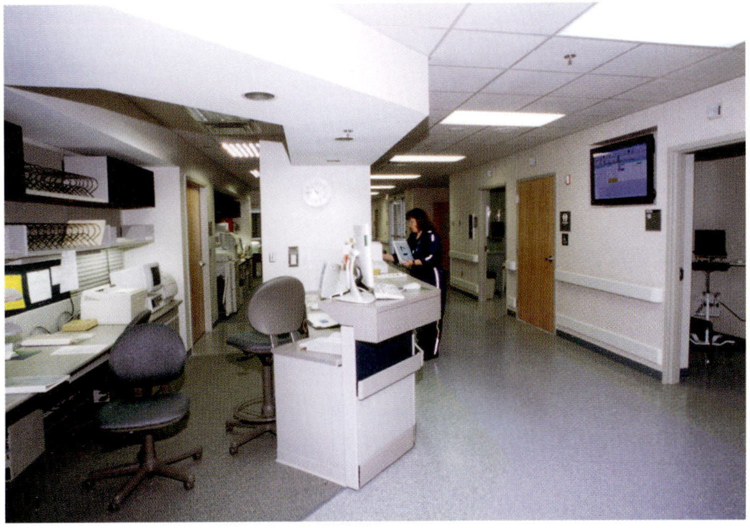

The construction of the Critical Care Tower in 2000 resulted in the move of the Emergency Room entrance from River Road to Jefferson Highway.

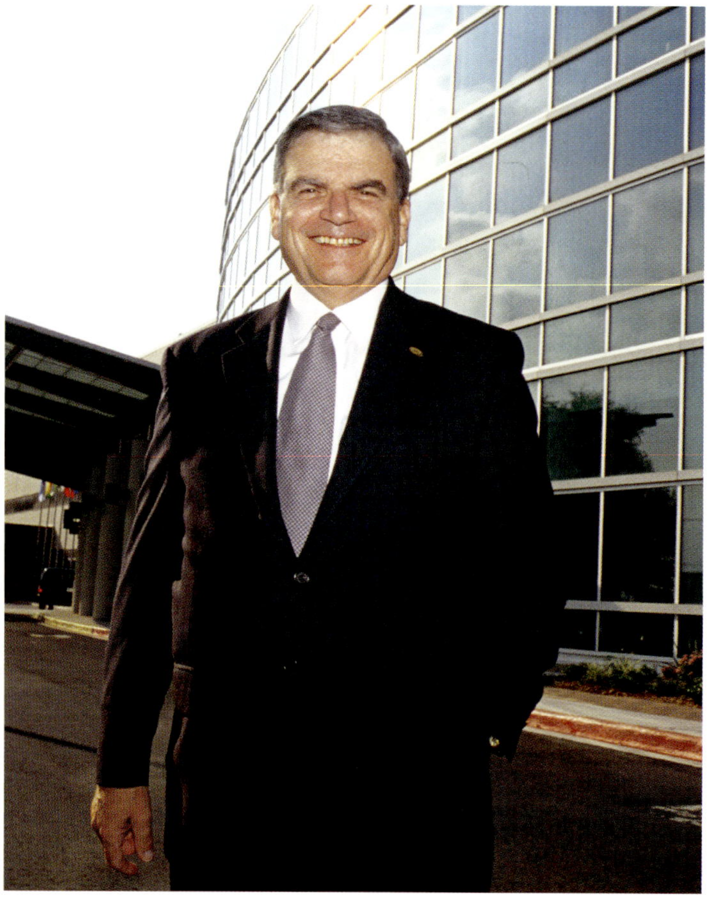

Charles Heim directed philanthropy initiatives at Ochsner from 1981 to 2008.

Heim was constantly on the lookout for ideas to help Ochsner raise money. In 1984, he received a telephone call from a contact at the Touchdown Club of New Orleans. The caller wanted to know if Ochsner did leukemia research. The call led to an association with leukemia patient Raymond Hester, a popular local football player for the New Orleans Saints.

Research has always been a favorite object of the Department of Philanthropy's affection. During the late 1980s, Heim repeatedly proposed to the Foundation that Ochsner needed to build a new research building. By the time the Ochsner Biomedical Research Building opened in 1993, Heim and his staff had raised $12 million for the building and $3 million for the endowment.

Since the building opened, it has been used as a model for those who are considering giving to Ochsner. The success of the campaign to fund the construction of the Ochsner Biomedical Research Building led to the Initiative for the New Century, a campaign designed to address facilities' needs. To date, the Initiative for the New Century has garnered almost $9 million in commitments.[8]

THE GOLDSTEIN YEARS

Michael Tooke's departure during the winter of 1995 left Ochsner scrambling to find a successor for Frank Riddick, who had retired as head of the Clinic but continued to lead the Foundation. Riddick was an integral part of the committee searching for Tooke's replacement.

After several false starts, the Ochsner Clinic Board selected Dr. Gary Goldstein, an Obstetrician from California, who had been operating managed care systems in the West since the late 1980s.

Goldstein's background in health plan management loomed all the more important in light of the challenges the Ochsner Health Plan faced by 1996. Managed care systems across the nation were losing money by the mid-1990s, and the Ochsner Health Plan was no exception.

In 1995, the Ochsner Health Plan secured a large State of Louisiana contract. Goldstein realized that Ochsner had underpriced its product but reasoned that the statewide approach offered the quickest way for the health plan to recoup its losses. He negotiated an agreement with the Sisters of Charity to use their statewide hospital network to support the Ochsner Health Plan.

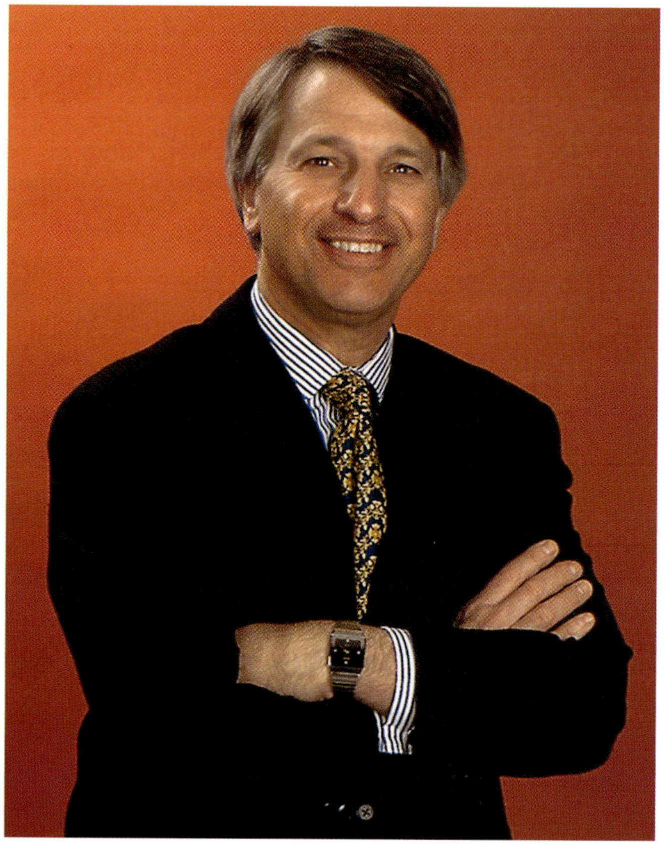

Gary Goldstein, M.D., headed the Clinic at a time when the Ochsner Health Plan was losing significant amounts of money.

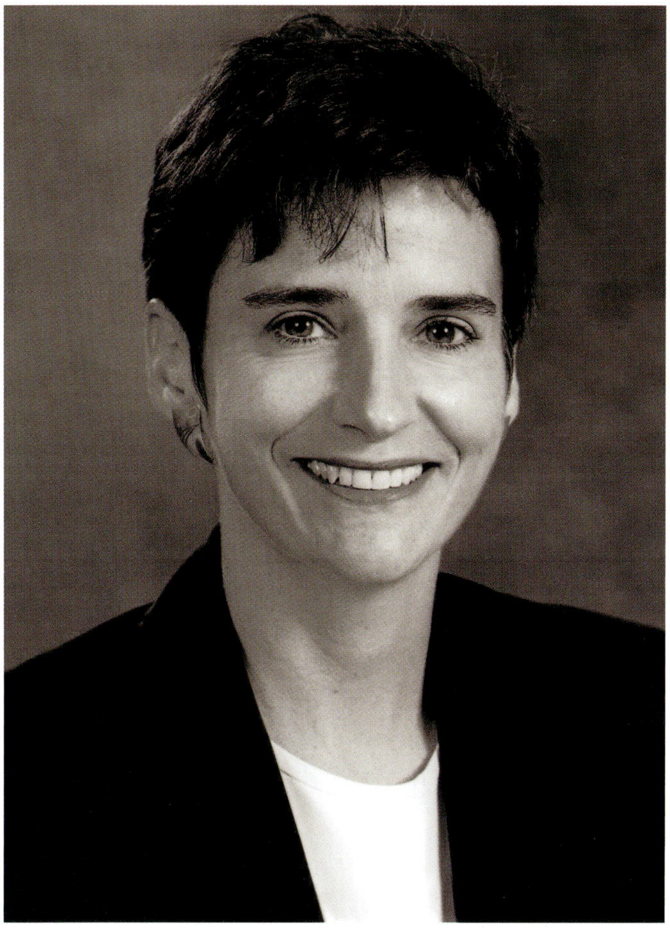

Mary Brown was Director of the Foundation Hospital during the late 1990s.

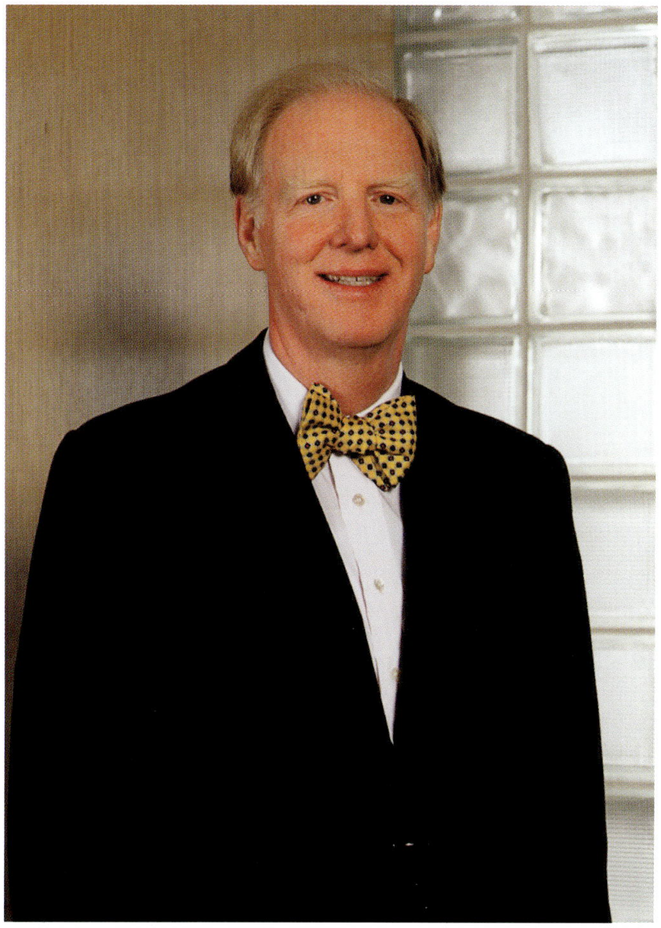

Richard Freeman Jr. succeeded his father on the Foundation Board of Trustees and became the longest serving board member.

TROUBLE AT THE PARTNERSHIP

The other difficult situation that Goldstein stepped into involved the Ochsner Clinic partnership. The Clinic hired Goldstein to be its Medical Director and CEO, with the idea that he would in time also become the Foundation CEO, as he did in January 1998. The Clinic Partnership, however, continued to be faced with financial obstacles. In addition, the partnership realized that the health plan was creating losses it couldn't afford.[9] The new corporate realities were in conflict with the original design. It was a formula for inertia.

During much of the period of upheaval, Mary Brown was the Administrator of Ochsner Foundation Hospital. She had trained in hospital administration under David Page, the longtime Foundation Hospital Administrator, and had taken the position when Phillip Robinson, Page's successor, left to work for the major for-profit hospital chain, HCA.

In 1998, Brown left Ochsner Foundation Hospital, and Goldstein followed shortly afterward, in 1999. "Richard Freeman, Chairman of the Foundation Board, called me at my hotel in Chicago and asked if I'd resume leadership of the Foundation as CEO," Riddick said. "My marching orders were to merge the Clinic and the Foundation."[10]

Riddick would spend the next two years accomplishing that goal, achieving success at a task that Ochsner administrators were unable to accomplish for nearly 20 years. He would be greatly assisted in the task by new administrators.

'THERE WERE GOOD THINGS GOING ON'

The organization that Alton Ochsner and the other founders had created in 1942 had been nurtured by succeeding generations of physicians and administrators who took the care and improvement of the New Orleans institution entrusted to their oversight seriously.

All of Ochsner took time in December 1999 to pay tribute to one of those physicians and administrators who had meant so much to the organization. The death of Dr. Merrill Hines at the age of 90 was a reminder of the patient care legacy that earlier generations of Ochsner physicians had left their successors.[11]

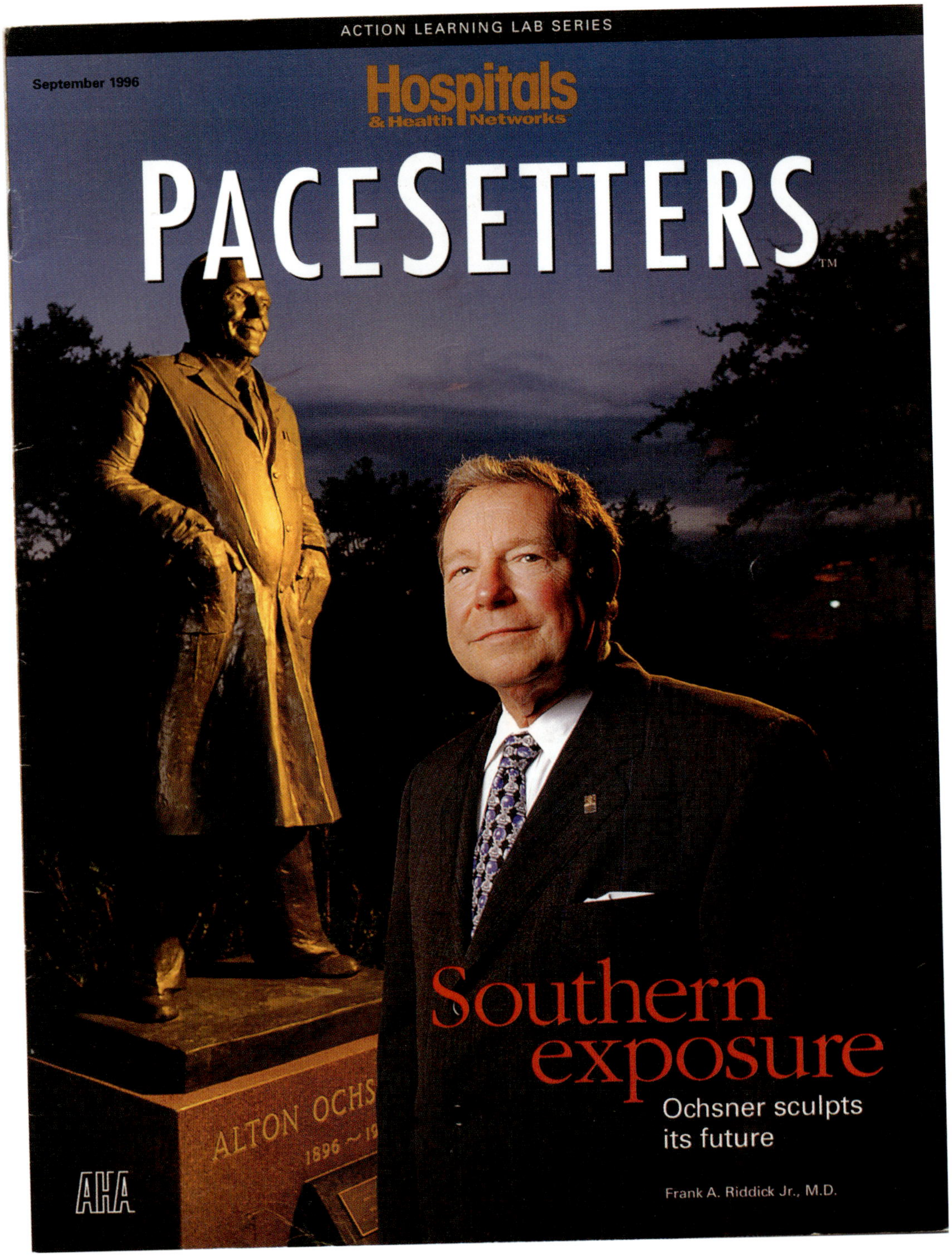

The strong hand of Frank Riddick, M.D. at the helm of the Clinic helped guide Ochsner through the difficult years of the 1980s and 1990s.

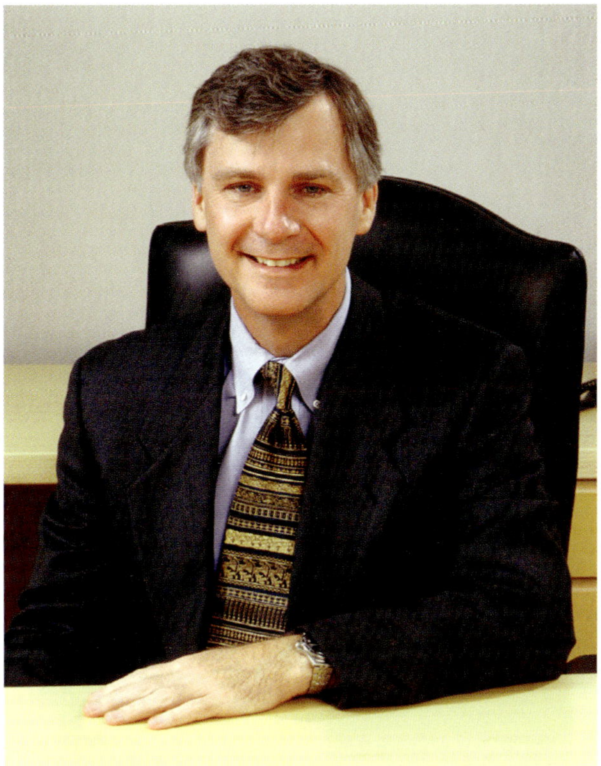

Patrick Quinlan, M.D., came to Ochsner in 1999 from Lovelace Clinic in Albuquerque, New Mexico, and was quickly promoted to Interim CEO when Gary Goldstein left.

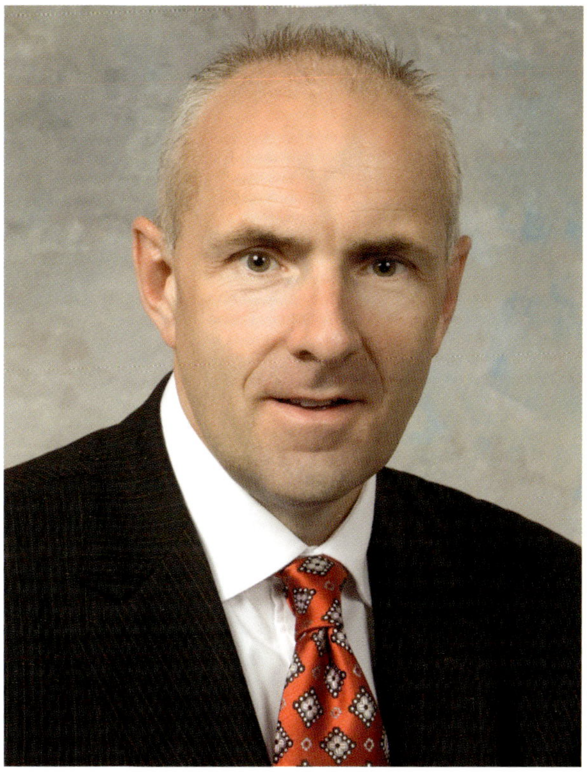

Warner Thomas arrived at Ochsner about the same time as Patrick Quinlan and immediately began to seek solutions to the financial problems with the Ochsner Health Plan.

"There were good things going on," said Mary Brown. "Ochsner had a very strong culture of quality care. They were always excited about innovations on the clinical side. That was the positive that kept them going. Some companies have a 'bland culture.' Ochsner Hospital never had that. It was a team mentality."

"There were good things going on," said Mary Brown. "Ochsner had a very strong culture of quality care. They were always excited about innovations on the clinical side. That was the positive that kept them going. Some companies have a 'bland culture.' Ochsner Hospital never had that. It was a team mentality."[12]

Goldstein, for all of the difficulties he faced during his short tenure at the helm of the Clinic, made some key decisions that have been paying dividends ever since. He took steps early in his years at Ochsner to change the pricing structure of the Ochsner Health Plan.

In 1998, with the strong encouragement of the Ochsner Clinic Board, Goldstein recruited Dr. Patrick Quinlan as Chief Medical Officer of Ochsner Clinic from Lovelace Clinic in Albuquerque, New Mexico. A native of New York, Quinlan had earned a degree in medicine at the University of Texas and had spent 13 years at Lovelace as a clinician with a growing role in administration, a clinic setting that was much like that of Ochsner. Quinlan arrived in New Orleans in late 1998, about the same time Warner Thomas, another Goldstein hire, started work. Thomas, a Vermont native with an MBA from Boston University, began tackling a mountain of challenges as the Clinic's new Chief Operating Officer (COO). Three months into 1999, Goldstein was gone.

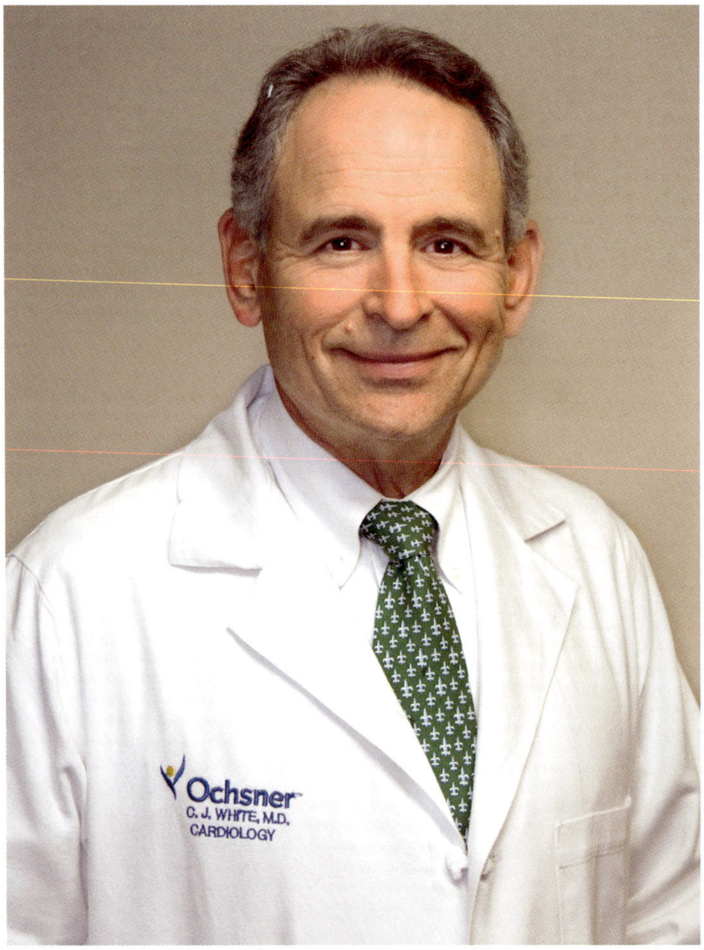

Nationally known Cardiologist Christopher White, M.D., is the Chairman of the Department of Cardiology and the Director of the John Ochsner Heart and Vascular Institute.

Riddick, in one of his first actions as Goldstein's replacement as the Foundation CEO, recruited Dr. William Pinsky from Wayne State University to be the Chief Academic Officer to turn around a coasting academic program. Pinsky understood that academics had always been important at Ochsner, and that Dr. Alton Ochsner and his colleagues had every intention of maintaining that academic atmosphere. The clinical side of the institution, however, assumed a dominant role at Ochsner during the 1980s. Pinsky knew that for the academic program to flourish, things had to be changed. There was an opportunity for him to establish accountability, raise standards and help redefine the identity of Ochsner.

• WHAT OCHSNER MEANS TO ME •

"One of the things I really appreciate about Ochsner is that I've been able to practice medicine the way I wanted to practice medicine – to a very HIGH STANDARD, and without having to compromise the quality of treatments or the way we would treat patients."

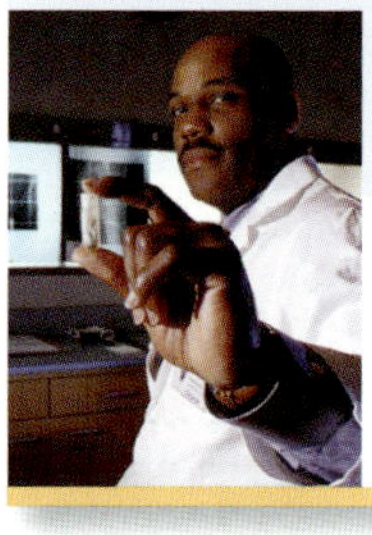

Dr. Troy Scroggins, Chairman of Radiation Oncology, Ochsner Medical Center

To watch the full interview with Dr. Troy Scroggins, visit **ochsner.org/history**.

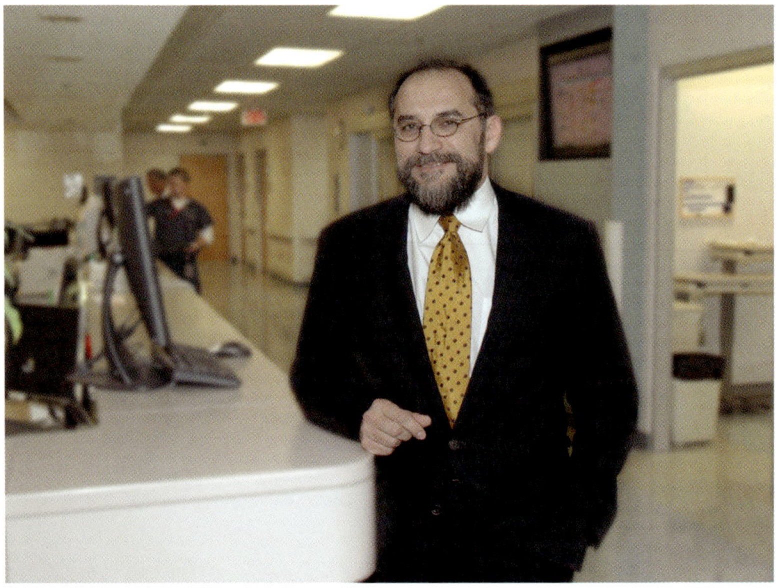

Joe Guarisco, M.D., Chairman of the Department of Emergency Medicine, led the revitalization and state-of-the-art computerization of Ochsner Medical Center's Emergency Department and now heads all of the Emergency Departments across the System.

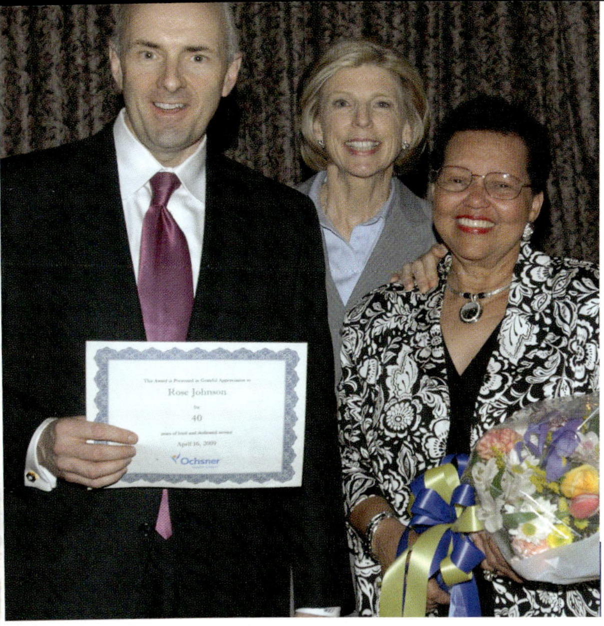

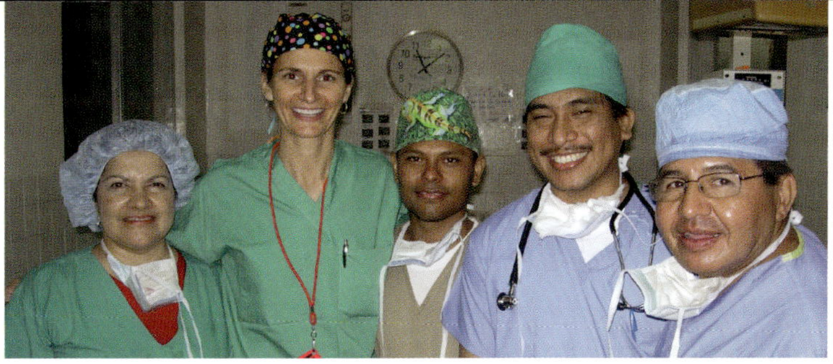

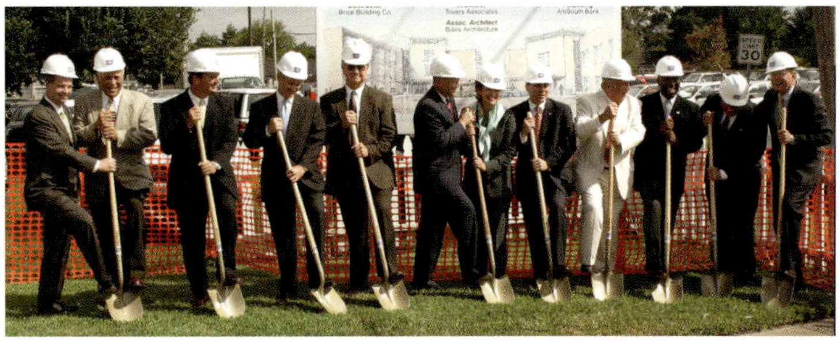

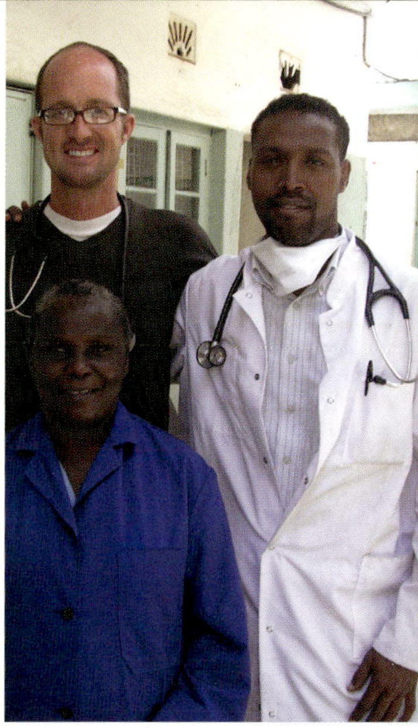

WE SERVE

OCHSNER IS DEDICATED TO PROVIDING A HIGHER LEVEL OF SERVICE TO OUR PATIENTS AND THE COMMUNITIES WHERE WE LIVE AND WORK. Through gifts like the Hope Lodge and Trace Playground properties, through the devotion and long years of service of our outstanding employees and volunteers, through our commitment to local organizations who share our goal of better healthcare, and through the mission work of our physicians and programs, Ochsner expands our service area to serve people in need.

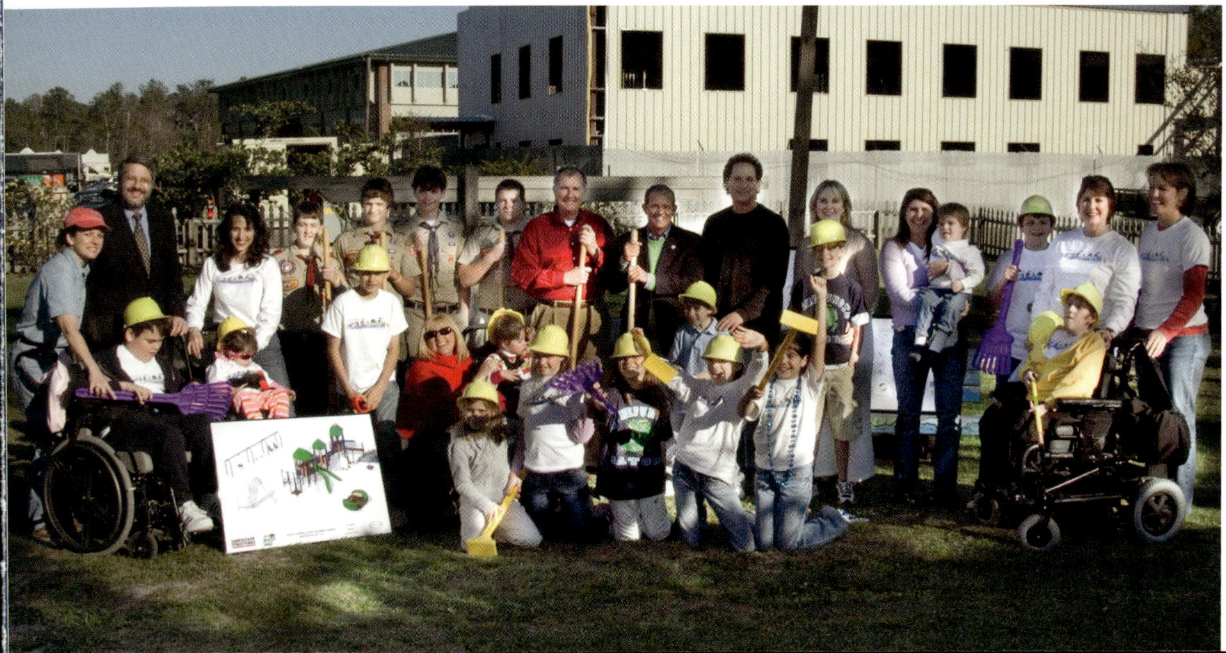

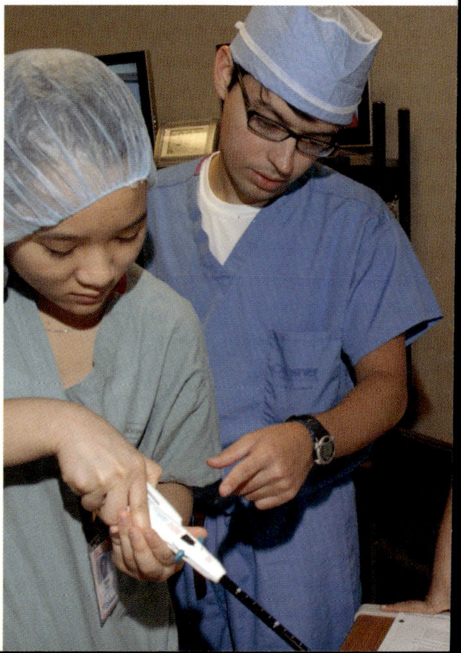

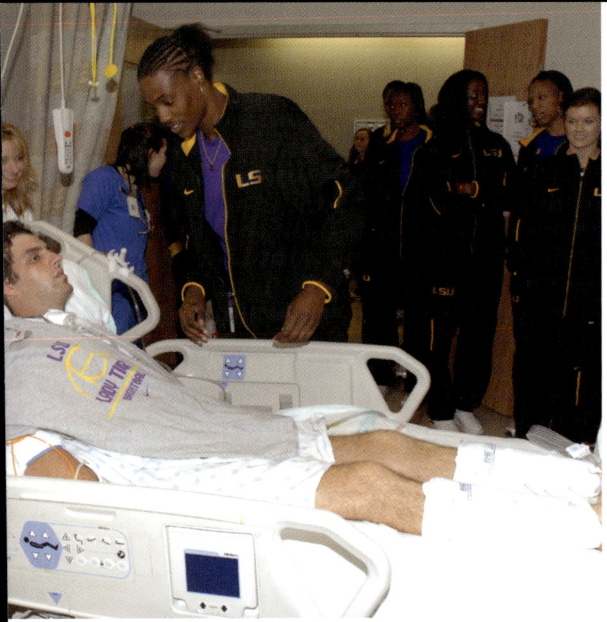

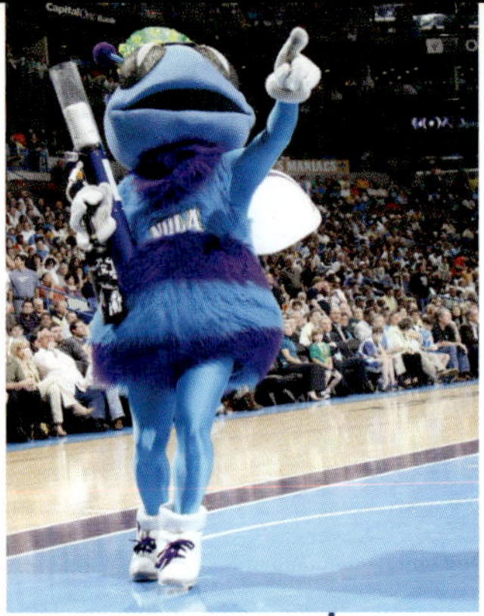

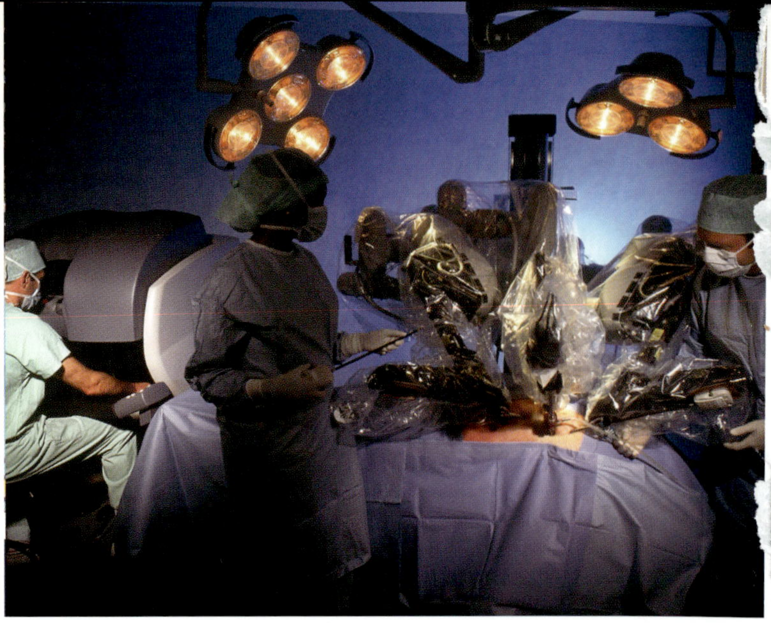

WE LEAD

BY SUPPORTING SPORTS ACTIVITIES AND ORGANIZATIONS THAT PROMOTE FITNESS AND HEALTHY LIFESTYLES, through a commitment to improving emergency care throughout our service areas, by raising the public's awareness of the importance of diet and exercise to health and through use of the most advanced surgical technologies like the robotic da Vinci® Surgical System, Ochsner takes a leadership position in our communities by advancing the quality and level of care.

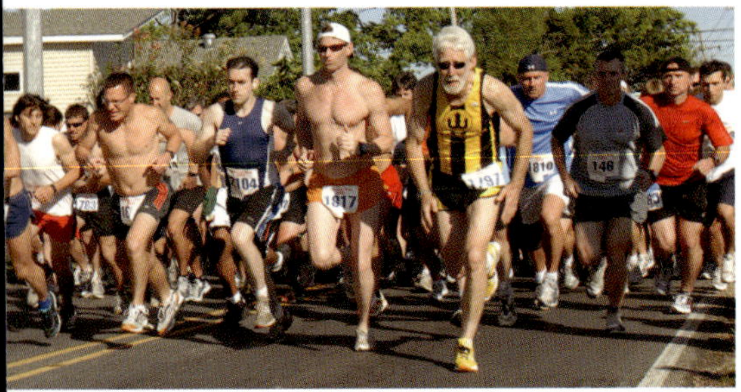

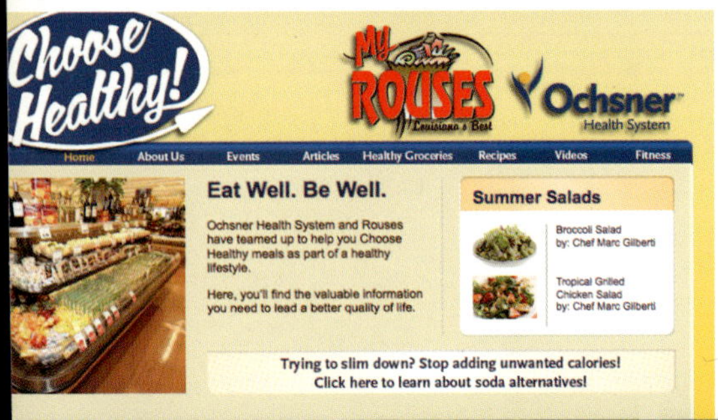

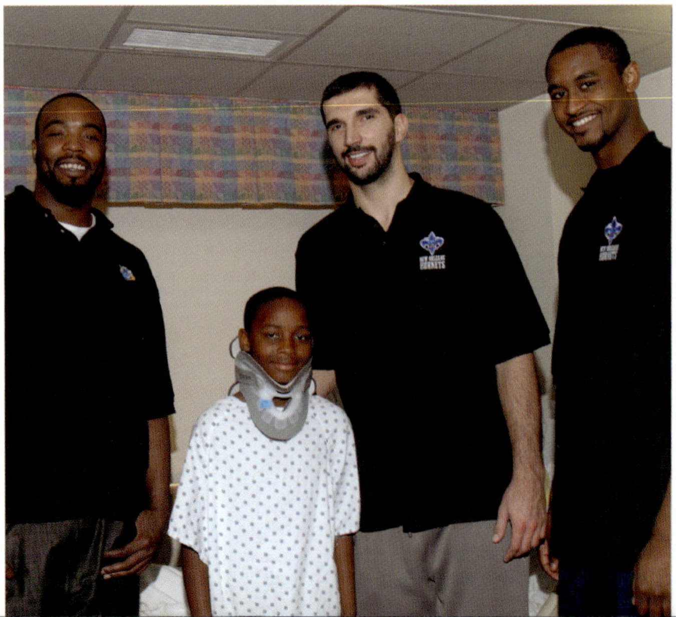

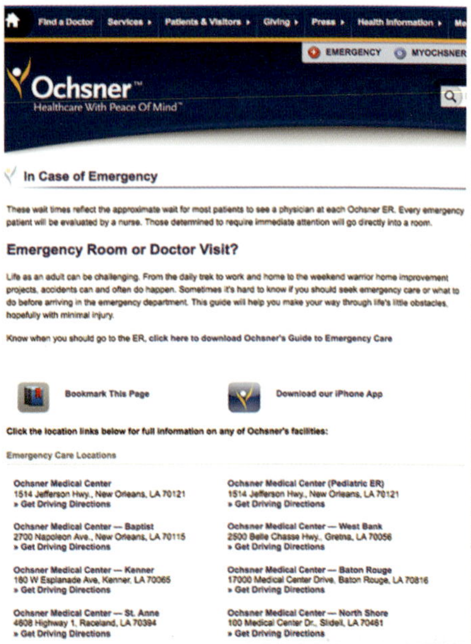

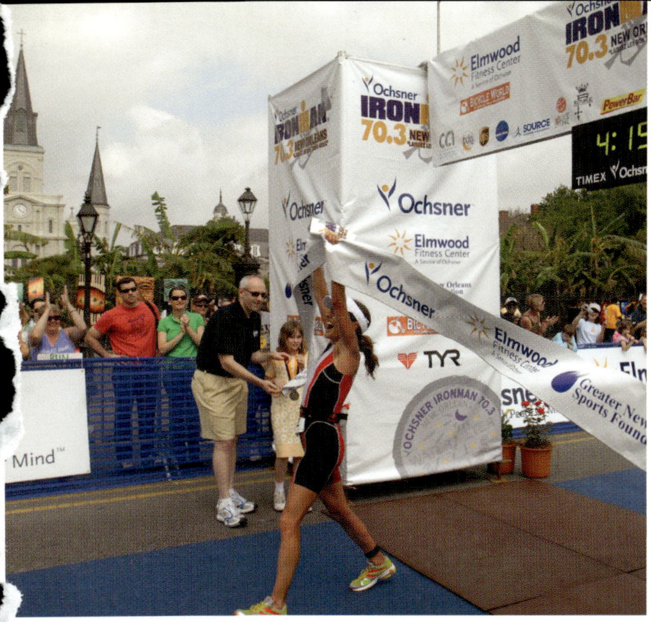

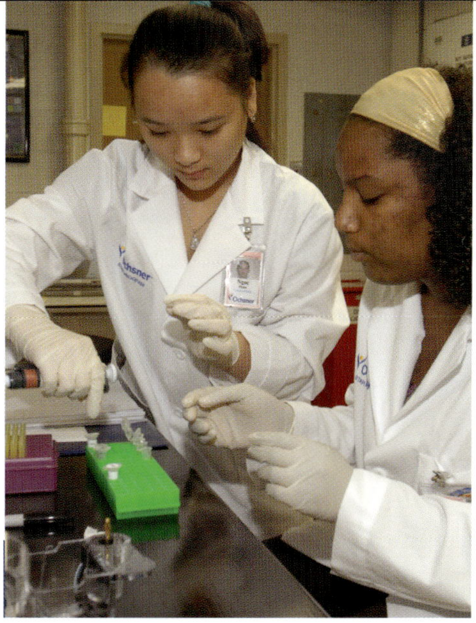
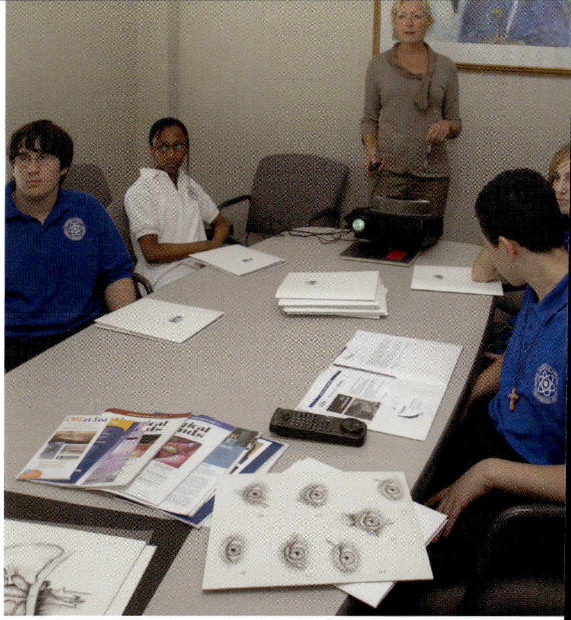

WE EDUCATE

OCHSNER IS COMMITTED TO EDUCATING MEMBERS OF OUR COMMUNITY, OUR EMPLOYEES AND THE PHYSICIANS OF TODAY AND TOMORROW through the STAR Program, the Girl Scouts Science Discovery Day, partnerships with local schools, Nursing and Allied Health education, our medical student and residency programs, *The Ochsner Journal* and medical conferences.

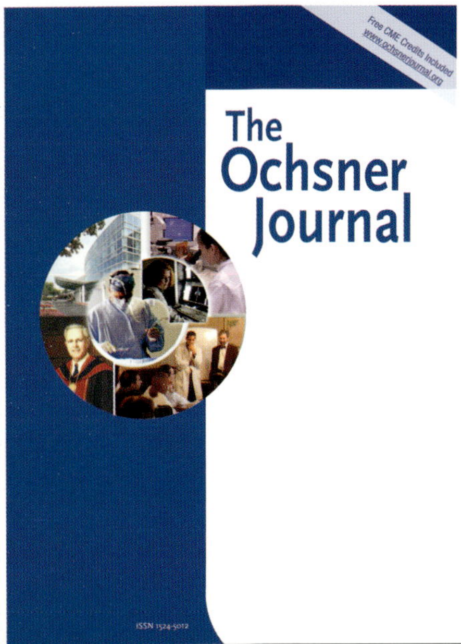

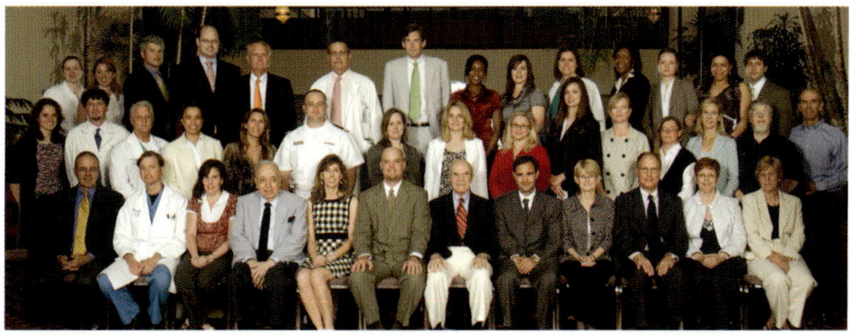
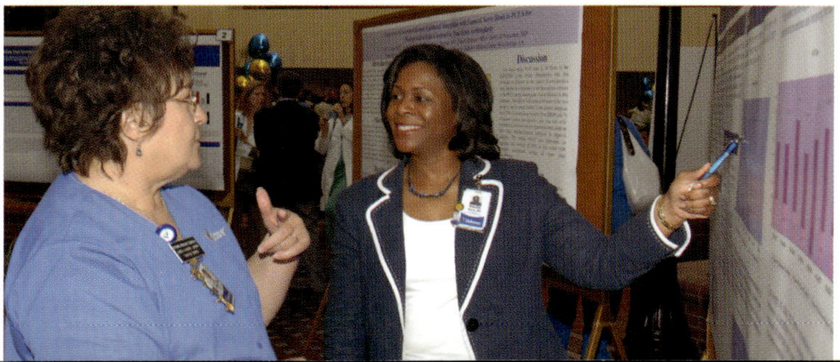
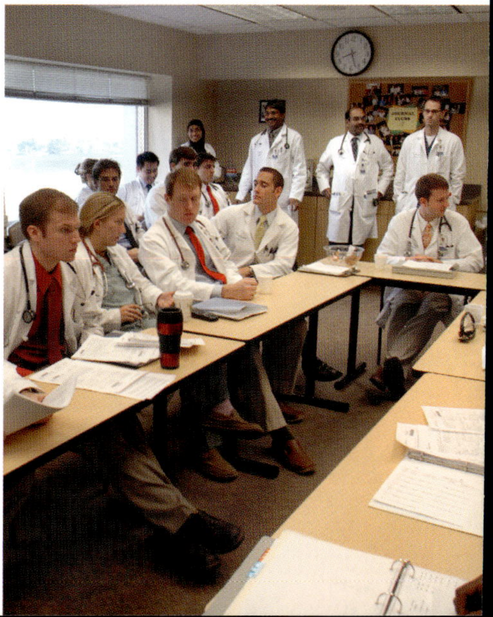

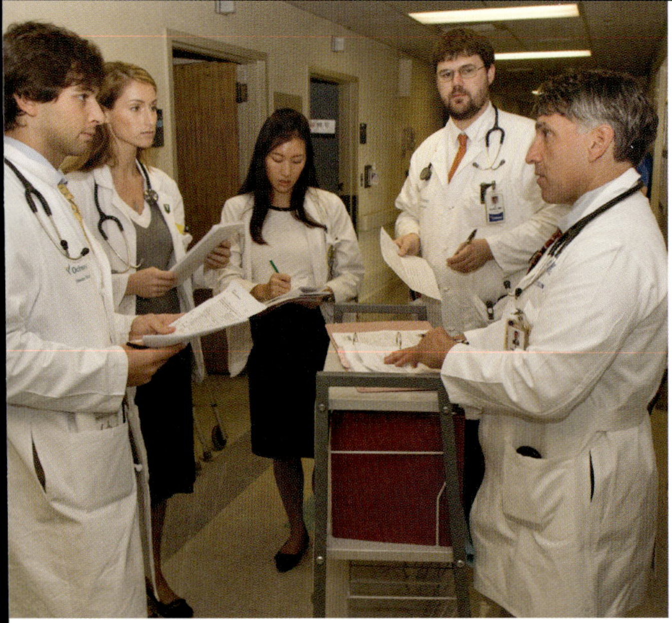

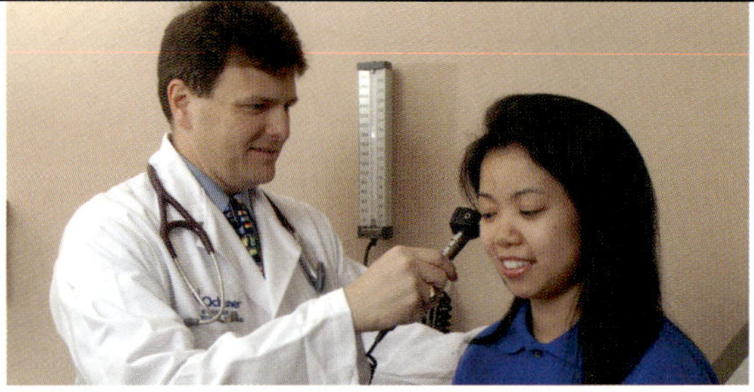

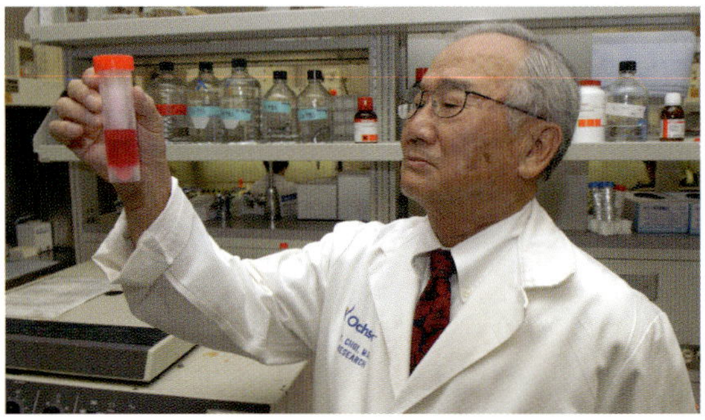

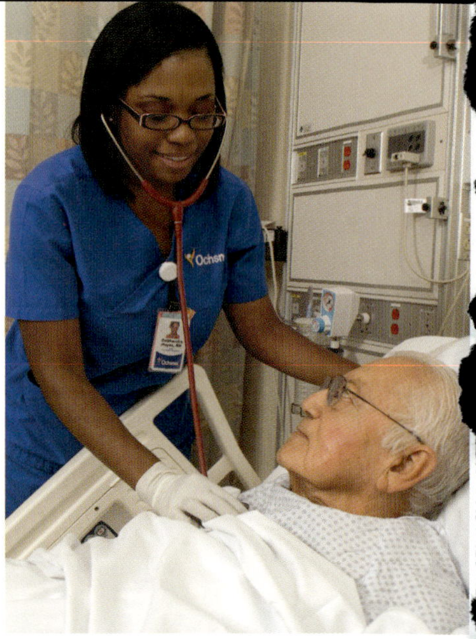

OUR MISSION

We Serve, Heal, Lead, Educate and Innovate.

OUR VISION

Ochsner will be a global medical and academic leader who will save and change lives. We will shape the future of healthcare through our integrated health system, fueled by the passion and strength of our diversified team of physicians and employees.

Ochsner™
Healthcare With Peace Of Mind™

Throughout Ochsner's long history, the health system has received generous support, financial and otherwise, from many corporate and individual donors as well as our own employees. Their selfless gifts and tireless work support Ochsner's mission to serve, heal, lead, educate and innovate, and go far to help shape the future of healthcare locally, nationally and globally.

SOME OF OUR MAJOR DONORS:

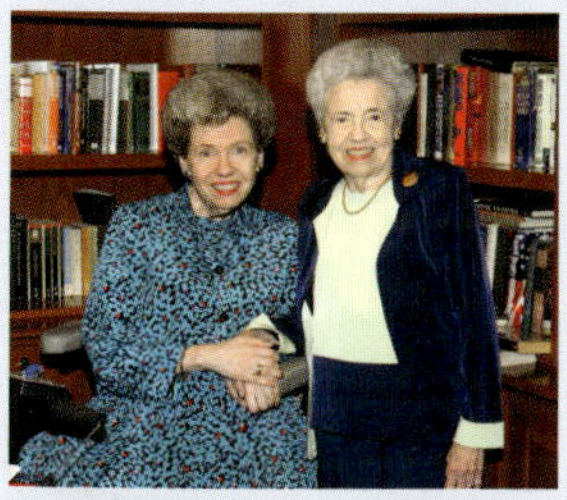

JANE AND KATHERINE GAGE

The Ochsner Foundation is honored and pleased to have Jane and Katherine Gage as members. These longtime supporters and patients have contributed their valuable time, talents and generous financial support through the years. Jane Gage has also served as a Trustee of Ochsner Clinic Foundation and is an Emeritus Member of the Board of Councilors.

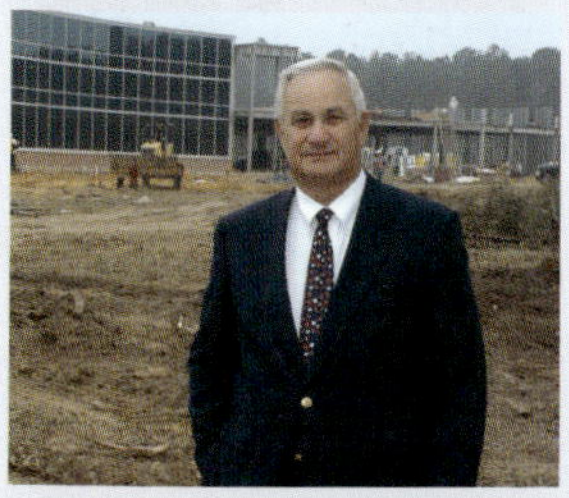

DOYLE COATNEY

Doyle Coatney underwent a life-saving liver transplant at Ochsner in 1995. Since then he has been a generous benefactor. Before his transplant procedure, he made a vow, "I promised myself, if I live through this, I'm going to help Ochsner." Now he's keeping that promise. His enthusiasm is contagious, his gratitude to Ochsner is genuine and his love of life affects everyone he meets.

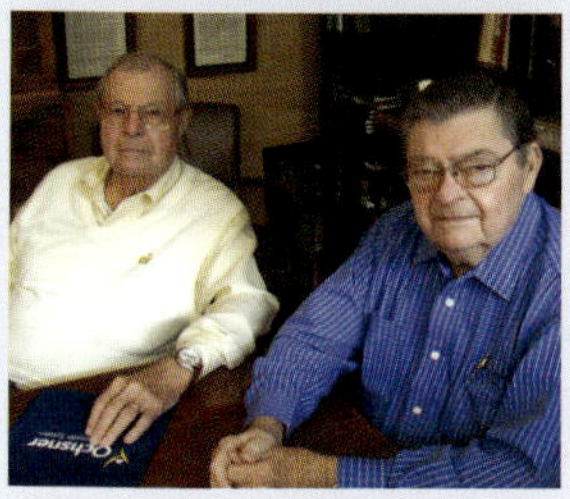

FRANK AND CHARLES GODCHAUX

Frank and Charles Godchaux have been devoted supporters of Ochsner for more than 20 years. Their commitment to Ochsner's mission and their philanthropic efforts on our behalf have been unwavering. Most recently the Godchaux Family Foundation and Charles and Frank individually provided major support toward the John Ochsner Heart and Vascular Institute.

Each year, Ochsner employees, board members, volunteers and physicians provide financial support to the Health System's research, education and care-giving programs through individual contributions made to the Ochsner Employee Giving Program. Their generous personal gifts demonstrate their personal commitment to Ochsner's mission to provide healthcare with peace of mind to the communities we serve.

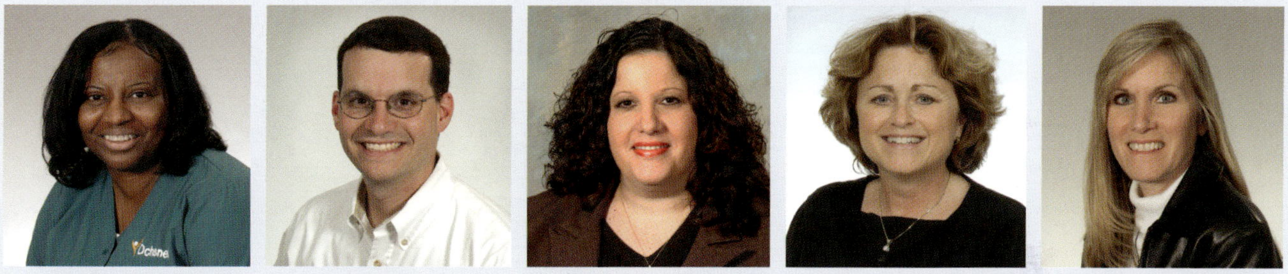

Many Ochsner employees participate in the Ochsner Employee Giving Program annually. Left to Right: Carmon Valinda, Michael Heim, Laura LeBlanc, Vicki Kaplan and Melanie Roques

To learn more about giving to Ochsner, visit Ochsner.org, or call 504-842-7110.

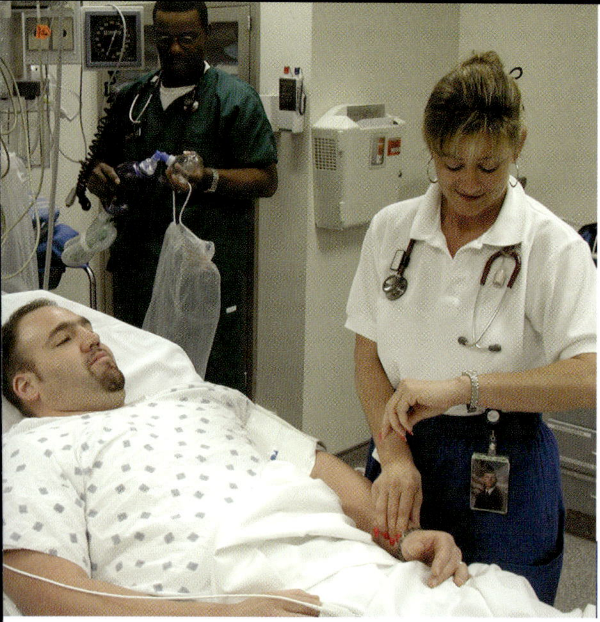

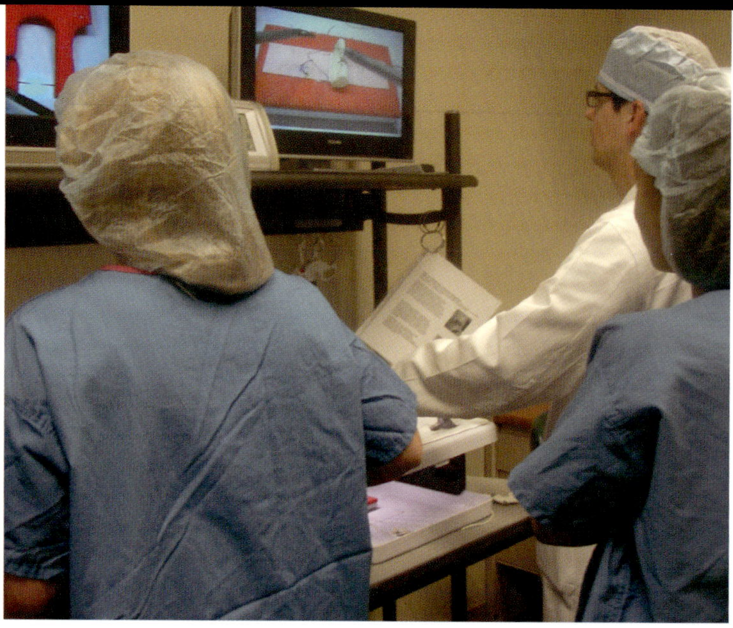

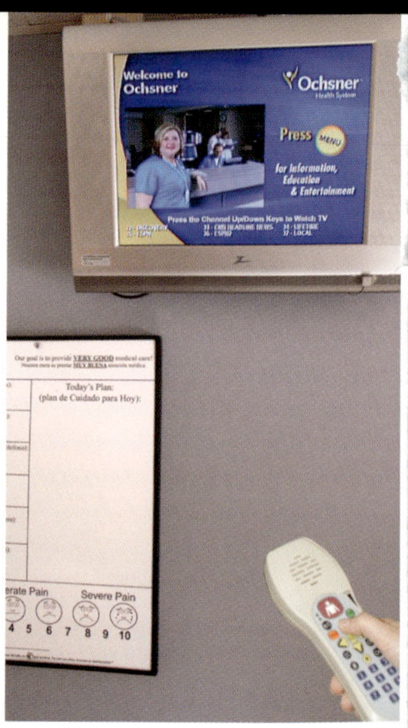

WE INNOVATE

OCHSNER CREATES AN ENVIRONMENT THAT SUPPORTS INNOVATION AND ADVANCES PATIENT CARE. Through programs like the Clinical Librarian Rounds or the Interactive LodgeNet TV system, patients can access quality health and medical reference information in their hospital rooms. And through extensive investments in technology and information systems like Ochsner's state-of-the-art electronic medical records system, we ensure that physicians and staff have the most complete picture of a patient's medical history to deliver the most efficient and effective care possible. Ochsner was recognized as one of the "most wired" hospitals for our extensive Internet and Intranet communications networks.

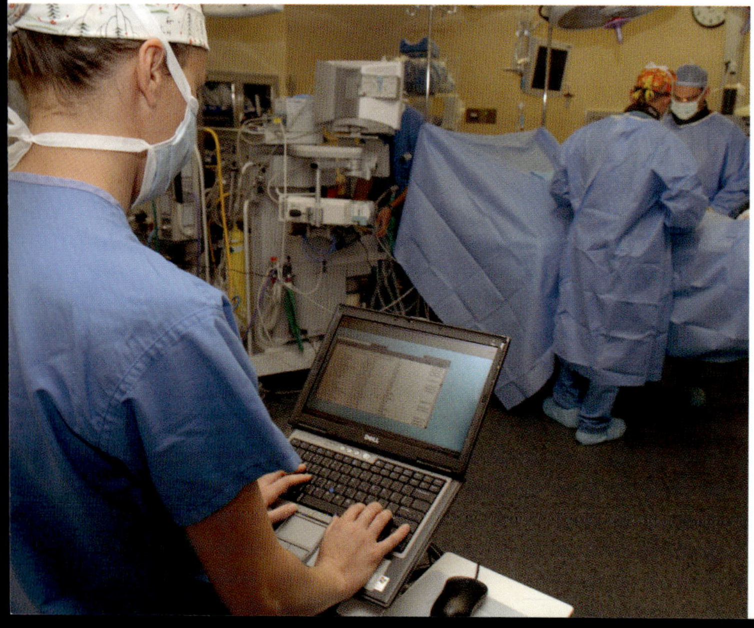

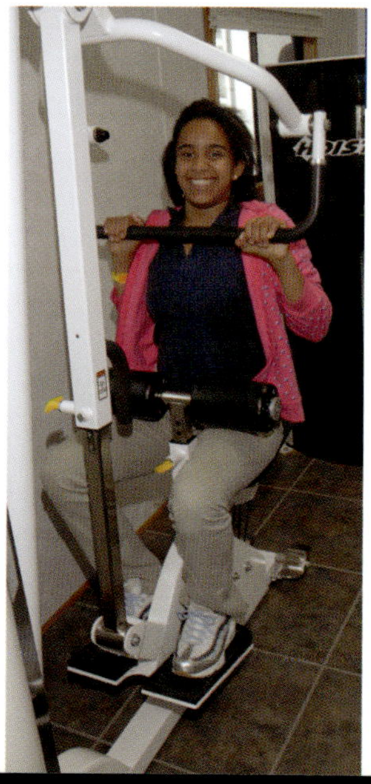

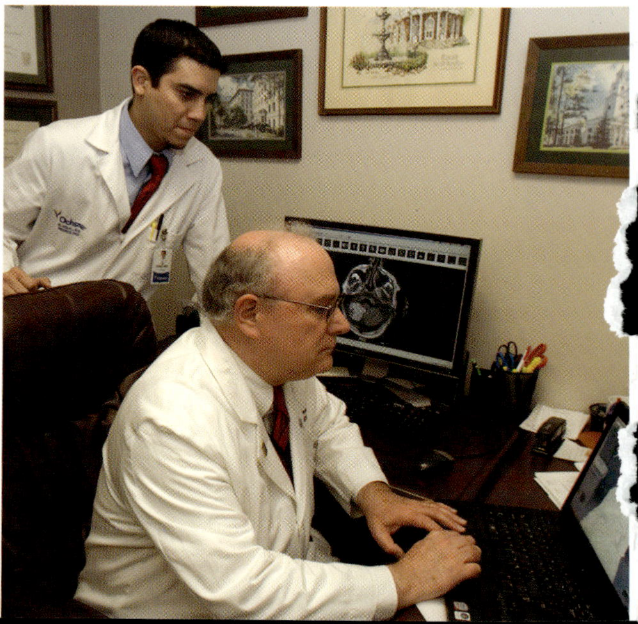

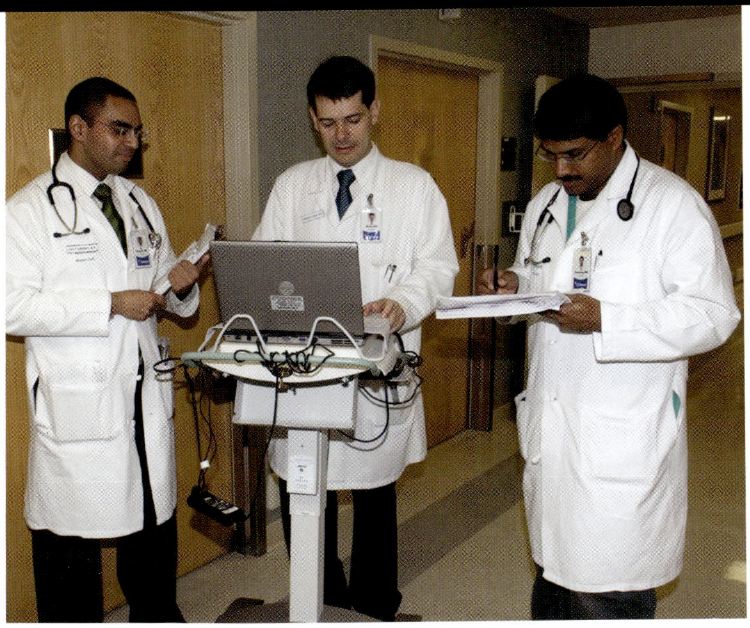

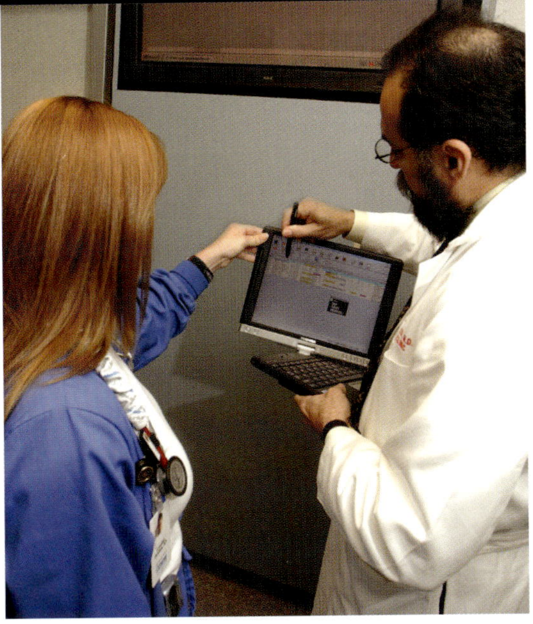

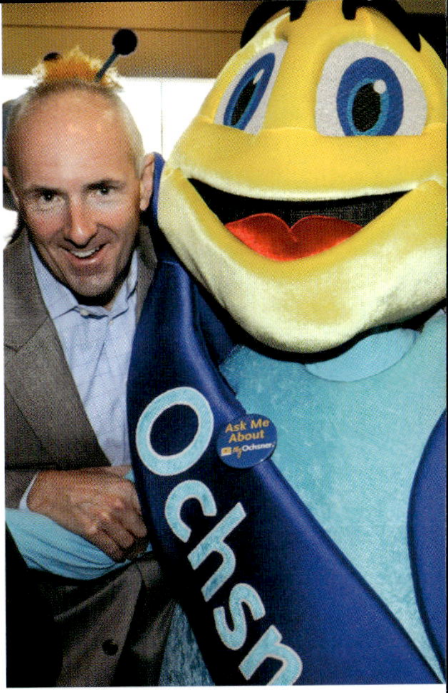

Ochsner™
Healthcare With Peace Of Mind™

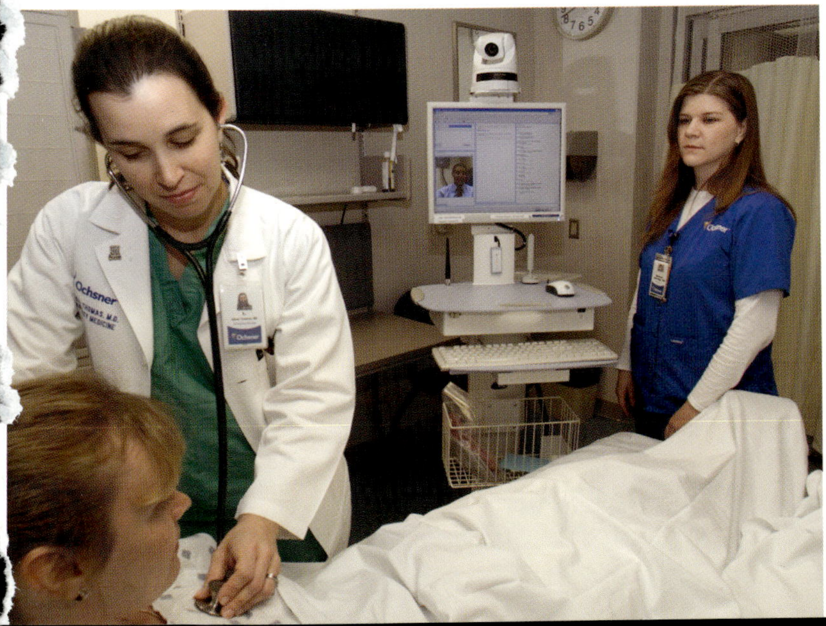

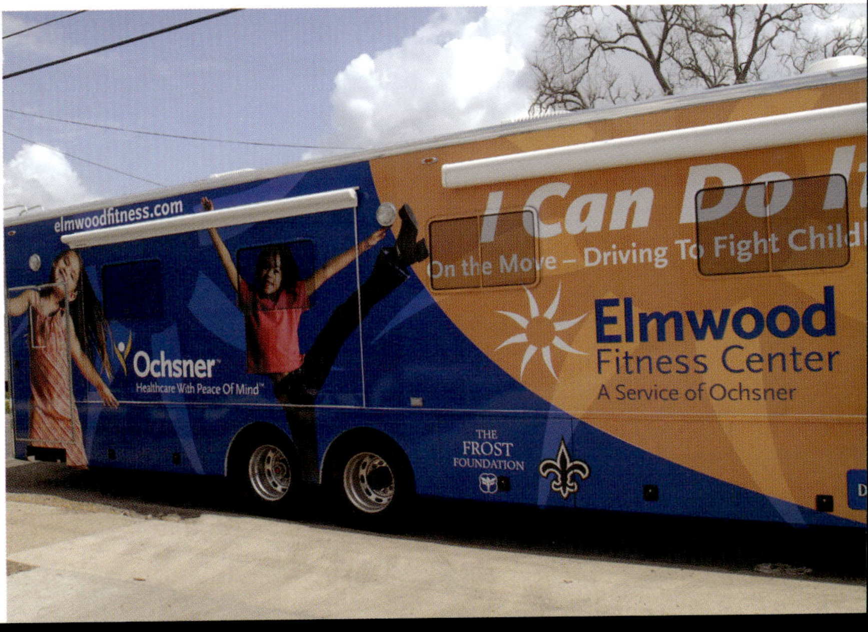

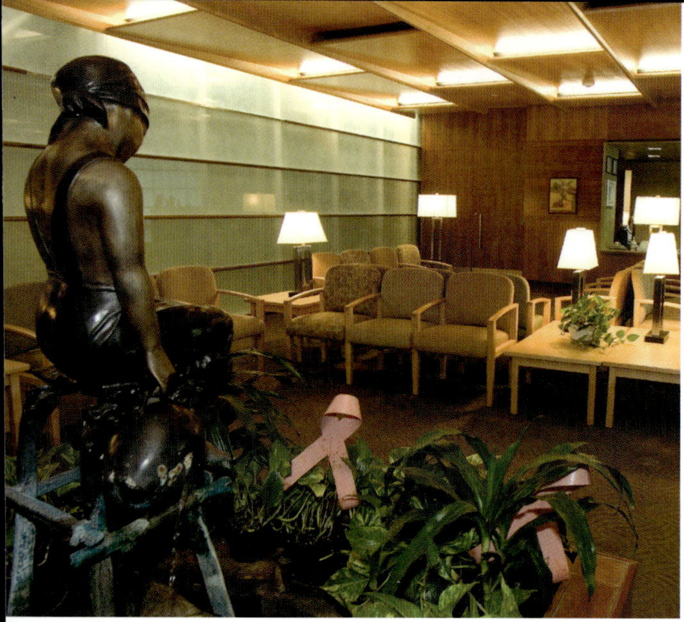

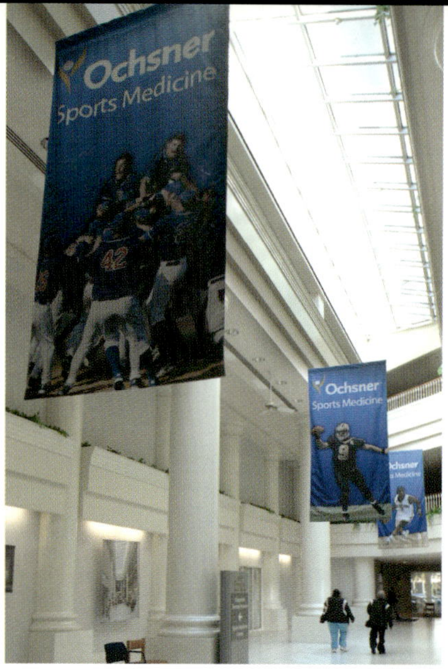

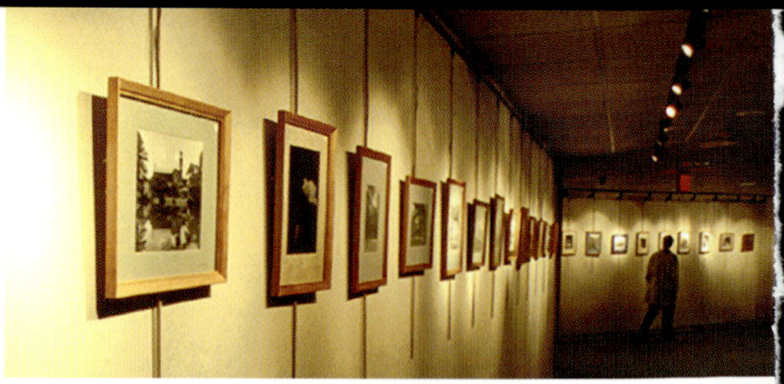

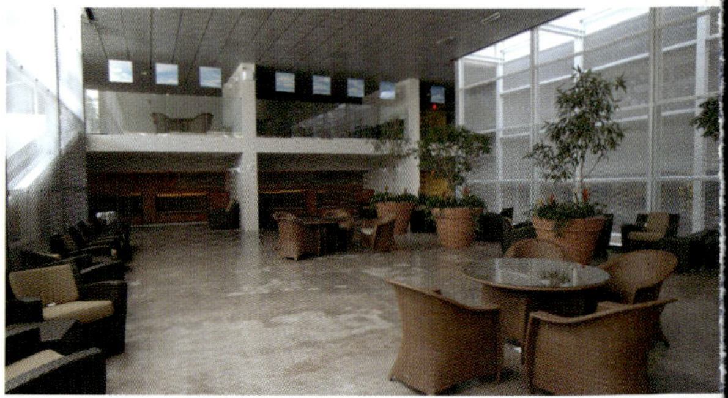

WE HEAL

MEDICAL RESEARCH HAS PROVEN THE HEALING POWER OF ONE'S ENVIRONMENT. In our role as a health system, we are committed to creating environments and spaces that enable and enhance the healing process of our patients, their families and our staff. From the underwater theme of our Children's Health Center to our Winter Garden and Art Walk, Ochsner is committed to creating nurturing and healing spaces within our facilities. From the serenity of our non-denominational chapel to the Ochsner Lieselotte Tansey Breast Center's European spa atmosphere and our Sports Medicine Institute, Ochsner takes a holistic approach to providing healing environments for all aspects of our patients' lives.

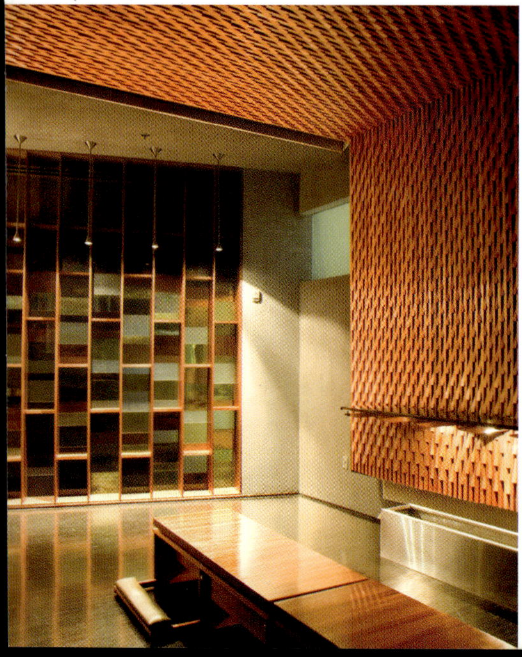

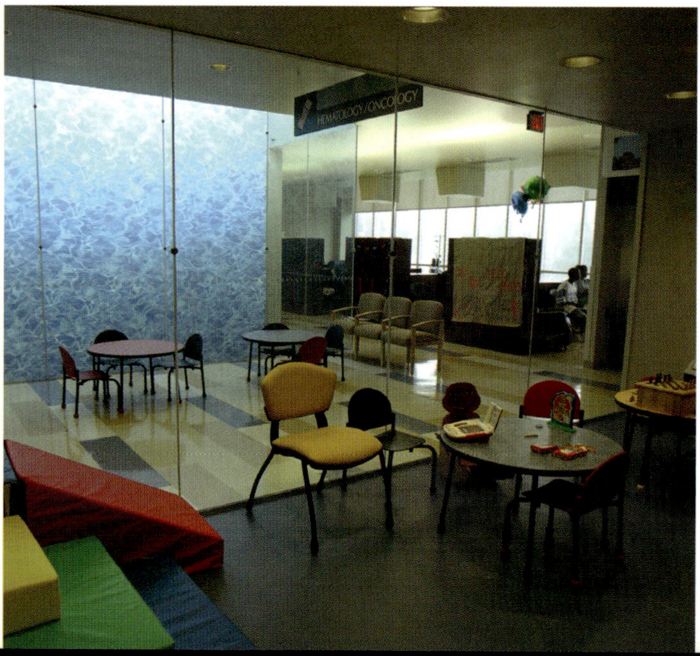

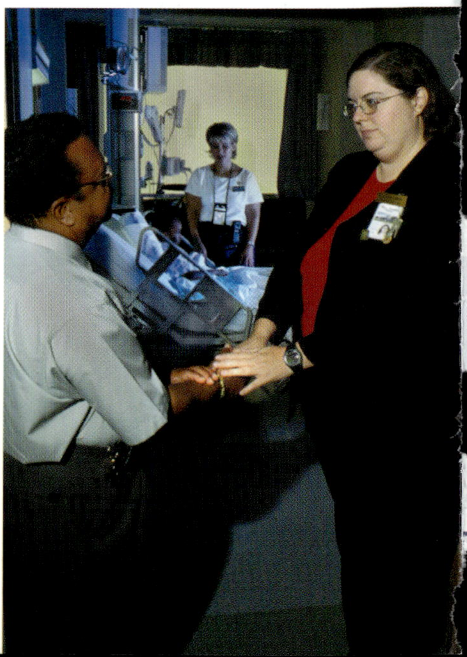

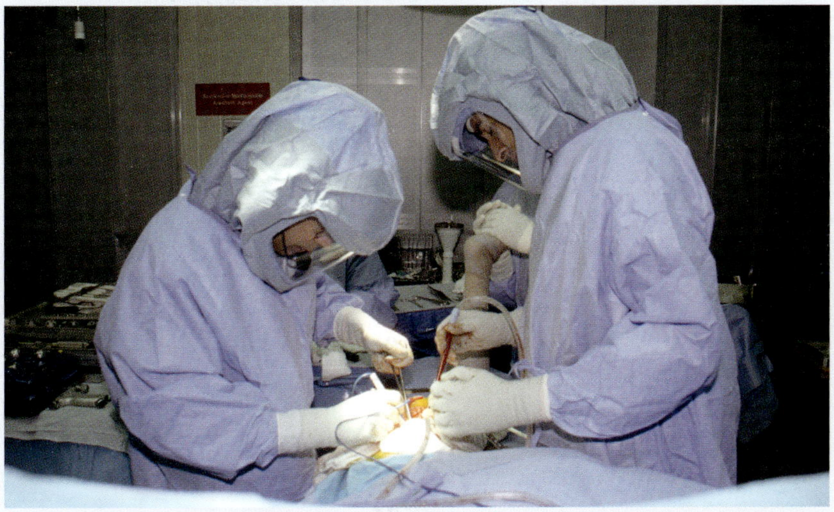

John Lockwood Ochsner returned to the Clinic his grandfather helped found. He almost left New Orleans after Katrina, but the lure of the place the Ochsners had called home since 1927 remained strong.

THIRD GENERATION

Dr. John Lockwood "Lock" Ochsner has carried the standards of the Ochsner name into the third generation at the medical institution named for his grandfather. The son of Dr. John Ochsner, the Cardiovascular Surgeon who performed the first heart transplant at Ochsner Foundation Hospital in 1970, Lock Ochsner knew growing up the pressures he would face if he chose medicine as a career.

He resisted those pressures in college, opting to major in economics rather than biology or organic chemistry. "I was a little bit of a Pollyanna," he said. "I didn't appreciate medicine until I saw how other people lived their lives."[13]

Urged by his father to take as much non-medical instruction as possible, Lock Ochsner came to medicine late. "Medicine wasn't something I really wanted to do," he said. "I wasn't following in the family's footsteps. Dad encouraged me to study more science outside medicine."[14]

Unlike his father and grandfather, Lock Ochsner decided not to go to Tulane. He attended Vassar College in Poughkeepsie, New York, for undergraduate work and went to LSU for medical school. From 1981 to 1986, he trained in Orthopedics at the University of New Mexico in Albuquerque and then spent a year in a fellowship in Los Angeles.

"I absolutely thought about coming back," Ochsner said, adding that his decision to practice Orthopedics was because he "wanted to do something different than my father and grandfather. I was never going to do what they did. I didn't think I had that commitment."[15]

Lock Ochsner values the close relationship he has with his father. "On more than one occasion," he said, "Dad and I were operating at the same time. We could visit and chat, yet we were independent of each other. To this day, he comes around and visits my patients. Dad can't help but give me medical advice, and I can't help but listen to it."[16]

After more than 20 years at the hospital that bears the family name, Lock Ochsner still marvels at "how little it has changed since 1987. There's a special pride among the employees. People really feel a bond with each other. They feel they have something special."[17]

Lock Ochsner is one of five grandchildren of Alton Ochsner practicing medicine. Alton Ochsner Jr.'s daughter J. Coller Ochsner is a Dermatologist, and daughter Isabel "Missy" Ochsner is an Emergency Room physician. Mims Ochsner's son Gage is a Surgeon, and Lock Ochsner's younger sister Catherine is an Ophthalmologist.

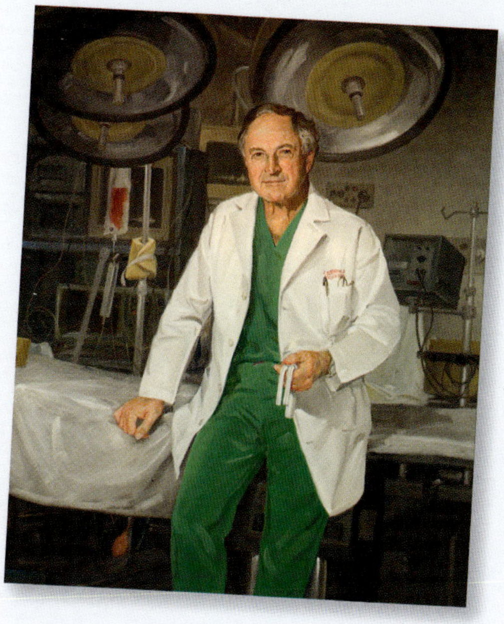

John Ochsner studied under Michael DeBakey and brought his surgical skills back to the Clinic his father had helped found.

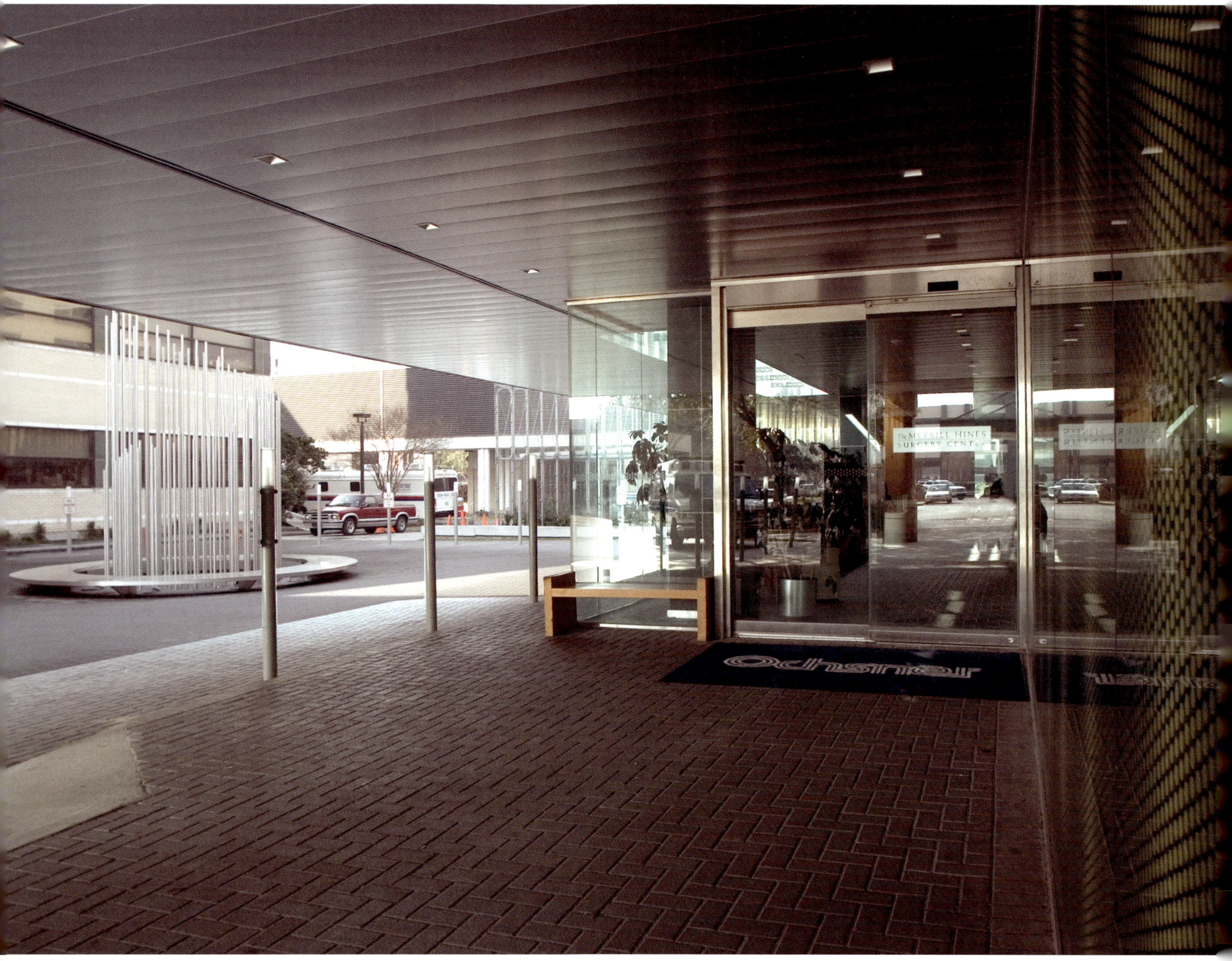
The MERRILL HINES
SURGERY CENT
ochsner

CHAPTER 9:

ECONOMIC FREEFALL

WHEN GARY GOLDSTEIN LEFT OCHSNER CLINIC IN 1999, Dr. Patrick Quinlan was appointed interim CEO. His goal was to work with the senior management team at Ochsner Clinic and Ochsner Foundation to forge a unification agreement that would be meaningful and capable of being approved by the Clinic Board of Management and the Foundation Board of Trustees. Quinlan and his team—Foundation CEO Dr. Frank A. Riddick Jr., Ochsner Clinic COO Warner Thomas, Foundation Director of Finance and Treasurer Bobby Brannon and Foundation Hospital Director Eileen Skinner—had their work cut out for them.

Quinlan, who had come to Ochsner Clinic the previous year from Lovelace Clinic in Albuquerque, understood instinctively what he and his team were up against. "The merger was a very difficult period," he said. "We owned a health plan in economic freefall. Lovelace had run a similar health plan in New Mexico. A health plan can lose a fortune, and it was busy doing just that."[1]

Quinlan and his team approached the unification from several perspectives. "We didn't want a standard holding company," he said. "We organized the merger around the way a patient would see it. We organized it around the patient. Continuity of care was so important. It was a different model. We wanted to make it new, not something old living on with a new name."

Quinlan and his team would help create something new with an established and very respected name.

The Merrill Hines Surgery Center opened on the main campus in 2004 in honor of one of Ochsner's longtime leaders.

"We professionals take pride in the quality of care we provide: making the correct diagnosis, providing appropriate services, assuring scientific content and the latest advances, and achieving the best outcomes. Excellence in patient care has always been the hallmark of services at Ochsner."

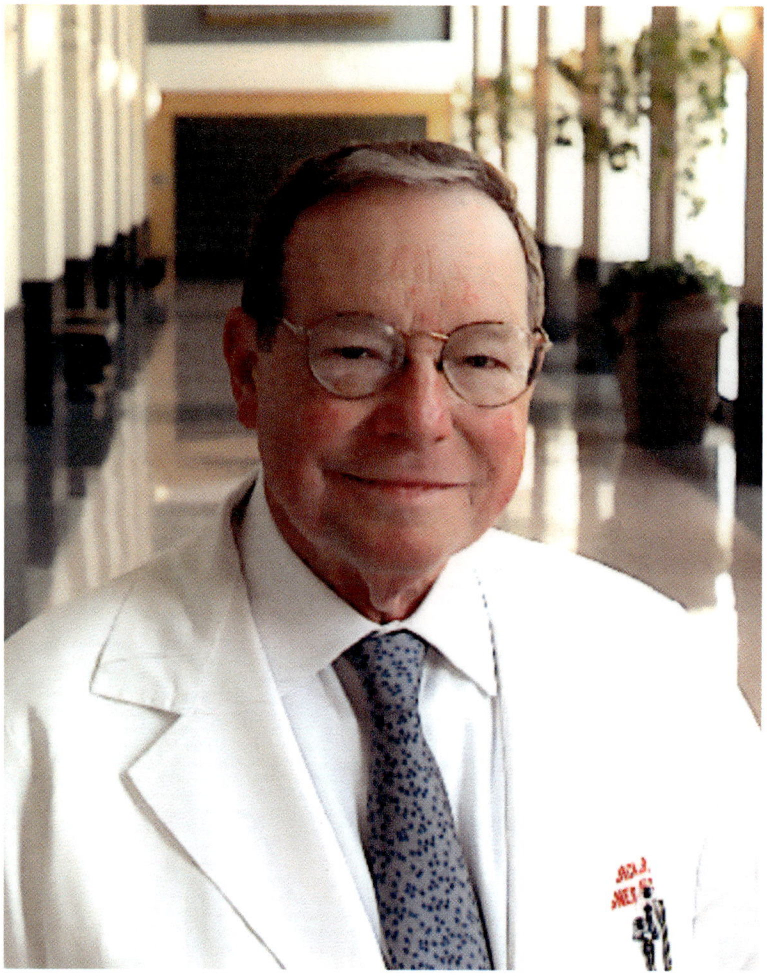

Riddick considered the unification between the Foundation and Clinic to be the most important accomplishment in his later years of management.

Frank Riddick summed up the team's philosophy when he said that "we professionals take pride in the quality of care we provide: making the correct diagnosis, providing appropriate services, assuring scientific content and the latest advances, and achieving the best outcomes. Excellence in patient care has always been the hallmark of services at Ochsner."[2]

The second perspective governing the eventual success of the unification involved the Clinic Partnership structure, critical because of the partnership's 70 percent ownership of the health plan. "An important aspect of the unification was that two conditions had to be met," Quinlan said. "The partners had to vote. And a very high threshold of approval had to be achieved."[3]

SERVANT LEADERSHIP

Quinlan credits a great deal of the success of the unification to the quiet, behind-the-scenes leadership of Richard Freeman, Chairman of the Foundation's Board of Trustees. "There remained a fair amount of disagreement between the Clinic and the Foundation," Quinlan said. "Some on the Clinic Board of Management had very different points of view."[4]

Freeman was an island of calm and reason. "Richard Freeman got everybody into one room and said 'This is a Board decision. What do you want to do?' It was a great example of servant leadership." Quinlan said. "I remember one of his sayings that captured the transition: 'Let's do this right. Let's be thorough and persistent.'"[5]

Freeman, for his part, credited newcomer Quinlan with pointing out the obvious. "There was a compelling argument that we needed to be unified," he said. "That was best summed up by Pat Quinlan at the first background meeting."[6]

TWO YEARS OF NEGOTIATIONS

The Clinic Board of Management and the Foundation Board of Trustees each chose a small group to begin consolidation discussions. It would be two long years before the two sides could agree to a workable plan of unification.

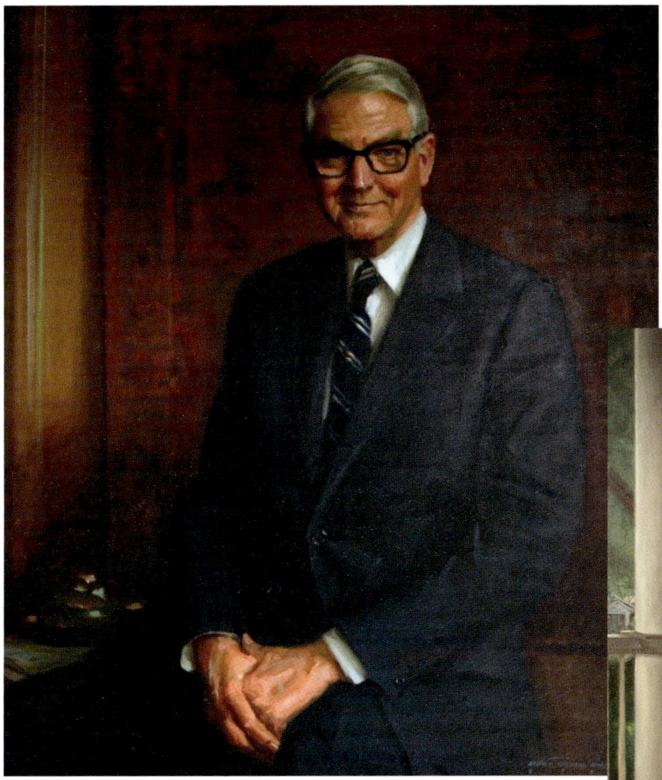

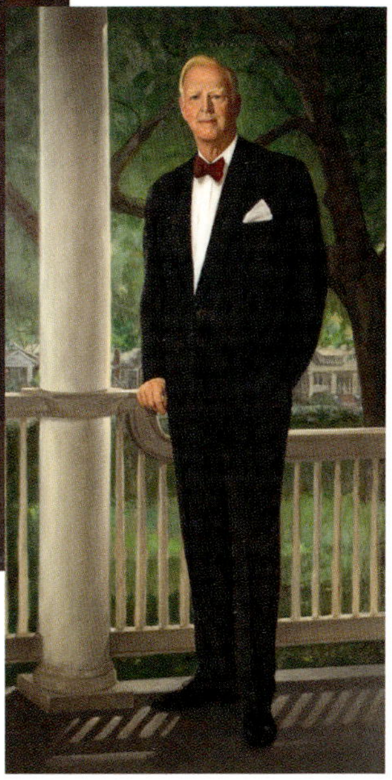

Richard Freeman Sr. and his son, Richard Freeman Jr., provided business acumen and discipline to the leadership of Ochsner for decades.

• WHAT OCHSNER MEANS TO ME •

"Ochsner stands for commitment to quality healthcare. It stands for dedication to the work we do. It stands for being there for our patients, our physicians and our employees. It means being of SERVICE to the community."

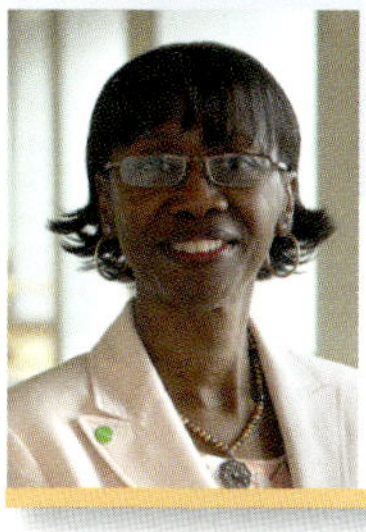

Audrey Jack,
Former Manager of Business Offices,
Ochsner Medical Center – Kenner

To watch the full interview with Audrey Jack, visit **ochsner.org/history**.

"We purposely called it unification instead of merger," Freeman said. "It was two years of intense negotiations. I have been involved in acquisitions and labor negotiations, and these were the most complex I have ever seen."[7]

The groups negotiating unification realized early on that they needed an outside, third party facilitator to coordinate meetings, set agendas and establish ground rules. "We hired Tom Kale, an attorney from Cincinnati, Ohio," Freeman said, "and he was quite helpful."

Quinlan was adamant that employees and physicians of the Clinic and the Foundation Hospital needed to have a voice in the unification talks. "We worked it hard and met with numerous groups for their feedback," he said. "It was an open decision-making process. It took a few years for employees to get used to the idea that we were actually listening to their input."[8]

One group whose input was critical was the 240 members of the Clinic Partnership. "The big thing from the doctors' perspective involved employment assurance," Freeman said. "They also had a fear that whoever was leading the organization might not be a physician. There had been a tradition in the Clinic that the management person would always be an M.D. We approved that concept early on."[9]

Quinlan was a champion of appealing to the best instincts of everyone involved in the negotiations. "It was a sense of higher purpose," he said, "of obligation to serve. We needed to tap the beliefs in people that attracted them to medicine in the first place. And we needed to preserve the legacy of the founders."[10]

A medical resident reviews the previous evening's admissions with staff at morning report.

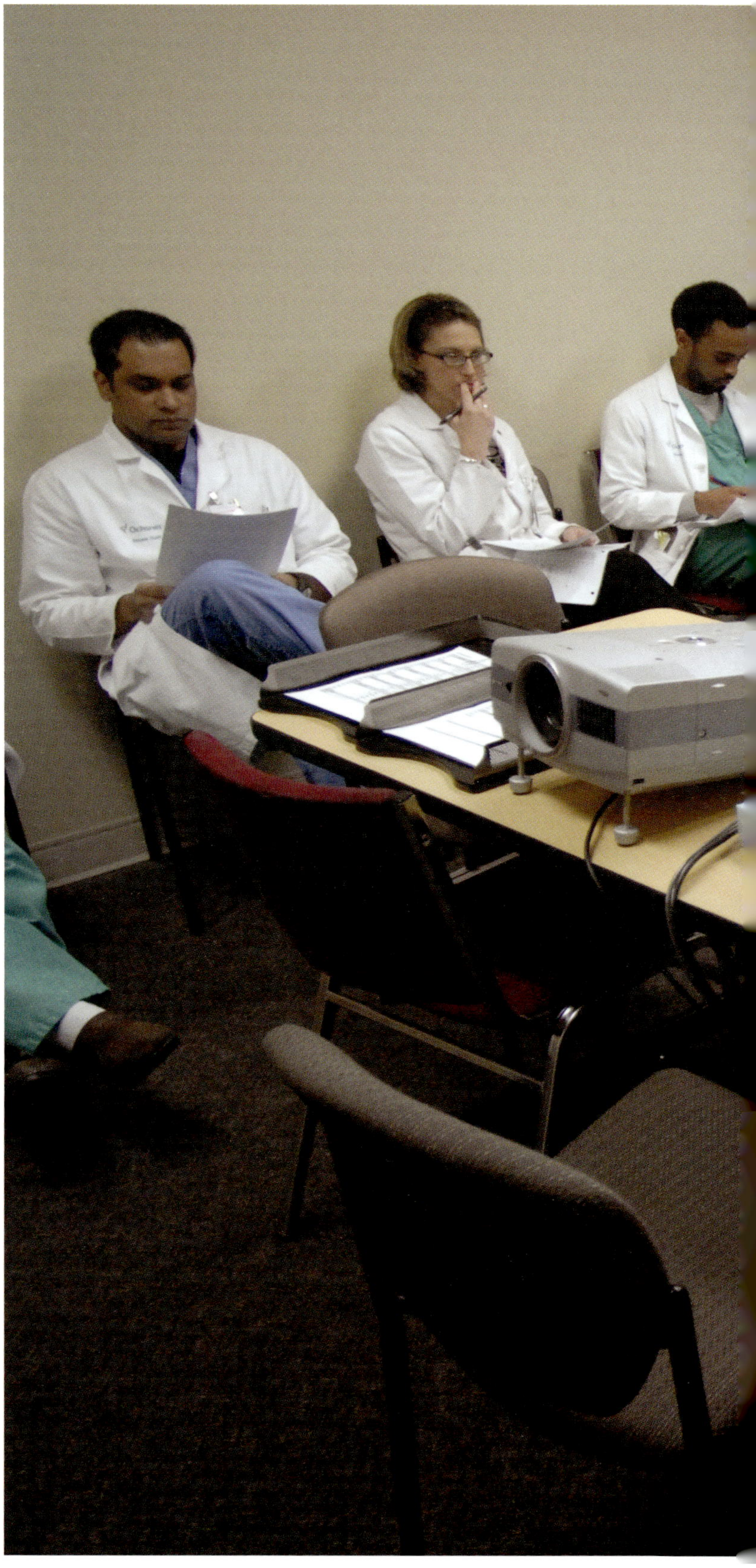

THE HEALTH PLAN DRILL

For the Clinic Partnership, whose members owned 70 percent of the Ochsner Health Plan, a financial rescue of the HMO was paramount if the unification was to ultimately succeed.

"So we went through the health plan drill," Quinlan said. "Our task was turning a potential disaster into a positive outcome."[11]

Warner Thomas took on the challenge of turning around the health plan. "The health plan was worth zero in 1999," Thomas said. "We were on track to lose $25 to $30 million. We didn't have the leadership we needed."

Thomas, who had come to Ochsner from New England, knew people at a medical group in New Hampshire who had sold their health plan to Cigna, the big Philadelphia health insurer. "They came down and looked at Ochsner's Health Plan," Thomas said of his New Hampshire colleagues. They said it was very serious. The health plan had overly focused on growing membership, and as a result, the premiums were seriously underpriced.

The Clinic changed management at the health plan and repriced the premiums. "We priced premiums 30 to 40 percent higher," Thomas said, "and nobody canceled. The plan was profitable by 2001. We were profitable until we sold it in 2004."[12]

AGREEMENT IN PRINCIPLE

In early 2001, Quinlan announced to the Ochsner community that the Clinic and Foundation had a unification agreement in principle. Both the Foundation and Clinic signed a non-binding memorandum of understanding that initiated the first formal step toward unification. "If both Boards approve," Quinlan said, "the final vote toward unification then goes to the physician partnership. If both Boards agree and the physician partnership votes the merger into effect, we will become an organization similar to the Cleveland and Mayo Clinics, much as our founders had initially intended."[13]

Richard Freeman continued to shepherd the agreement through to its ratification by both Boards and the physician partnership. Right up until the partnership vote. "My main concern was that details not derail the operation of the merged entities," Freeman said.[14]

There was still a great deal of work to do before the final documents could be signed and approved. Quinlan checked off a list of tasks that had to be accomplished before Ochsner Clinic Foundation could truly be considered one organization. "Human Resources has spent countless hours creating a benefits plan, Marketing and Public Affairs has been working on new logos, and Facilities and Security on signage and employee badges," Quinlan said. "We want Ochsner Clinic Foundation employees to feel the pulse of the organization, to know what is going on and to have a sense of ownership."[15]

The two Boards and the physician partnership voted during the late summer of 2001 in near unanimity to unify the Clinic and the Foundation Hospital as Ochsner Clinic Foundation under the

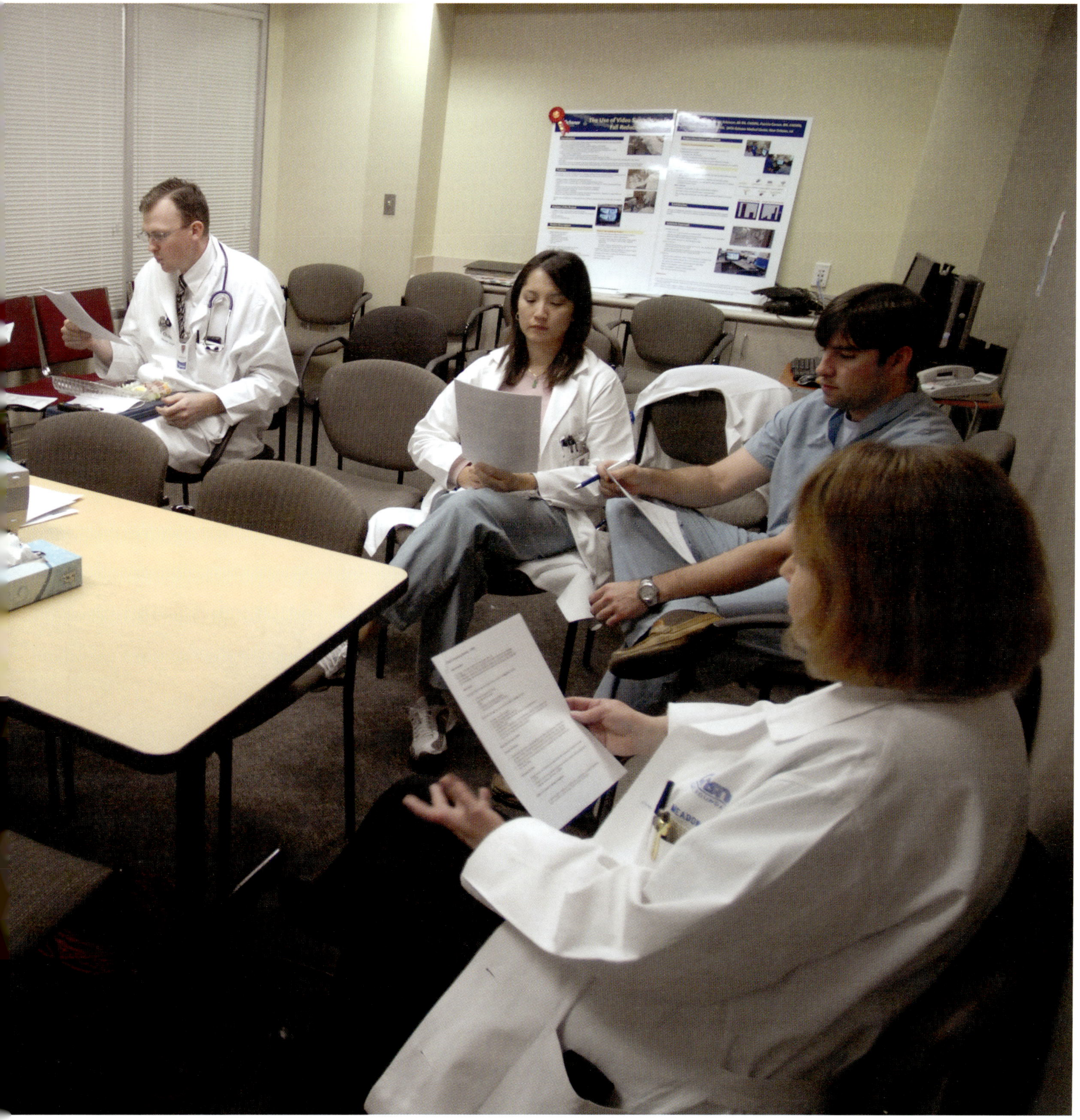

Foundation's tax-exempt status. The vote by the partnership was particularly gratifying. On August 9, 2001, 97 percent of the Ochsner Clinic physicians voted in favor of the proposal to unify.[16]

Quinlan, who was named Chief Executive Officer of Ochsner Clinic Foundation, explained in a series of media interviews in late August and early September that dissolving the Clinic Partnership and establishing a single tax-exempt entity would bring property and income tax advantages to the newly unified organization to fund their mission.[17] Quinlan also made sure to point out that the unification would first and foremost bring benefits to patients. "We want to become fully flexible as to how we deliver services," he said, "without discussing whether it's in the Hospital or Clinic."[18]

'TIME TO HANG THE DOOR'

By early September, the unification documents were ready for final signatures. Several Ochsner Clinic board members suggested one final round of checks that would not take more than two or three weeks. Quinlan and Kale argued that the deal needed no additional scrutiny. "He said, 'It's time to hang the door,'" Quinlan recalled the discussion.[19] Board members acquiesced, signed the definitive unification documents and scheduled a press conference to announce the creation of Ochsner Clinic Foundation.

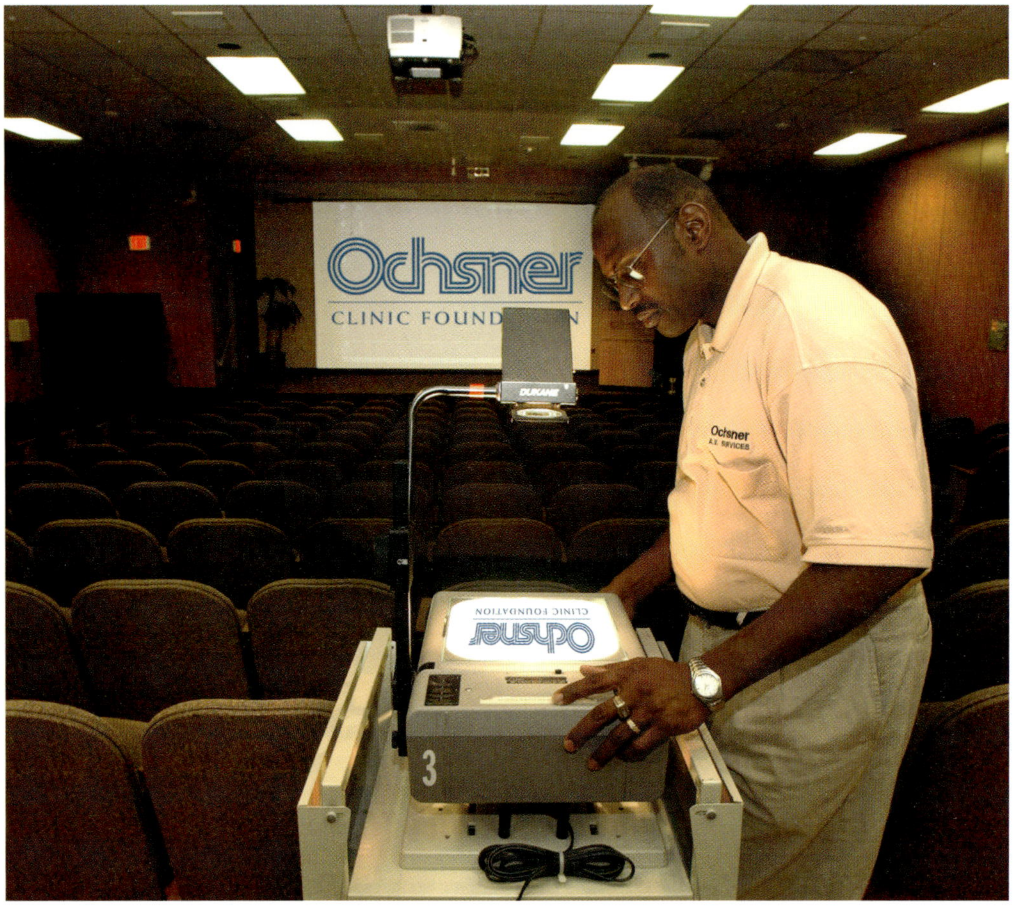

Longtime employee Floyd Grayson, Audio-Visual Specialist, prepares a slide introducing the newly unified Ochsner Clinic Foundation in 2001.

At that September 6, 2001, press conference, Frank Riddick, who was stepping down from his post as Chief Executive Officer of the Foundation, gave an eloquent assessment of medical accomplishments and progress at Ochsner since he arrived at the Clinic in the early 1960s, over 40 years earlier. "Growth gave complexity in direction, strategic planning and management of resources. Over the past decade or more, it became apparent that the often-competing interests of education and research versus patient care, of ambulatory versus inpatient care, of one geographic area against another, of the insurance company against the providers of care could not be evolved effectively in the configuration of management and governance which existed at Ochsner. The presence of two or three governing boards, duplicative or sometimes triplicative management structures, and governmental restrictions on the movement of funds between not-for-profit and taxable entities were major impediments to effective strategic planning, growth and smoothly flowing systems across the spectrum of patient care. Simply put, we reached a point where the Clinic and Foundation had to unify or drift apart and seek their separate destinies. I am happy that we chose unification."[20]

Riddick reassured his audience that Ochsner would continue to make patient care a priority. "Our mission remains the same," he said, "meeting the patient's overall needs with the best practices so that we improve the health of the population we serve."[21]

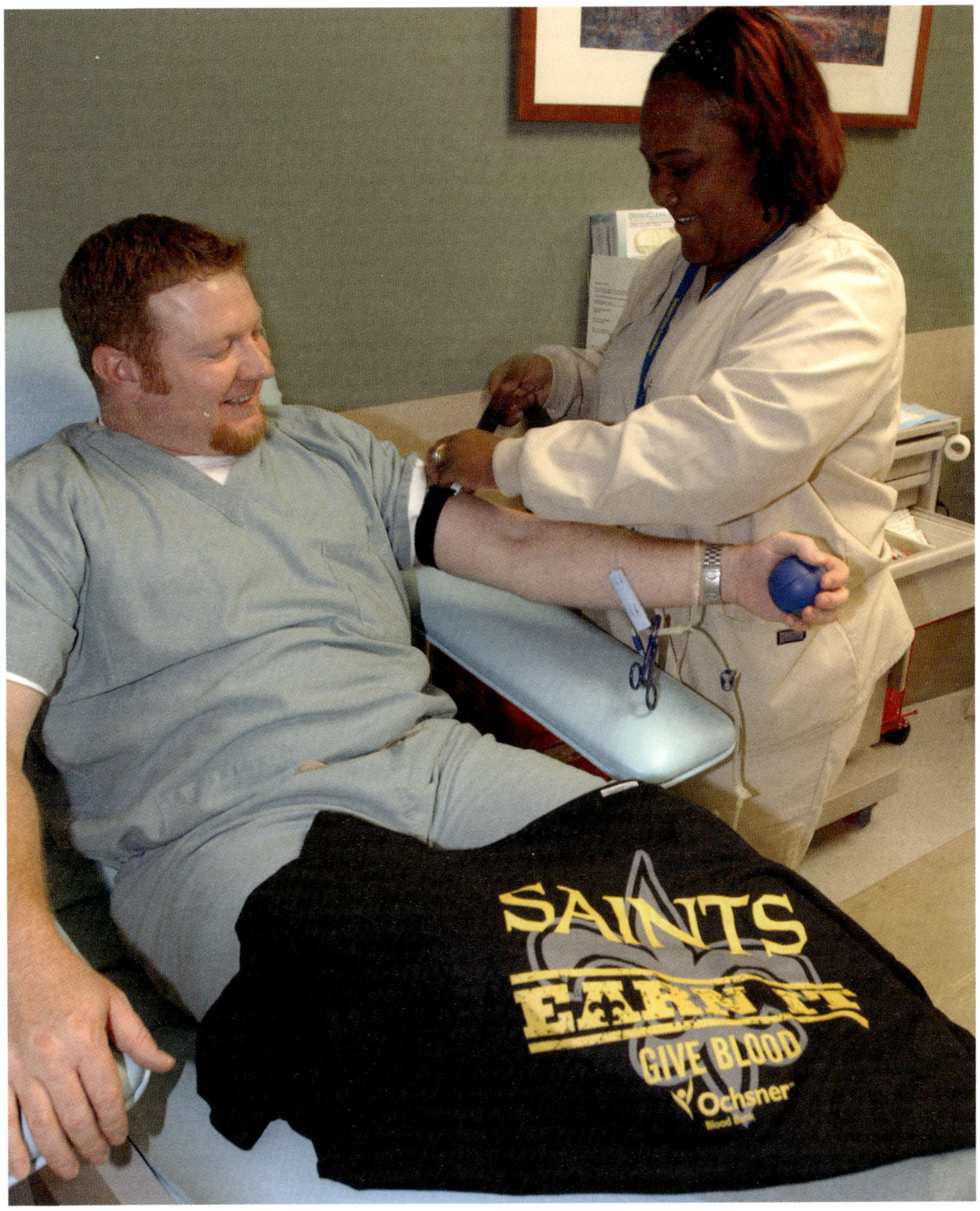

The Ochsner Blood Bank has multiple collection centers for employees and communities to donate blood.

DR. PATRICK QUINLAN

Dr. Patrick Quinlan arrived at Ochsner in late 1998 from Lovelace Clinic in Albuquerque, New Mexico. Quinlan had spent 13 years at the clinic, which in many ways was similar to Ochsner. The clinic was governed by a foundation, and it operated a very large health plan in New Mexico. Unlike Ochsner, Lovelace Clinic had become a part of Cigna Corporation in Philadelphia, which sold the group practice, hospital and health plan to the for-profit Ardent Corporation in 2002.

"I learned how things really worked—and didn't work," Quinlan said of his years at Lovelace.[22]

Born in New York City, the son of a construction engineer, Quinlan earned an undergraduate degree in economics from the University of Texas-Austin and earned his M.D. at the University of Texas' Medical Branch in Galveston. He did his residency in Dermatology at the University of Alabama-Birmingham and practiced in Selma, Alabama, before moving to Albuquerque.[23]

Quinlan and Warner Thomas arrived in New Orleans within weeks of each other, and Quinlan was asked to become the interim CEO of Ochsner Clinic in January 1999. The timing was not what he expected, but Quinlan took the reins and skillfully guided the fortunes of Ochsner into the twenty-first century. "I feel very lucky to have had Warner Thomas as my partner through all of these years."

With the Clinic and Foundation unified in 2001, Ochsner became one of New Orleans' most impressive success stories during Hurricane Katrina, and Quinlan presided over a major Ochsner acquisition initiative after 2005.

"We need to finish the job," Quinlan said. "We need to find out how good we are and get as good as we can be. We need to be a great place for our patients."[24]

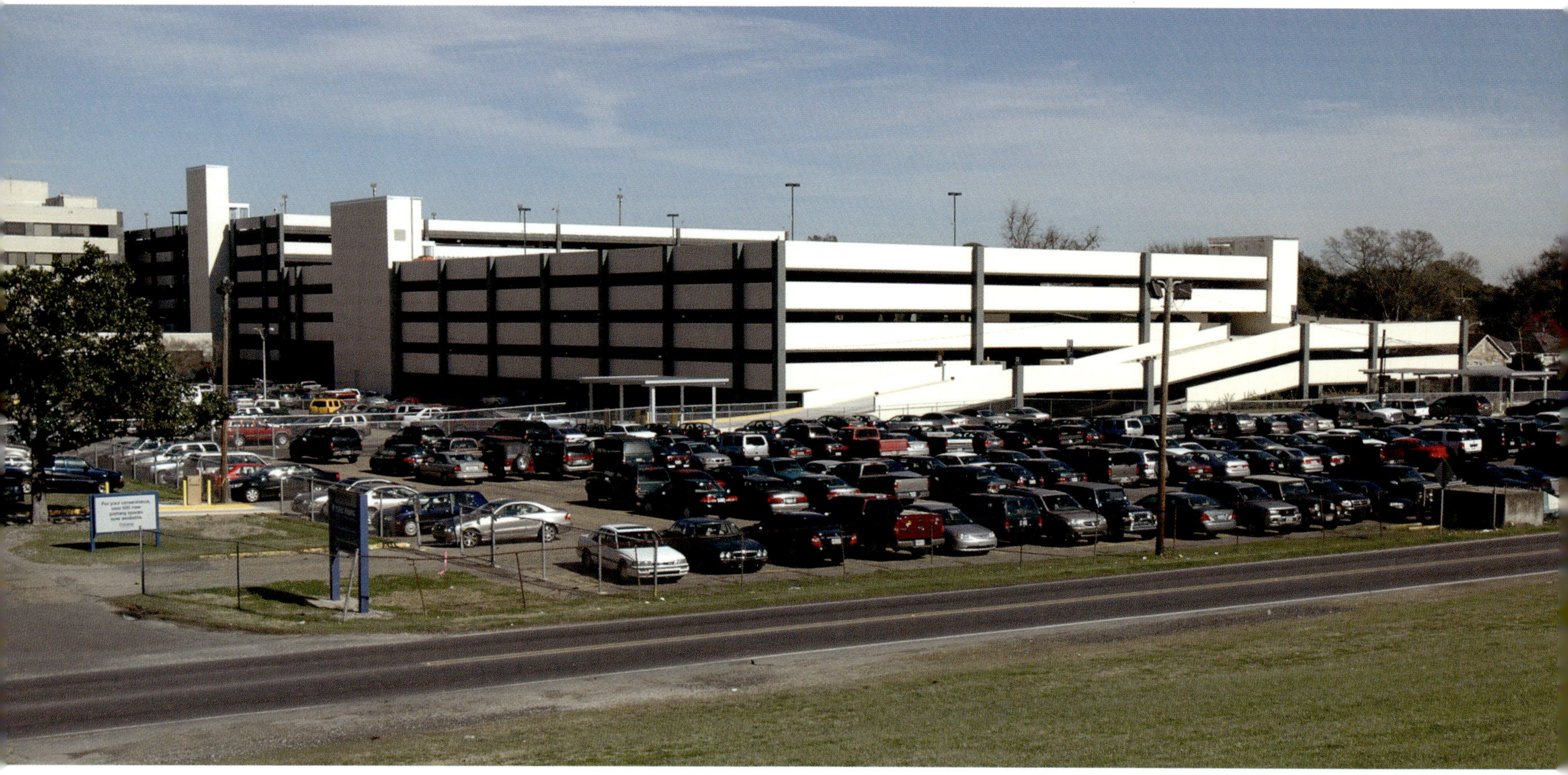

9/11

The press conference on the Thursday of Labor Day week 2001 was the culmination of two decades of unification discussions and studies. The following Tuesday, the more than 7,000 employees of Ochsner Clinic Foundation watched in horror as hijacked jetliners plowed into the World Trade Center towers in New York City, the Pentagon in suburban Washington, D.C. and a rural farm field in Pennsylvania.

Those at Ochsner who invested so much time and energy into the unification effort couldn't help but think of what might have been. "If they had checked it one more time, it would have been 9/11 and the deal would have been off," said Patrick Quinlan. "A good idea that's late is a bad idea. We made it by the skin of our teeth."[25]

Like most of the American healthcare system, Ochsner Clinic Foundation was involved with the response to 9/11. In the weeks following the attacks, employees donated to relief funds and gave more than 2,000 units of blood. Ochsner Clinic Foundation management worked with local and federal law enforcement agencies to implement new bioterrorism efforts in the wake of October's anthrax scare on the East Coast.[26]

The years of attempting to unify the organizations had taken a financial toll on Ochsner. There was a great deal to do to bring the unified organization to a level where it could offer top-flight patient care for the twenty-first century. "We had gotten significantly behind in the age of plant and equipment," Quinlan said. "Once unified, we renewed the place."[27]

One facility that had been needed desperately for years was an increased parking garage. "People want a place to park," Quinlan said. "You go back to the basics, parking and service. We decided to spend more on the frontline services, and that increased productivity."[28]

Ochsner Clinic Foundation continued to pay close attention to patient care. In the years following the unification, the organization implemented a new Pediatric Emergency Care section, created the Endovascular Operating Suite and opened the Merrill Hines Ambulatory Surgical Center on the Jefferson Highway campus, where surgeons and other physicians can practice primary care and specialty care together in one site convenient for the patient and family. At its neighborhood centers, Ochsner grew its Internal Medicine physician base in Metairie and expanded its OB/GYN presence in the community when it added the specialty group from Baptist Memorial Hospital in 2002.

During the four years following unification, Ochsner Clinic Foundation made tremendous strides. However, it would face its greatest challenge just one week shy of its fourth anniversary as a unified organization.

The new parking garage contains spaces for thousands of patients and visitors who arrive at Ochsner each day.

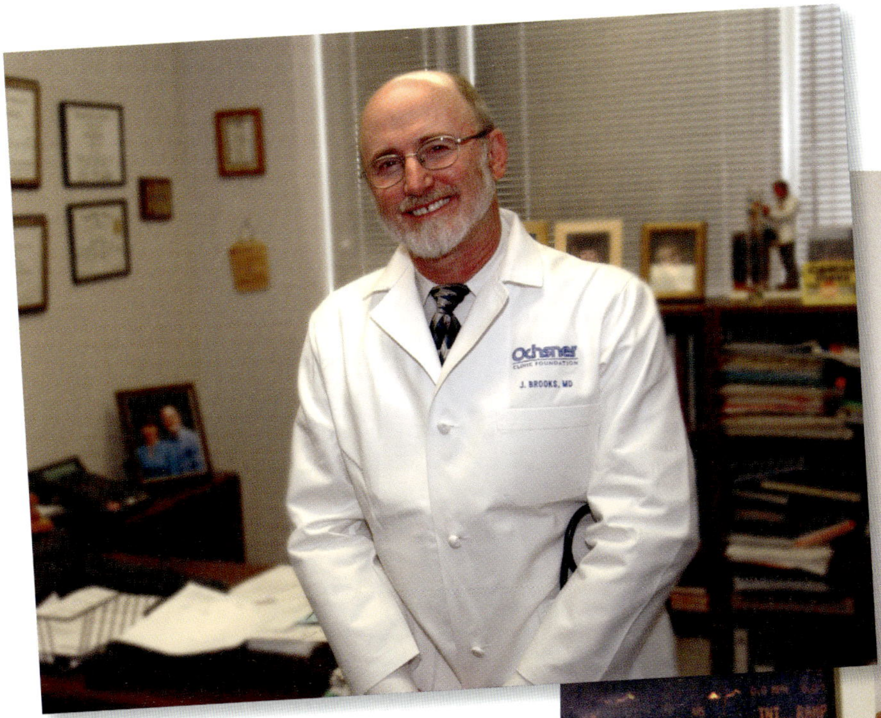

B. Jay Brooks Jr., M.D., longtime Board Member and Chairman of Ochsner's Department of Hematology/Oncology in Baton Rouge, brings expertise in lung cancer, breast cancer treatment and prevention and cancer genetics.

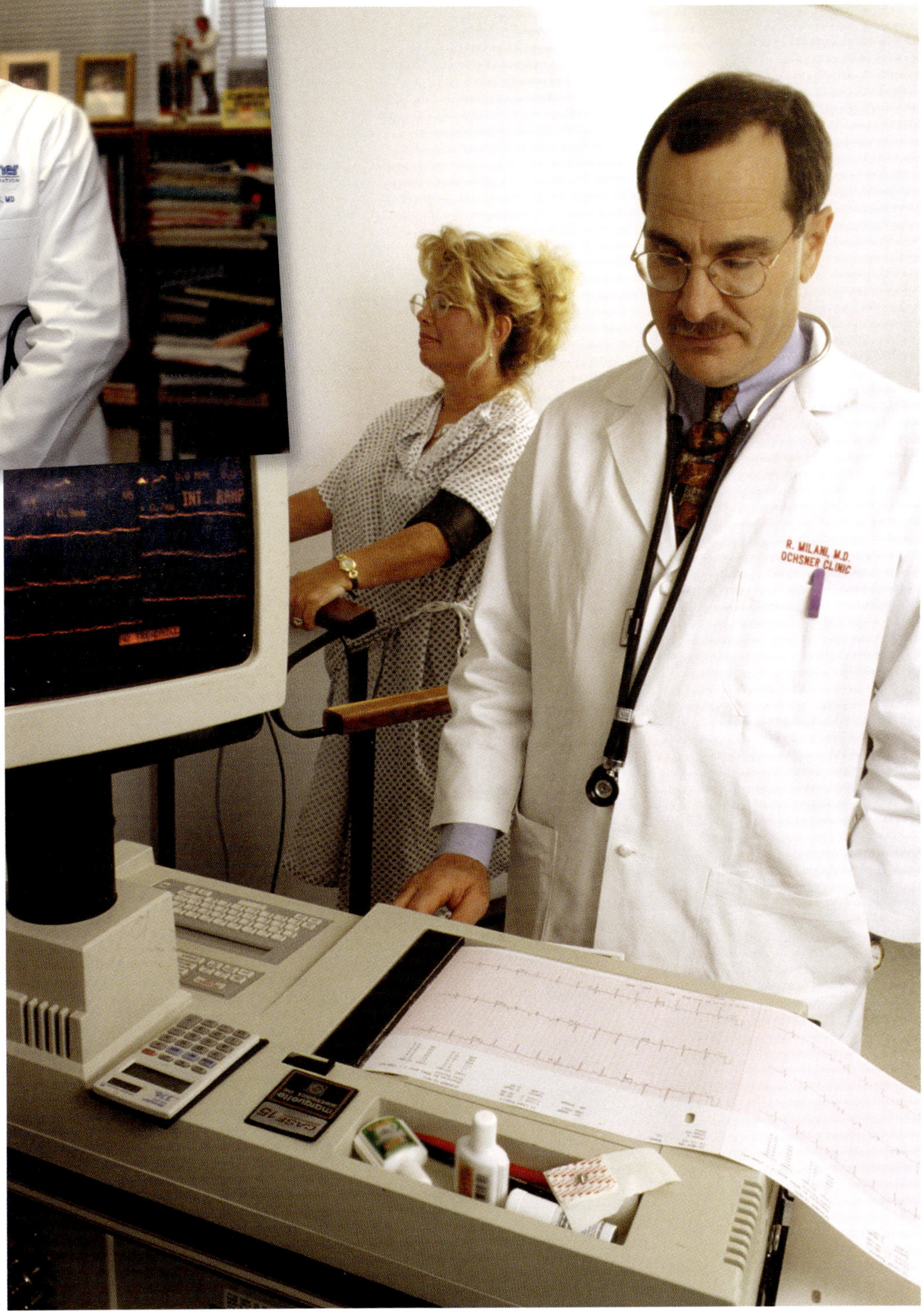

Dr. Richard Milani performing a stress electrocardiographic procedure.

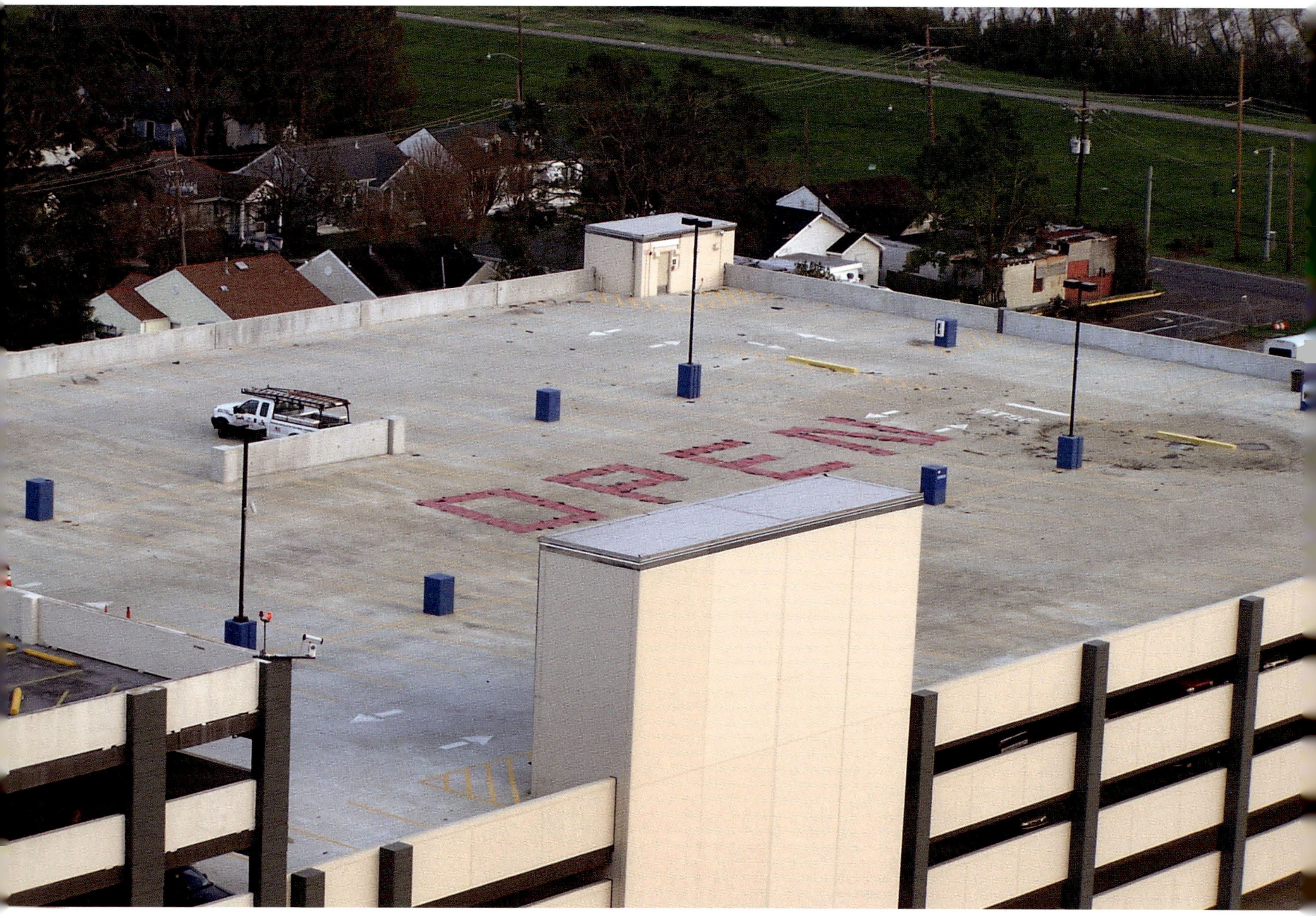
OPEN

CHAPTER 10:

HURRICANE KATRINA

WHEN HURRICANE KATRINA ROARED out of the Gulf of Mexico in the early morning hours of Monday, August 29, 2005, the Category 4 storm changed life in New Orleans like no event in the city's 250 years of existence.

The powerful storm made landfall southeast of the city and sent a surge of water 15 feet high inland for miles. Much of the Louisiana and Mississippi coasts were devastated, and 120 mph winds lashed areas as much as 75 miles inland. Katrina left much of southeastern Louisiana without power, and electricity was not restored for many residents for weeks or months.

For New Orleans itself, the storm's landfall east of the city initially appeared to be a blessing. While the city was spared the full impact of the winds and storm surge, more than 10,000 people were trapped on rooftops and the upper floors of buildings when levees protecting the city ruptured, spilling floodwaters into city streets. A breakdown in civil order played out on national television and the Internet, giving the city a reputation for lawlessness.

Team A employees of Ochsner's Radiology Department made a sign on the rooftop from trash bags to let the world know that Ochsner remained open to care for patients.

Through it all, Ochsner was a shining example of calm and business as usual. Ochsner personnel had used the lessons of Hurricane Ivan the year before to implement a meticulously rehearsed hurricane plan that was a model of competence. True, floodwaters did not inundate the Jefferson Highway campus. The lights stayed on. There was potable water. Patients received the outstanding care they had grown accustomed to, even though that care was made available in trying circumstances.

"Katrina was a big turning point in Ochsner history," said Warner Thomas. Ochsner had dealt with hurricanes before; when Hurricane Betsy slammed into the city in September 1965, staffers at the Jefferson Highway campus remained at their posts in spite of power outages and flooding. Katrina, with its devastation, was a whole different order of magnitude when it came to legendary New Orleans hurricanes.

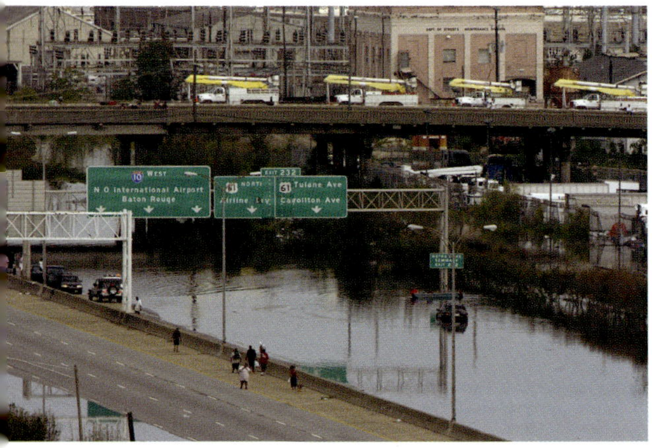

Photo by Kathy Anderson © 2005 The Times-Picayune Publishing Co., all rights reserved. Used with permission of the *Times-Picayune*.

Overall storm damage from Katrina amounted to billions of dollars, and extensive flooding nearly destroyed the city.

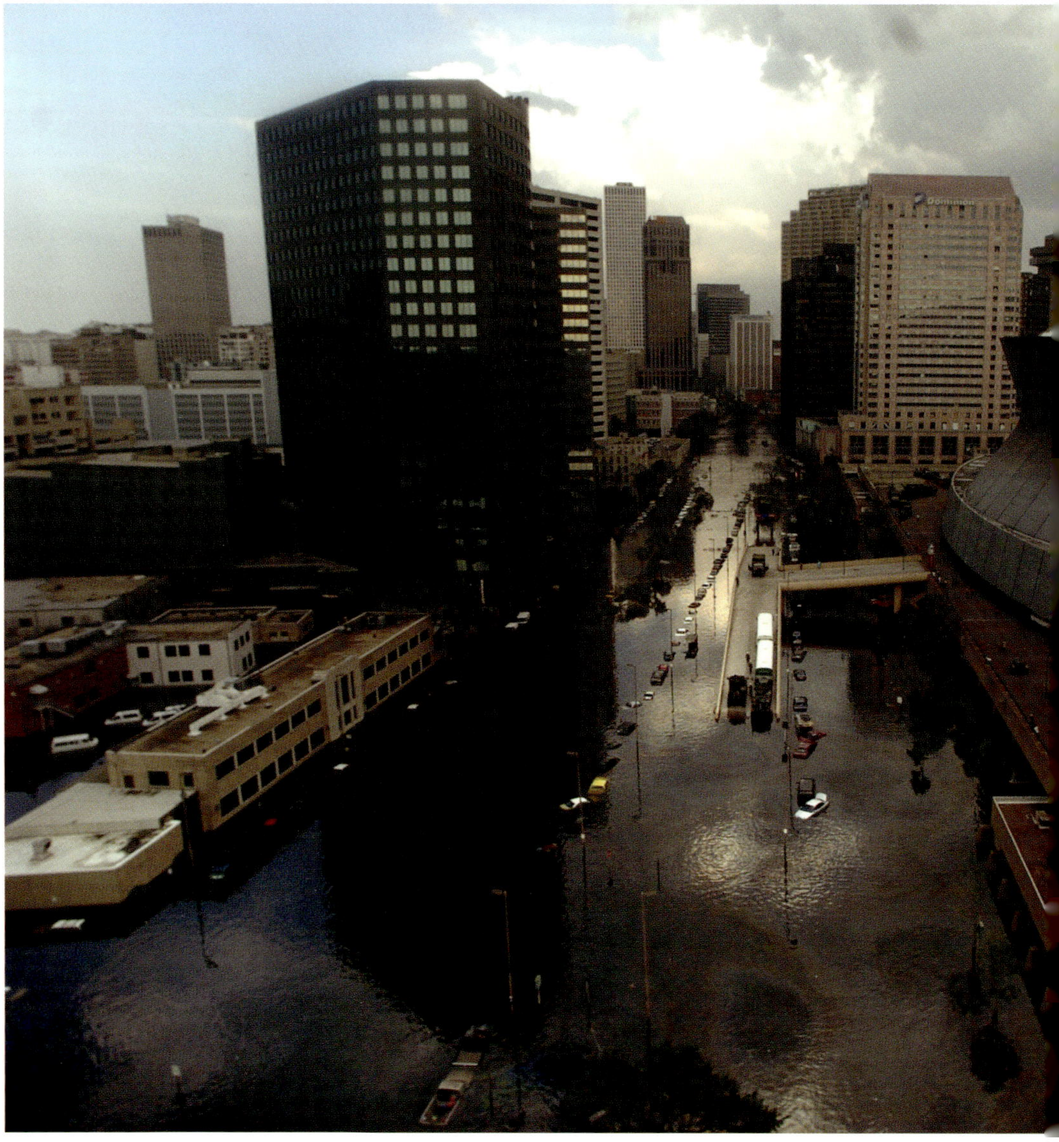

Photo by Ted Jackson © 2005 The Times-Picayune Publishing Co., all rights reserved. Used with permission of the *Times-Picayune*.

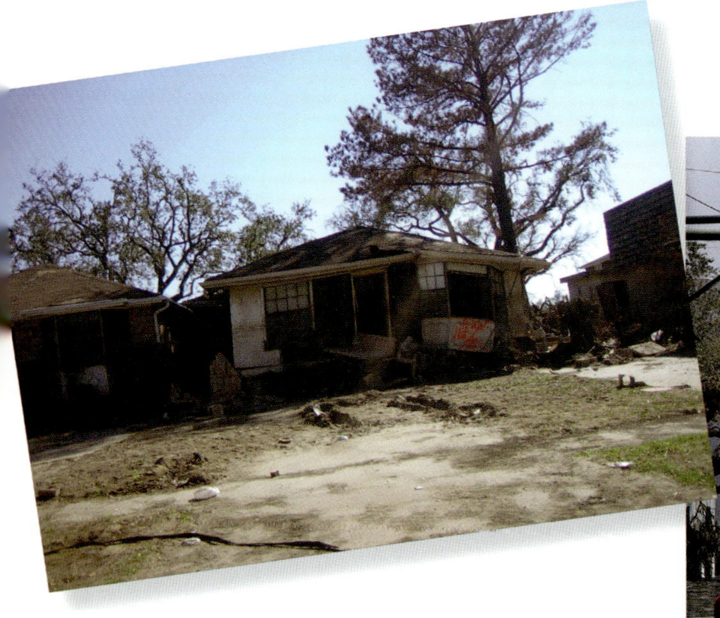

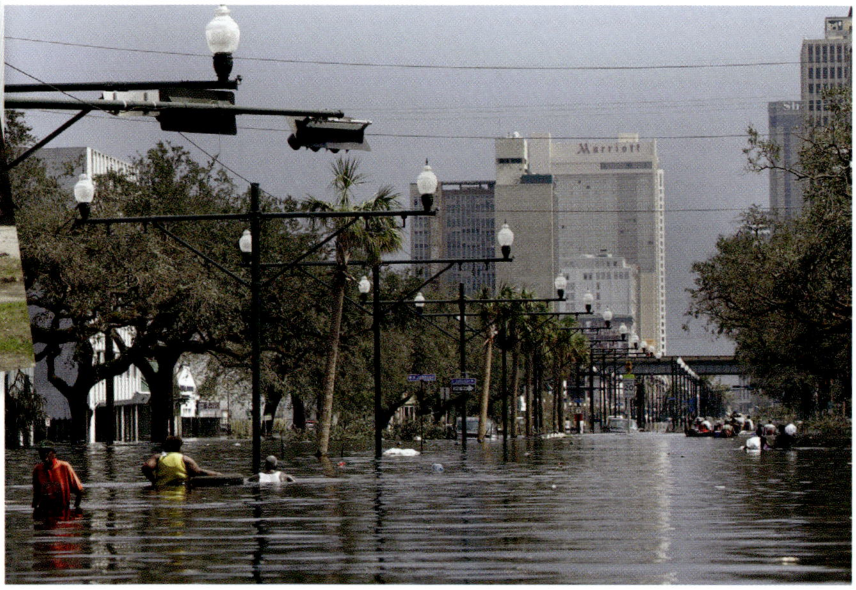

Photo by Alex Brandon © 2005 The Times-Picayune Publishing Co., all rights reserved. Used with permission of the *Times-Picayune*.

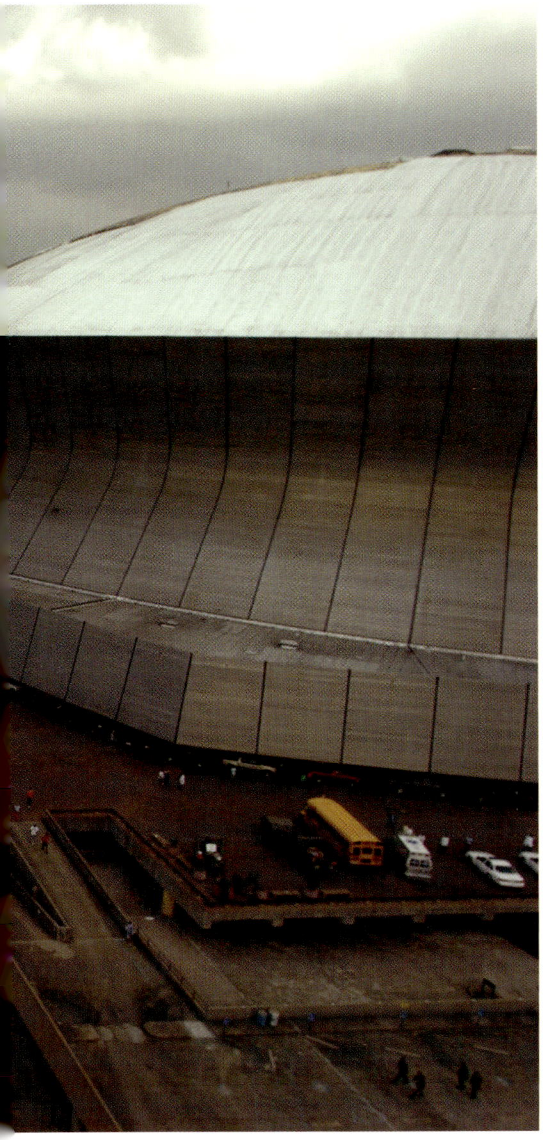

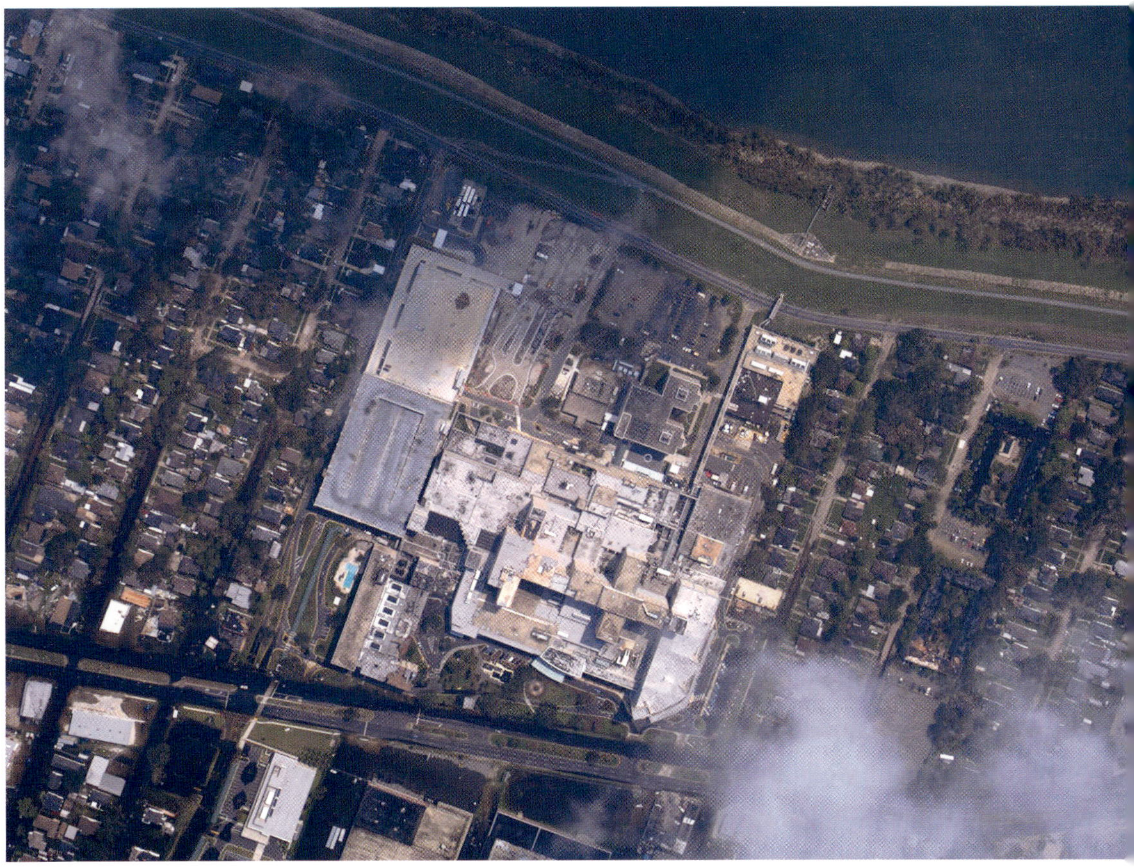

Flooding from the wake of Katrina came close but did not inundate the Jefferson Highway campus (NOAA).

A DEFINING MOMENT

For Dr. Patrick Quinlan, CEO of Ochsner Health System, Hurricane Katrina "was a defining moment for Ochsner. It was an extreme challenge, one in which you find out what you're made of. It gave us new insights into our own capabilities."[1]

Those capabilities were tested to the maximum, and Ochsner was not found wanting. While the rest of the world watched in horrified fascination as the city and many of the residents who were left behind descended into chaos—despite the best efforts of U.S. Navy and Coast Guard rescue teams—Ochsner went about its 60-plus-year mission of providing care to the people of New Orleans with its typical efficiency. Ochsner doctors, nurses, employees and administrators manned the Jefferson Highway campus in the face of what sometimes seemed to be insurmountable odds.

"Their view of themselves was confirmed," Quinlan said of the Ochsner employees who shut out the havoc and chaos around them—even while worrying about families and homes—and focused on things that have always been important to Ochsner: patients, the team, excellence, trust, care and competence.[2]

"It looks real easy in hindsight," Quinlan said. "It wasn't."[3]

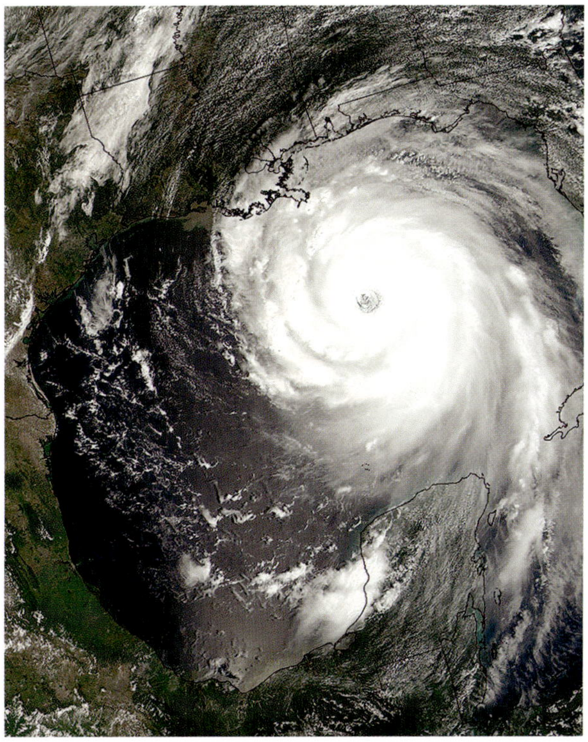

Hurricane Katrina, the greatest disaster in Louisiana's history, approaches the coast (NOAA).

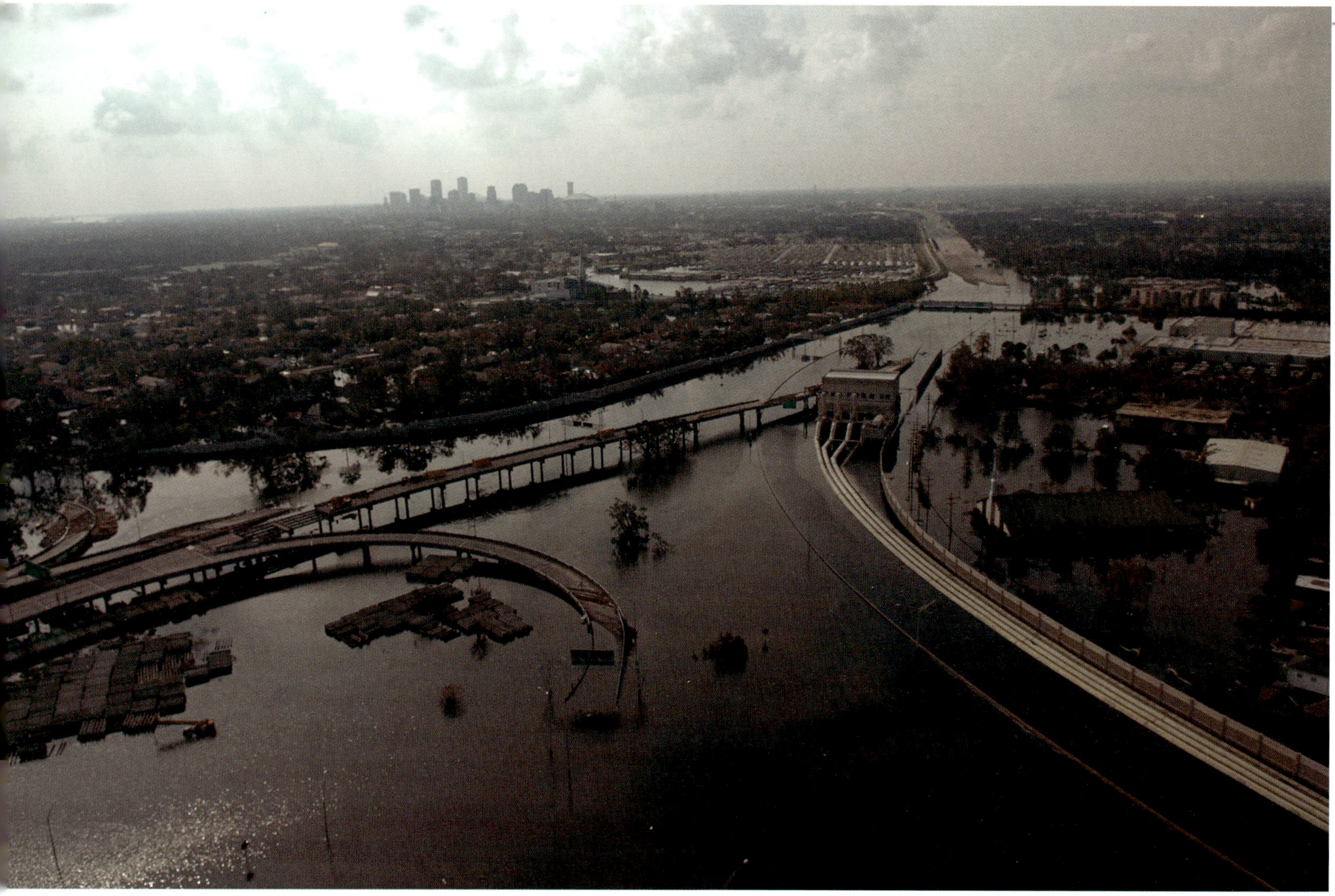

Photo by David Grunfield © The Times-Picayune Publishing Co., all rights reserved. Used with permission of the *Times-Picayune.*

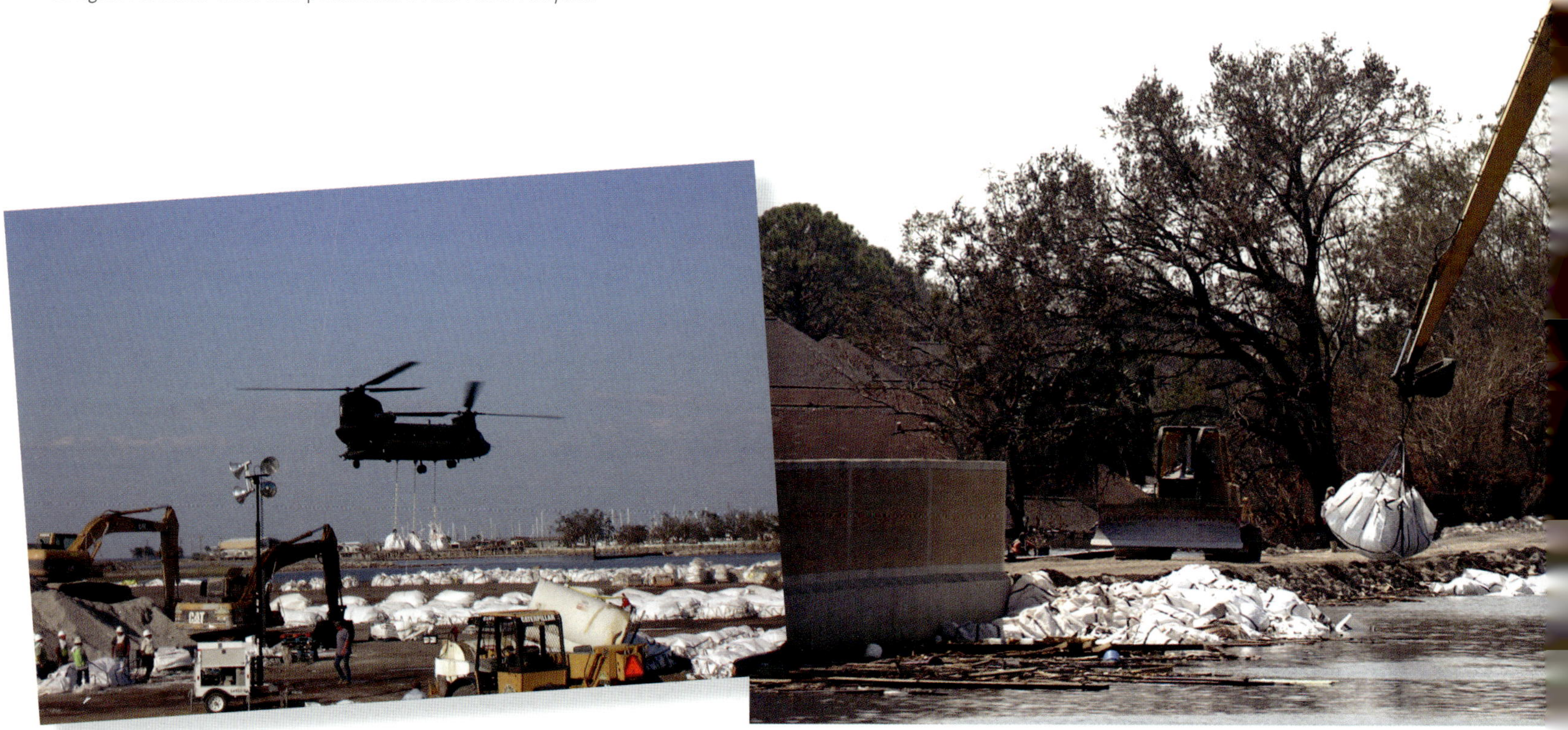

Residents thought New Orleans had avoided the worst of Katrina, but when levees in the city breached the Monday morning following the storm's passage, chaos quickly ensued. Photo by Ellis Lucia © 2005 The Times-Picayune Publishing Co. all rights reserved. Used with permission of the *Times-Picayune.*

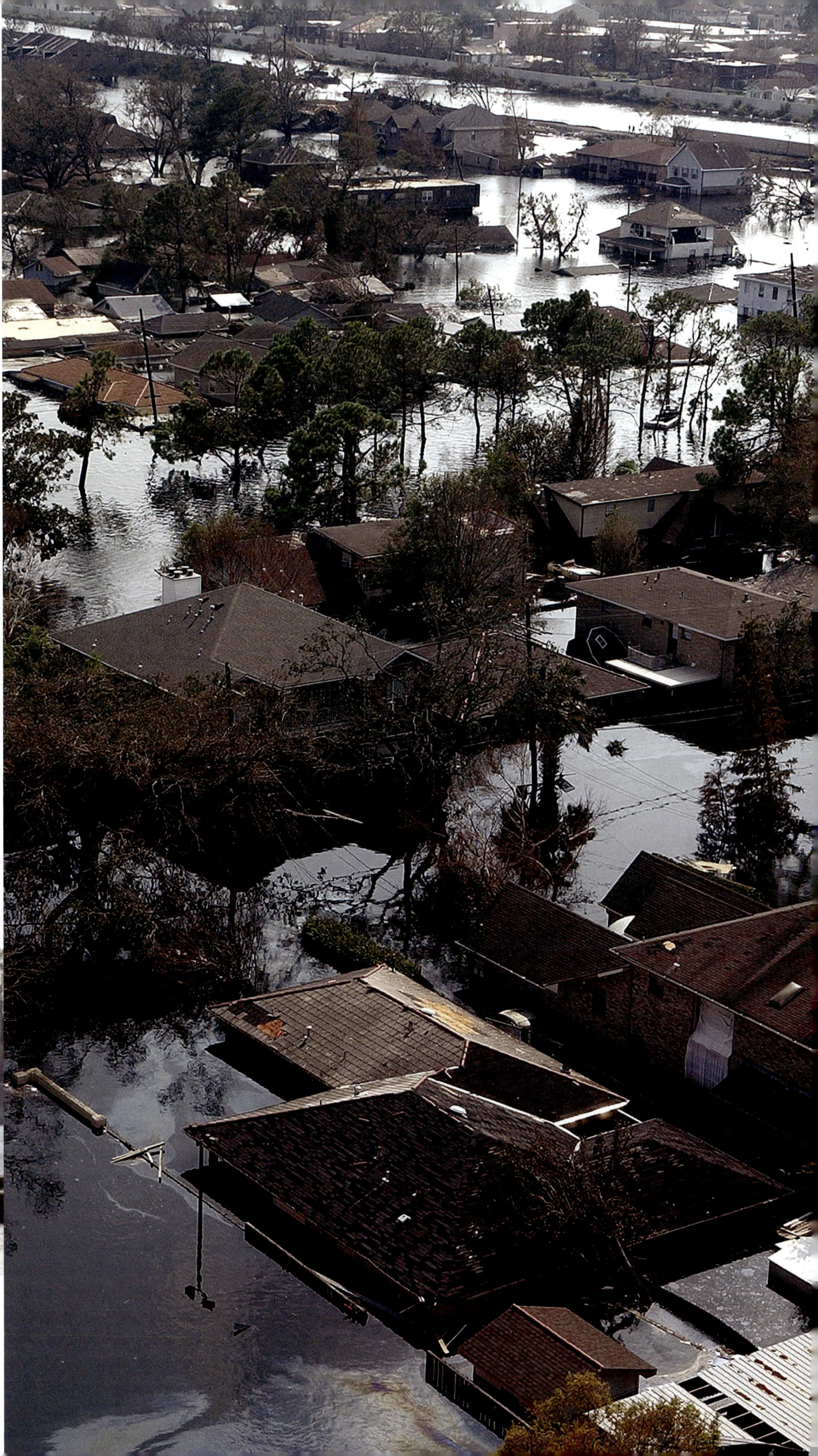

Thousands of residents were stranded on rooftops as floodwaters inundated entire neighborhoods.

Photo by Alex Brandon © 2005 The Times-Picayune Publishing Co., all rights reserved. Used with permission of the *Times-Picayune*.

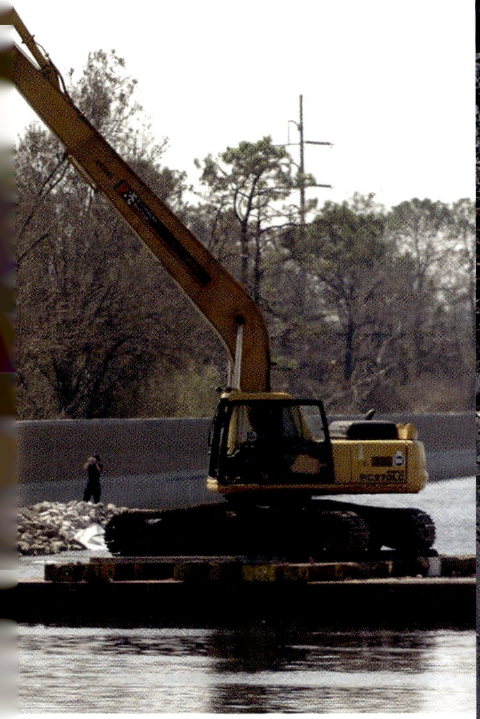

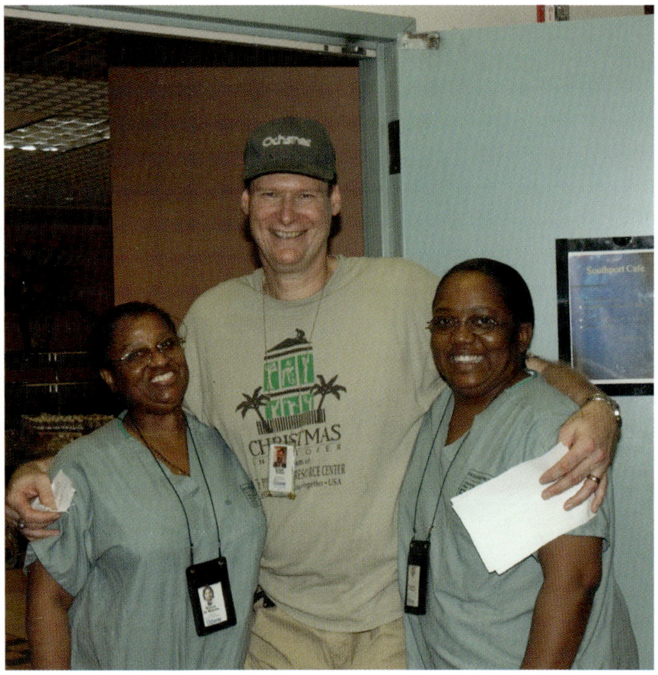

Grant Walker, seen here with Ochsner staffers, used his U.S. Army training to help prepare Ochsner for the trials it would face in the wake of Katrina.

PREPAREDNESS

Ochsner was fortunate that it had prepared for the eventuality of a catastrophic weather or terror event. Much of that planning had been led by Vice President of Support Services Grant Walker, a Pennsylvania native who came to Ochsner in 2000 as the organization's Facilities Manager.

Walker, who spent 10 years in the U.S. Army running combat support hospitals and 14 years with a Pennsylvania hospital system, immediately felt at home at Ochsner. While still interviewing for the Ochsner job, Walker found he could relate to the employees who made the Clinic and Hospital tick.

"I would go to the cafeteria and just sit with people," he said. "I wanted to see what the culture was like. The staff was like a family. They'd sit and talk like they were at a 100-bed hospital with 250 employees. Every time an employee had a crisis, word got out. People were already bringing supplies in to help out. I called it the Ochsner family. It has held true since day one."[4]

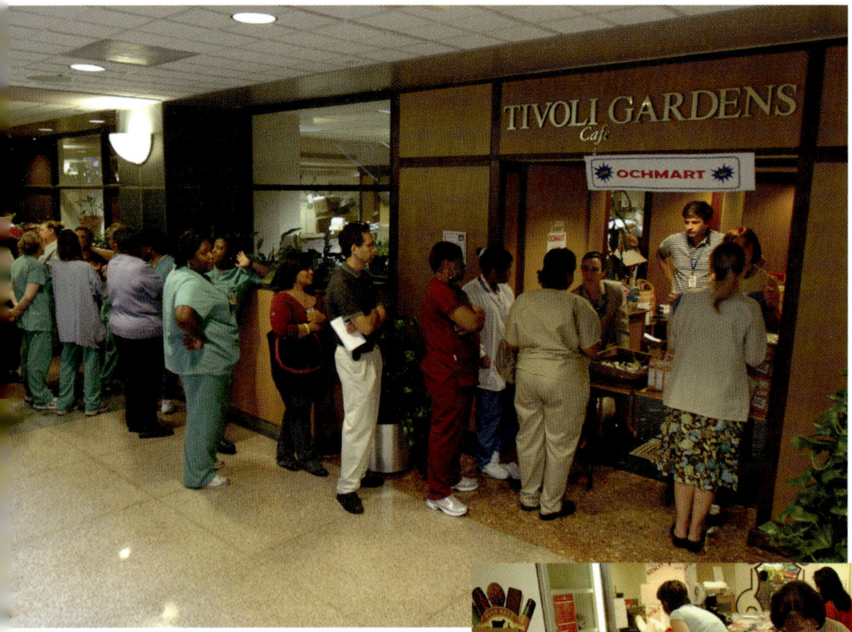

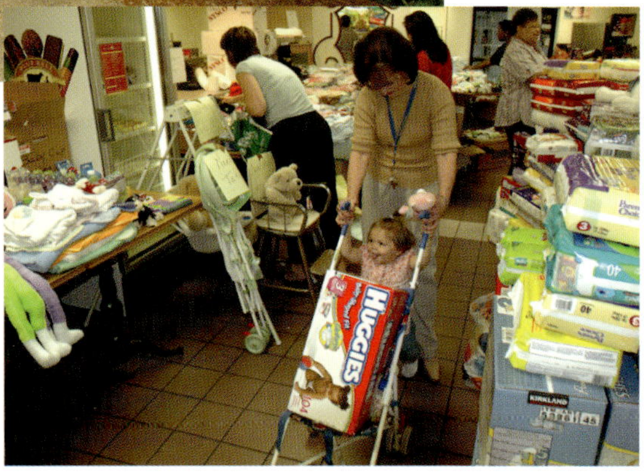

Ochsner set up Ochmart, a temporary "store" with all donated items for employees in need.

Walker noted that the 2001 unification of the Clinic and Foundation had a great deal to do with the preparedness that was so evident in the days after Katrina hit. With lessened internal competition for resources, the unified Board of Trustees agreed to "start replacing everything that was installed in the 1950s," Walker said.[5]

Perhaps Ochsner's biggest advantage in the critical hours after Katrina had devastated New Orleans was the simple fact that there were two functioning wells on the Jefferson Highway campus. Alton Ochsner had insisted on drilling the first well when the original Hospital was built on the site in the mid-1950s. A second well was drilled in the 1980s. These precautions would place Ochsner in good stead in the days and weeks following Katrina.

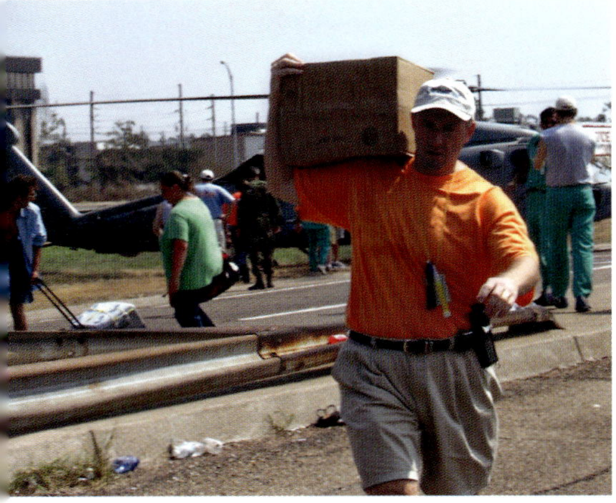

For Warner Thomas, Katrina was a turning point in Ochsner's history. Thomas was among the Ochsner executives who worked literally around the clock during the weeks following the storm.

The second factor that contributed to Ochsner's sense of preparedness was Hurricane Ivan in 2004. Ochsner had begun its hurricane preparedness planning during the 1990s. When Ivan came barreling out of the Gulf of Mexico on September 16 and slammed head on into the Florida Panhandle, Ochsner saw a chance to put its planning into practice. Seeing the devastation on television, Warner Thomas picked up the phone in his office and called the Sacred Heart Hospital in Pensacola. A woman who answered the call asked Thomas to not hang up because the hospital could receive incoming calls but could not make outgoing calls. Thomas held the line open the remainder of the day. By 8 p.m. that night, Ochsner had five tractor-trailers loaded with supplies rolling toward Pensacola's Sacred Heart Hospital.[6]

Ochsner took the lessons it learned from Ivan and "adjusted our own planning," Walker said. "We bought 200 fans, 450 extension cords, glow sticks, Meals Ready to Eat (MREs) and bottled water. As it was, during Katrina we didn't have air conditioning for five days. We did have emergency power for the West Tower. We had a diesel-generating unit with 60,000 gallons of fuel underground. The fans kept the perspiration off and made it livable."[7]

'THE STAIR DOOR WAS VIBRATING'

Grant Walker, Ochsner's System VP—Supply Chain, compiled a day-by-day journal recounting his experiences at Ochsner during Hurricane Katrina. Walker was at the Hospital when the hurricane came ashore during the early morning hours of Monday, August 29, 2005.

As the storm roared overhead, the generators kicked on and picked up the Hospital's electric power load. "Later in the afternoon," Walker said, "the hurricane ripped a hole in the roof of the generator building. Water leaked down on the generator that powers our air conditioning." The generator shorted out, causing Ochsner to lose cooling to the Jefferson Highway campus. "We always keep 1,000 fans on hand in our emergency supply," Walker explained as another example of the facility's preparedness.[8] Crews issued the fans to patients and staff Monday night and Tuesday morning.

While the storm raged outside, vice presidents and key directors from the A Team made continual rounds through the buildings, providing support and assistance to anyone who needed it. At the peak of the storm, about 11 a.m. Monday, Ochsner staff moved all patients into the hallways from the 7th floor up. Walker was in a patient room on the 11th floor when a window shattered.

"The storm was throwing the furniture around in the room," Walker wrote later. "The door vibrated loudly. Maintenance secured the door. The stair door was vibrating. I opened it, took a few steps up and looked up and saw nothing but black sky. The stairwell roof was totally gone. In a moment I felt my feet lifting off the ground."[9] Walker, who is tall and solidly built, struggled to regain his footing.

Two maintenance crewmembers helped Walker secure and lock the stairwell door. Walker worked his way down to the 6th floor, where patients and family members were sopping up water from the windows, all of which were leaking badly. He remembered climbing back up to the 10th floor and looking out a window to see the entire rubber roof of the adjacent building lift and fly off in the ferocious winds. Soon, pieces of brick and stone from the roof parapet wall were flying off, shattering windows below.

Within a half-hour, Walker watched his second roof of the morning blow away, this time from the Ochsner warehouse across the street. As wind gusts of 120 mph rocked the building, Walker made his way to the 2nd floor to inspect the bridge connecting the research building to the Hospital.

"At the far end I heard a loud sound like machine gun fire," Walker wrote, "and then a window shattered. Then the window next to me shattered, and I quickly ran across the bridge to the other side, covering my eyes."[10] Maintenance immediately secured the windows on the bridge, and Walker surmised later that a sound like gunfire came when a gust picked up gravel off one of the older roofs on the campus and threw the stones at the bridge.

Within a short time, the winds began to die down as the storm spent its force moving over land. A quick damage assessment revealed that all three boilers were out, there was no fresh water, the stacks were twisted (which meant that crews were unable to reheat or sterilize instruments) and the third generator used to provide air conditioning was disabled. In addition, water leaking through a hole in the roof shorted out some of the Hospital's circuitry.[11]

At noon that Monday, much of New Orleans' healthcare infrastructure was crippled or in ruins. Despite everything, Ochsner was open for business and would remain so throughout the crisis.

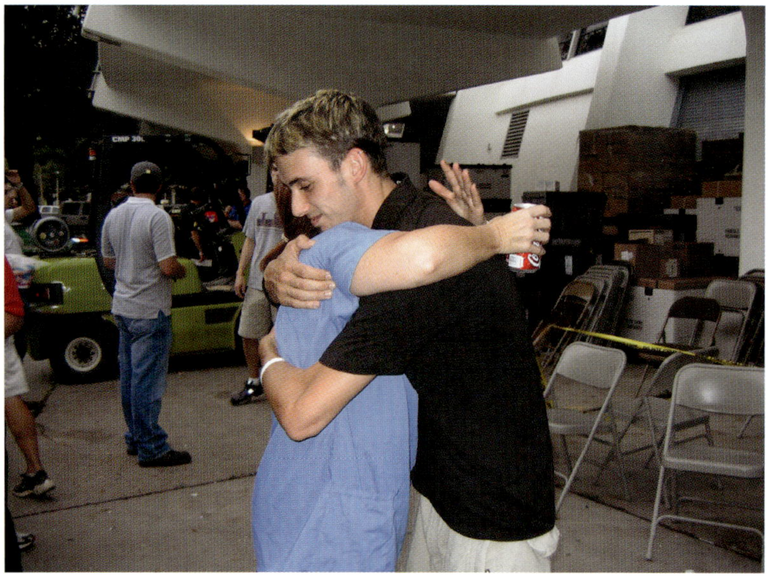

• WHAT OCHSNER MEANS TO ME •

"All of the research and all of the studies we do that result in publication serve as the FOUNDATION for the new discoveries, the new diagnostics and the new therapies that are ultimately invaluable to our patients."

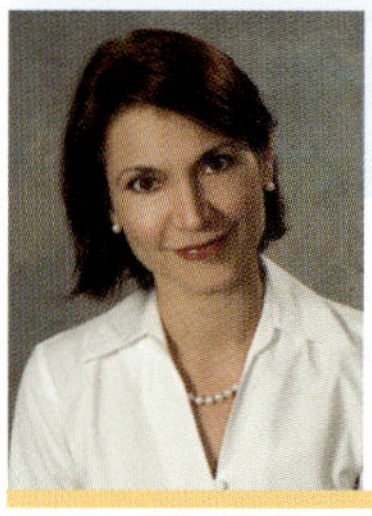

Julia Cook, Ph.D., Research Scientist and Director of the Laboratory of Molecular Genetics, Ochsner Medical Center

To watch the full interview with Julia Cook, Ph.D., visit **ochsner.org/history**.

FORMING A BOND

Ochsner employees have a loyalty to the institution that outsiders might find baffling. Betty M. Wells, a 30-year veteran of Environmental Services on the Jefferson Highway campus, never gave a thought to evacuating ahead of Katrina. Instead, Wells called her supervisor on Sunday morning to tell him that she was coming to the Hospital to ride out the storm. "There's one place I'm going," Wells said, "and that's Ochsner. I told him, 'I'm coming.'"[12]

Wells, like most of the other employees who were at the Hospital that Monday morning as Katrina roared ashore from the Gulf of Mexico, had no hint they would be there for 3-1/2 weeks. Wells was everywhere on the Jefferson Highway campus, from keeping restrooms clean and serviced to seeing to it that nurses' stations and wards were supplied with everything they needed to continue functioning during the ordeal. Wells joked that she had spent 30 years as a first-floor environmental services technician, but during Katrina she operated from the top floor of the Hospital all the way to the basement.

Betty Wells takes immense pride in the fact that "this Hospital never had to close. Just being here and offering my contribution meant a lot to me. Even though it was a traumatic situation, in my eyes it was fun and an experience. It taught me how to deal with circumstances when they are thrust upon you."[13]

Katrina also created bonds of friendship and respect that will likely never be broken. During the hurricane and the trying days after Katrina made landfall, Wells felt a closeness to the Ochsner community she had never felt before. "I saw how supervisors, management, doctors, nurses and employees all came together," Wells said. "We were all one. We bonded together as a family. We did whatever we had to do. We all pitched in. It made us better people."[14]

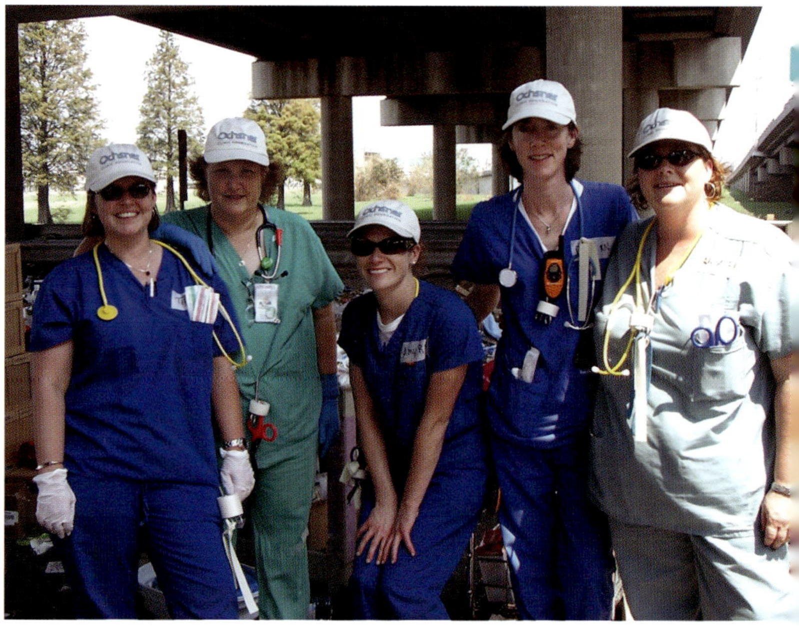

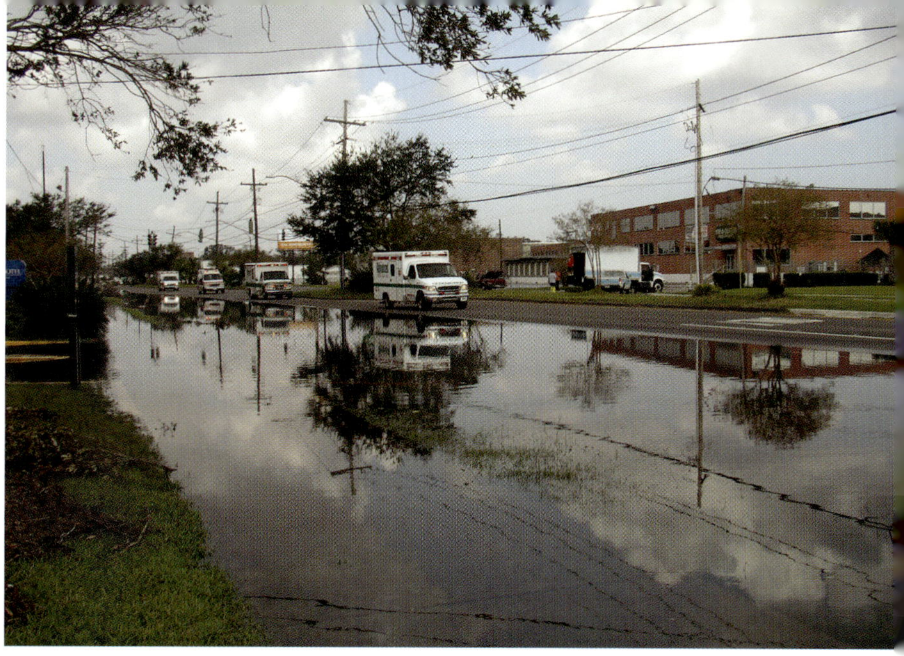

'WE THOUGHT WE HAD COME THROUGH IT JUST FINE'

Ochsner divided its response teams into two units. The A Team was assigned to ride out the storm at Ochsner facilities. The B Team was on call and assigned to rotate in to relieve A Team members.

Warner Thomas and all the top administrative and medical leaders were at an important management retreat in New Orleans when he received a telephone call from Grant Walker on Friday afternoon. Katrina was still gaining strength well out in the Gulf of Mexico, but the new projected path had New Orleans in the bullseye. Walker told Thomas that Ochsner needed to secure the previously identified emergency supplies and implement its hurricane plan immediately. Thomas did not hesitate. The hurricane plan was immediately initiated.[15] That decision Friday afternoon bought Ochsner valuable hours to prepare.

While New Orleans prepared for the hurricane that weekend, Ochsner put teams into place to keep the Clinic and Hospital operating during and after the storm. As Katrina strengthened from a Category 3 to a Category 5 hurricane that Saturday and Sunday, Ochsner was implementing its comprehensive plan to ride out the storm. Ochsner Clinic of Baton Rouge swung into operation as a backup for the Jefferson Highway campus and proved invaluable as a staging area for system support.

On Saturday morning, Quinlan gathered the leadership team for an 8 a.m. meeting at the Hospital. The group put the A Team on standby, with orders to report to the Jefferson Highway campus at 7 p.m. Sunday. Later that day, as storm tracks indicated that Katrina would come ashore very close to New Orleans, the leadership team put the A Team on full disaster alert; many team members began arriving at the Hospital that afternoon and evening to ensure they would be in place when the massive storm hit. Late Saturday morning, an industrial-sized generator arrived at the Brent House Hotel and was hooked up and running later that afternoon.[16]

That Sunday, crews staged 20 portable toilets around the Hospital and topped off the 60,000-gallon fuel tanks. Meanwhile, other A Team members moved through the Hospital corridors, placing 55-gallon drums of water on each floor for toilet-flushing and filling bathtubs and wastebaskets with water.[17]

By that evening, as Katrina reached its peak strength in the Gulf of Mexico south of the delta of the Mississippi River, Ochsner had established its command post on the second floor and had essentially locked the campus down. "We were ready for the storm," said Grant Walker that Sunday night.[18]

When the storm did come ashore as a Category 4 hurricane on Monday morning, August 29, power was lost and there was widespread tree and wind damage. Ochsner operated the lights and fans and all medical equipment in the West Tower with its diesel-electric generator. The peak of the storm moved across New Orleans that Monday morning between 8 a.m. and noon, and aside from 44 broken windows and one minor injury to a visitor who had been cut by a window blowing out in a waiting room, Ochsner had avoided major damage from flooding, wind and flying debris. Still, there was damage to the facility's roof and hundreds of leaky windows demanding attention from staff. That Monday night, Ochsner was operational and open for business. The same couldn't be said for much of the metropolitan area.

"When we woke up that morning, we thought we had come through it just fine," said Scott Posecai, Ochsner's Chief Financial Officer. "Nobody had any idea that the levees had broken. We didn't take on water at the main campus, but they did have water across the street."[19]

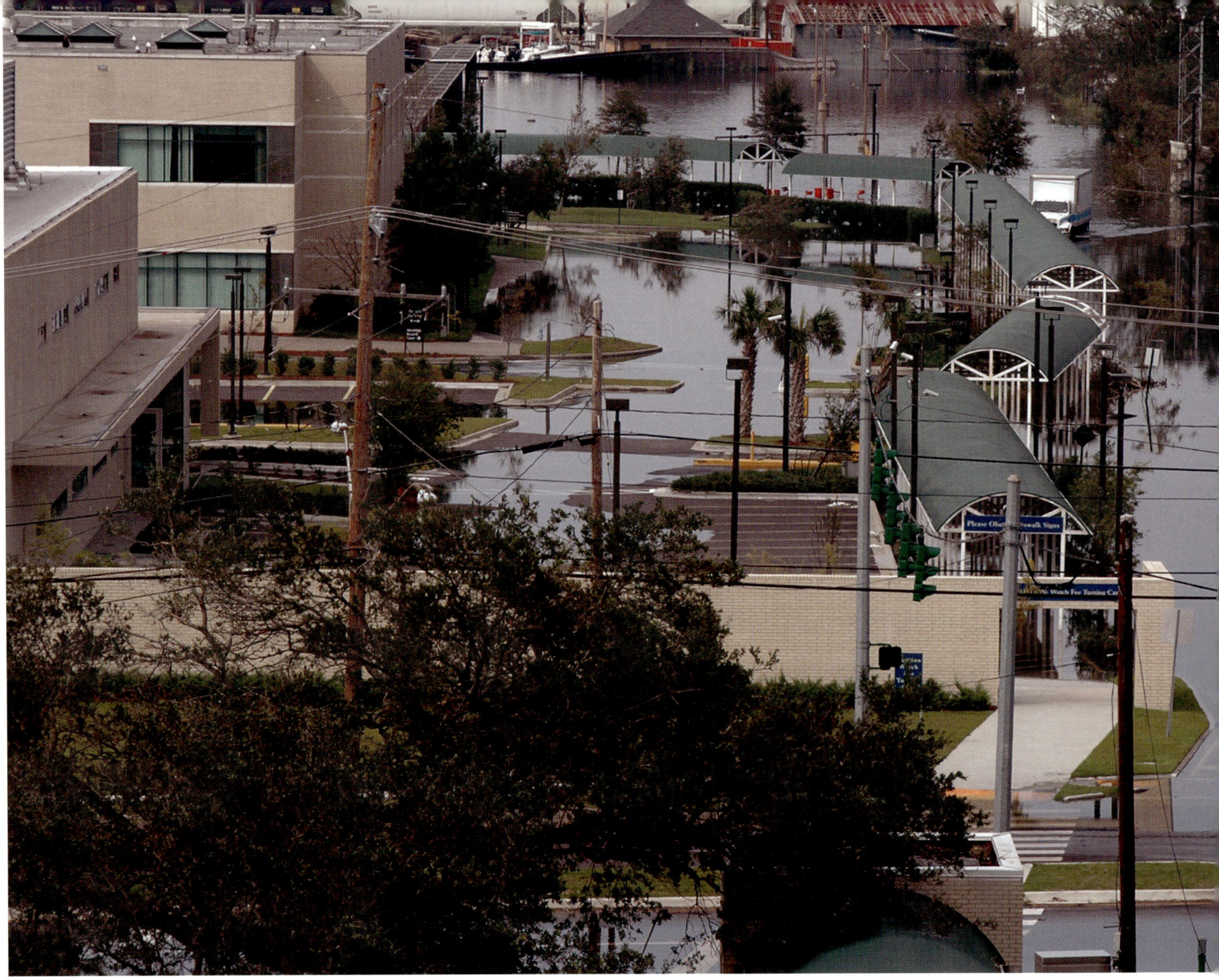

SIX MONTHS OF FOOD

Even though the immediate area surrounding the Jefferson Highway campus was still fairly dry, most of New Orleans was inundated Monday morning. A levee in the city's Ninth Ward breached that morning, sending 10 feet of muddy water cascading through the streets. Late that morning, a large section of the 17th Street Canal levee gave way. Much of the city filled with water. Tens of thousands of residents made their way on foot or in boats to the Louisiana Superdome. Media images broadcast to the rest of the world portrayed New Orleans in the grip of chaos.

Meanwhile, the A Team at Ochsner continued to do what it could to make Ochsner a beacon of hope in the growing crisis. Posecai, who was at the Jefferson Highway campus that Monday and Tuesday, recalled getting the assignment to visit a neighboring Walmart for supplies for patients and staff.

"The police let us in, and we got the supplies we needed," Posecai said. "The Walmart people met us in the store. They said just write down what you're taking, and we'll deal with payment later. We spent the next couple of hours filling up plastic garbage bags with deodorant, toothpaste, things like that. I don't know that Walmart ever came back to us for payment."[20]

Grant Walker had made arrangements with a Sav-A-Center warehouse in Jefferson Parish for Ochsner to be able to draw upon the store's food supply in case of emergency. It was essentially a six-month supply of food for the Jefferson Highway campus. Since the Brent House Hotel had electric power, Ochsner offered it to New Orleans public safety personnel as a safe haven in the storm. "We provided food and hot showers for all the cops and firemen," Walker said. "At one time, we were housing 75 police officers and 200 firemen."[21]

For most of the New Orleans area healthcare community, communication during Katrina was a nightmare. That was not the case for Ochsner, which had anticipated widespread communication failures as part of its emergency storm planning. Fully staffed disaster control centers at the Jefferson Highway campus and in Baton Rouge routed messages seamlessly by satellite phone. Realizing cell towers

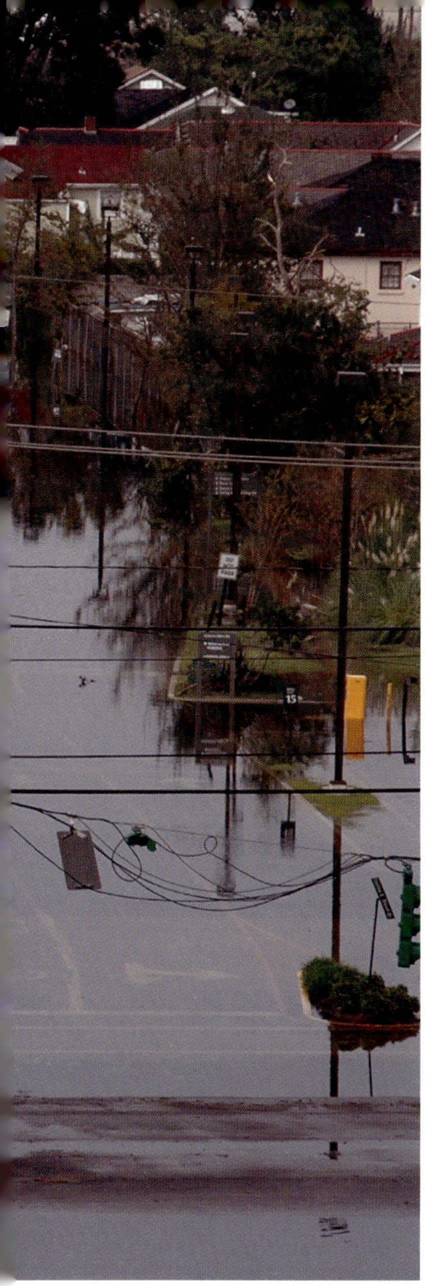

Muddy brown water 10 feet deep coursed through parts of the city in the wake of Monday's levee breaches.

could be out of service for an extended time in the wake of a hurricane, Ochsner had stocked up on cell phones with out-of-state area codes.[22] The Jefferson Highway campus served as the command center and as a central meeting place for various healthcare entities as the recovery developed.

Patrick Quinlan explained Ochsner's emergency planning always envisioned using Baton Rouge as a staging area and point of relief for the Jefferson Highway campus in case of a catastrophic hurricane in New Orleans. "The success and sustainability of the main campus depended on Baton Rouge for food, gas and supplies," he said. "It was a case of teamwork from the outside in. We had diversified geographically, and the organization came to appreciate the strength of that during Katrina."[23]

UNFORESEEN ISSUES

Dr. Richard Guthrie, Regional Medical Director in the New Orleans Region, who stayed in New Orleans during the storm, said the staff dealt with a number of unforeseen issues in typical Ochsner common-sense fashion. "We had to think of creative ways to pay people because they were dispersed around the country," Guthrie said. "It was unclear whether there would be massive pay cuts, or whether we'd have to downsize departments."[24]

What was immediately clear was that continuity of patient care was Ochsner's first priority. Patient electronic medical records were safe in Baton Rouge, and Ochsner's Board of Trustees never wavered in their support for doing the right thing, no matter the cost. The Board met by teleconference several days after the storm had passed and decided to spend whatever it took to keep Ochsner providing top quality medical care to patients.

"There was unanimous support from the Board for following that direction," Guthrie said. "We took our chances and believed in ourselves. It was a 'bet the company' decision to stay open and do right by the patients and the employees. It was a tribute to the Board's governance and the leadership of the organization."[25]

From the Board all the way to the maintenance worker who cleaned the building, the commitment to patient care was the same. Grant Walker will never forget bumping into a B Team member buffing the floor late in that first week after Katrina hit. "The guy was on the roof of his home for three days and was finally rescued in a helicopter and brought to the staging area at Causeway and I-10," Walker said. "When they flew over Ochsner, he tried to get the chopper to land him at the Hospital. He ran into an Ochsner doctor at the staging area, who dropped him off at Ochsner. He took a shower and started buffing floors." "Ochsner isn't Ochsner without shiny floors," he told Walker.[26] It was a manifestation of the Ochsner spirit.

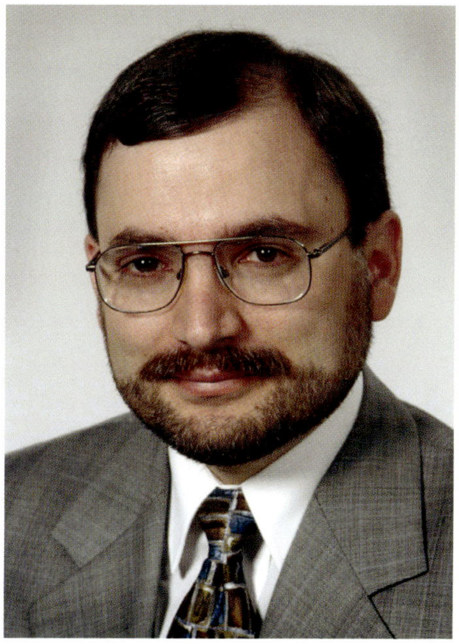

Richard Guthrie, Medical Director, New Orleans Region, stayed through Katrina and watched as Ochsner did the right thing by its patients and employees. Most members of the leadership team lived in their offices during the seven weeks following the storm.

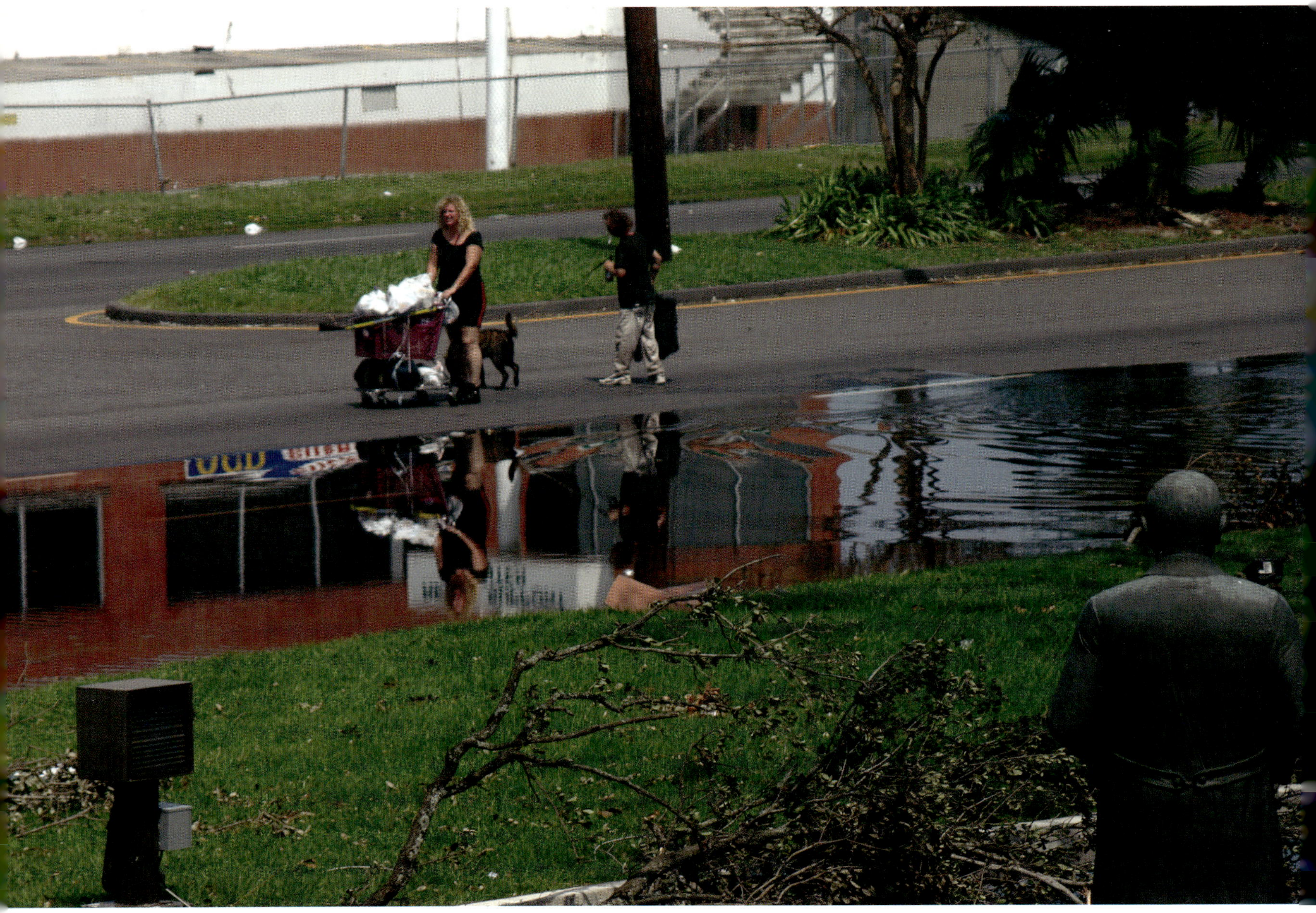

Residents escaping rising water pass in front of the Jefferson Highway campus.

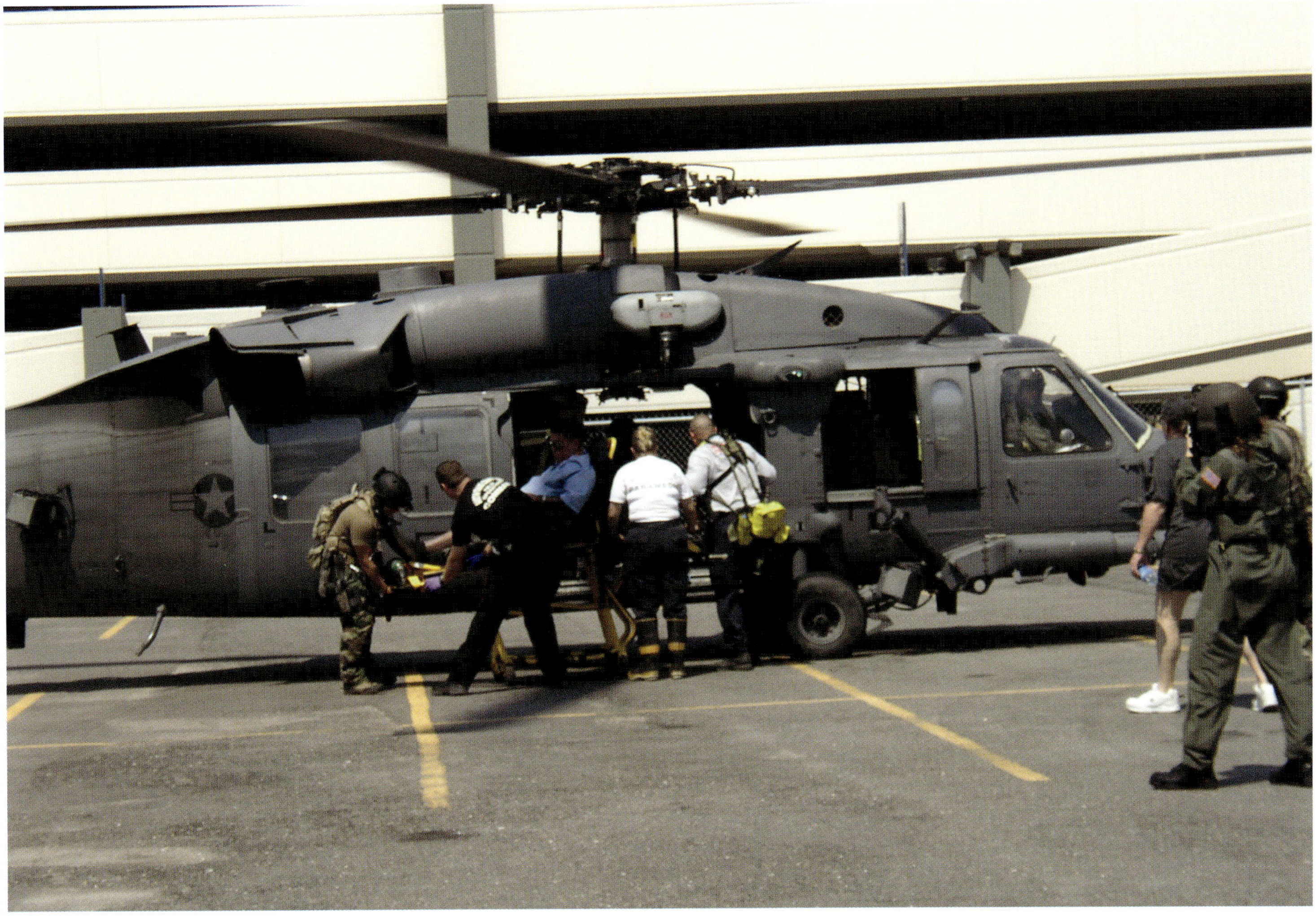

A U.S. Air Force MH-60G Pave Hawk Helicopter unloads patients on the roof deck of the parking garage at Ochsner Medical Center in New Orleans during the aftermath of Hurricane Katrina.

WATER AND AIR CONDITIONING

Necessity is the mother of invention, and Ochsner's A Team proved the point time and again in the days following Katrina's passage. The Hospital had lost one of its generators the morning of the storm, which was critical to powering the air conditioning system. Maintenance located a replacement part in Alabama and had the part and a repair crew flown to Lafayette on Wednesday, August 31, since the Baton Rouge airport was closed. The Ochsner helicopter picked up the part and a repairman on Thursday morning, and by that evening, the generator was operating and providing air conditioning.[27]

With electricity out across the metropolitan area, in some cases for weeks, fresh water was at a premium. Crews had stockpiled drums of water for flushing toilets and bottled water for drinking, but Ochsner also had an ace in the hole: the two wells that had been dug on the Jefferson Highway campus. The wells had not been used in more than a half-century, but maintenance crews had rebuilt the well pump in July 2005. By Wednesday afternoon, when those two wells were truly needed, the pump was feeding water to the hospital.

"We're the only place with flushing toilets and showers in the metro area," Grant Walker confided in his journal that evening.[28] By Thursday, crews had replaced the boiler stacks, which allowed the Hospital to provide hot water for showers. Ochsner quickly established a policy of offering free showers and meals for rescue, police, fire and military personnel, a fact that ensured the Hospital was well watched-over during the chaotic days of late August and early September.

For Patrick Quinlan, those first days after the passage of Katrina was an affirmation of what he calls "the Ochsner way." "The organization and the people supported each other. The theme was, 'we're all in it together'—patients, physicians, employees, the institution, families, pets," he said.[29]

The adrenaline that fueled Ochsner and the A Team in the immediate wake of Katrina would be even more severely tested in the weeks and months following the hurricane as the Hospital and the community of New Orleans struggled to come back from one of the worst natural disasters in American history.

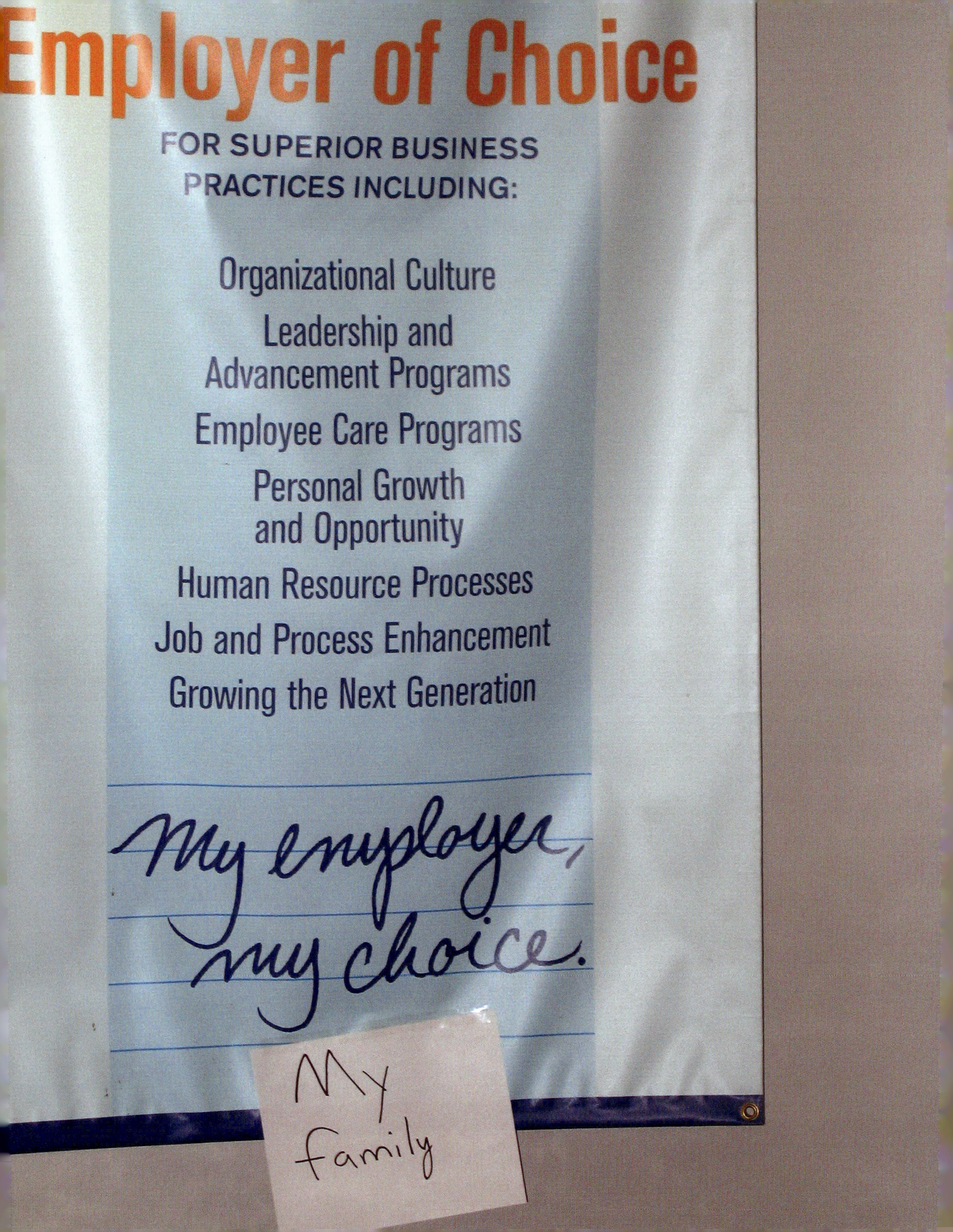
Employer of Choice
FOR SUPERIOR BUSINESS PRACTICES INCLUDING:
Organizational Culture
Leadership and Advancement Programs
Employee Care Programs
Personal Growth and Opportunity
Human Resource Processes
Job and Process Enhancement
Growing the Next Generation
My employer, my choice.
My family

CHAPTER 11:

AFTERMATH

THE EUPHORIA OF OCHSNER'S PERFORMANCE during Hurricane Katrina was tempered by the realization that the organization had a long, tough journey ahead of it in the weeks and months following the storm's passage. In the immediate aftermath of Katrina, doctors, nurses and employees were scattered from one point on the compass to another. Some would not return to Ochsner until 2006; others would never return.

The Clinic at the Jefferson Highway campus did not officially re-open for business until two weeks after the storm's passage. The Hospital itself remained open during the storm and after, a source of immense pride to Ochsner employees. Actor Sean Penn, one of the volunteer rescuers who brought patients to the ER in the week following the storm, told Ochsner employees that the place "looked better today than most hospitals would look on a typical Wednesday night."[1]

By late October, the Jefferson Highway campus facilities were operating at 80 percent of pre-Katrina volume, and when the New Year rolled around, the Jefferson Highway campus was operating at 100 percent of capacity. Ochsner neighborhood health center locations in the Greater New Orleans area also were operating at close to 80 percent, and Ochsner Clinic of Baton Rouge operated at more than 110 percent of normal activity.[2] Ochsner's relatively rapid recovery from Katrina would have significant implications for the New Orleans healthcare community in 2006.

An Ochsner employee appended a message to an "Employer of Choice" poster to reflect the spirit of togetherness that had permeated Ochsner in the wake of Katrina: My Employer, My Choice, My Family.

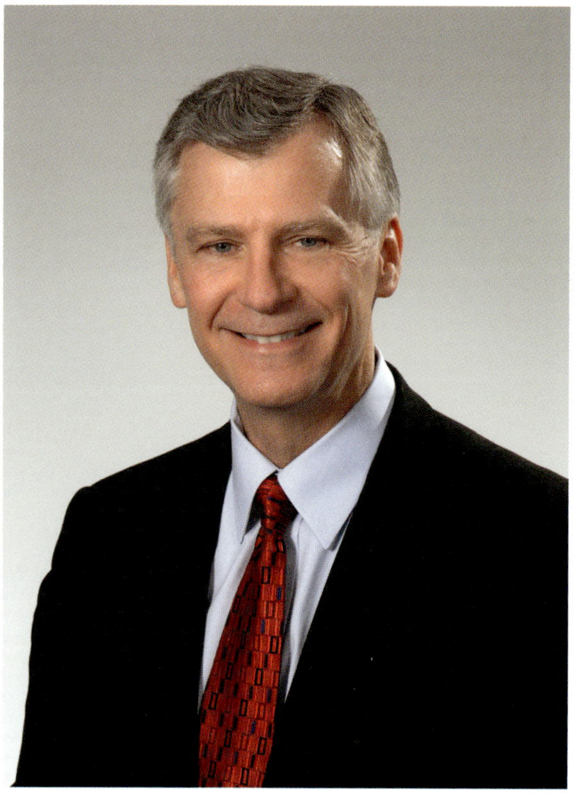

Patrick Quinlan called the purchase of three damaged New Orleans hospitals "a major positive step" in the city's recovery from Katrina.

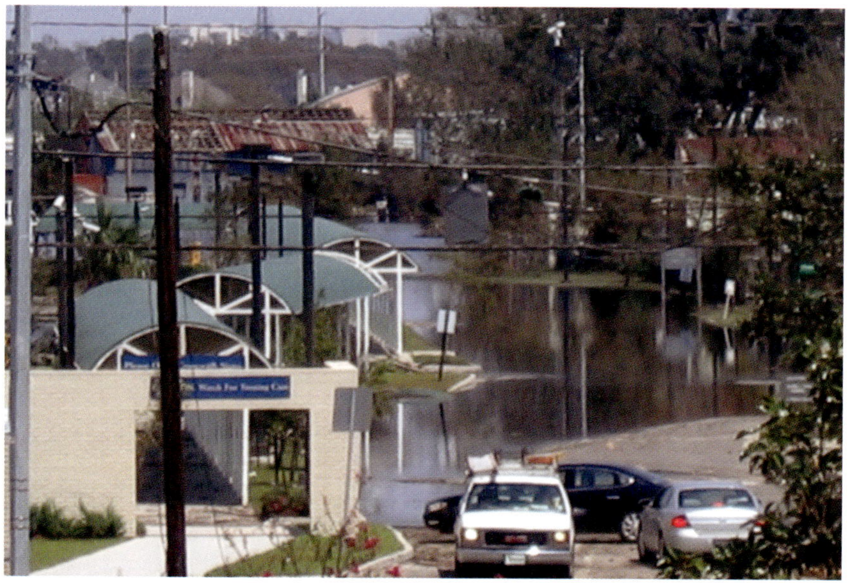

The parking lot and roads surrounding the pediatric ambulatory building—just across the street from Ochsner's main campus—were covered with water during the days after Katrina.

RUMORS

For Ochsner, the crisis following Katrina was in many ways worse than the actual storm. Most of the senior leadership lived in their offices for up to seven weeks and were on duty 24 hours a day, seven days a week. Patients had to be cared for, thousands of employees were coping with damaged or destroyed homes, and the city's healthcare infrastructure was barely functioning. Yet Ochsner went about doing what it had always done: serving the community.

By Thursday, September 1, however, one of the most difficult challenges facing senior leadership was quelling the rumors that swept the Hospital on a nearly hourly basis. National television news crews had descended on New Orleans like a swarm of locusts, making the chaotic conditions at the Louisiana Superdome an icon for the city's troubles. Unfortunately, much of what was being reported to the world was misleading or even worse.

Since Ochsner had electric power from early on, "the televisions were on all the time," said Dr. Patrick Quinlan. "We were in rumor control, non-stop. It was just sensationalist media. Much of it was just wrong."[3] Perhaps the most sensationalist reporting involved the perception that New Orleans and its residents were at the mercy of armed gangs of thugs. "Today," one A Team member said that Thursday, "the media made it look like all of New Orleans was burning to the ground."[4]

It wasn't. Ochsner maintained a fire watch on the roof of the Hospital, since visibility was easily 10 miles or more. Most of the fires being reported by the media weren't actually fires, and firewatchers could easily debunk the rumors. More widespread were the rumors of shooting and looting by armed gangs, from one end of the city to another.

To be sure, Ochsner had prepared for the possibility of a breakdown in civil order, and 30 security guards along with a contingent of National Guard soldiers had arrived at the Hospital on Thursday evening, September 1. The soldiers were only issued seven rounds apiece, so a security team member went home and returned with 1,000 rounds of his own

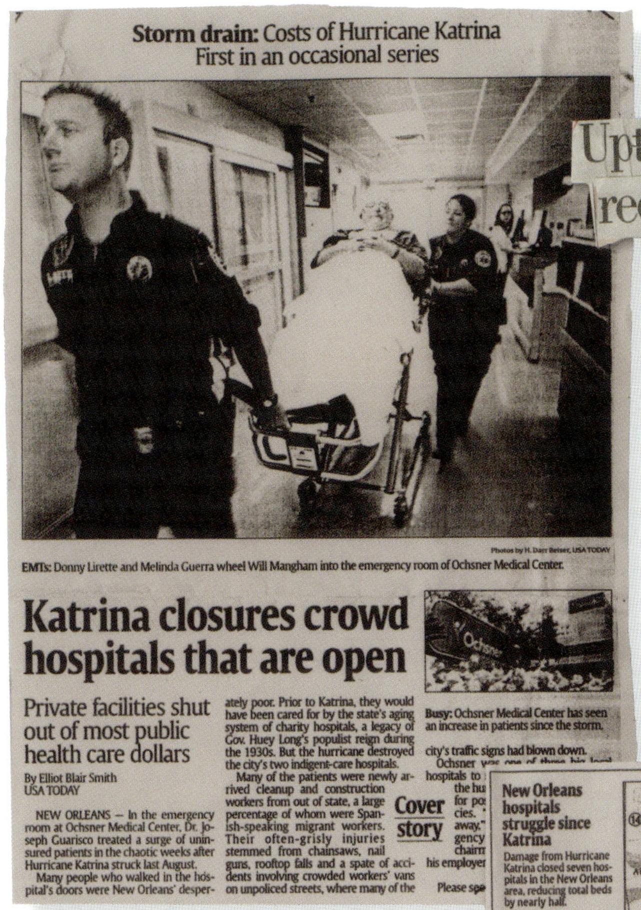

Storm drain: Costs of Hurricane Katrina
First in an occasional series

Photos by H. Darr Beiser, USA TODAY

EMTs: Donny Lirette and Melinda Guerra wheel Will Mangham into the emergency room of Ochsner Medical Center.

Katrina closures crowd hospitals that are open

Private facilities shut out of most public health care dollars

By Elliot Blair Smith
USA TODAY

NEW ORLEANS — In the emergency room at Ochsner Medical Center, Dr. Joseph Guarisco treated a surge of uninsured patients in the chaotic weeks after Hurricane Katrina struck last August.

Many people who walked in the hospital's doors were New Orleans' desperately poor. Prior to Katrina, they would have been cared for by the state's aging system of charity hospitals, a legacy of Gov. Huey Long's populist reign during the 1930s. But the hurricane destroyed the city's two indigent-care hospitals.

Many of the patients were newly arrived cleanup and construction workers from out of state, a large percentage of whom were Spanish-speaking migrant workers. Their often-grisly injuries stemmed from chainsaws, nail guns, rooftop falls and a spate of accidents involving crowded workers' vans on unpoliced streets, where many of the city's traffic signs had blown down.

Cover story

Busy: Ochsner Medical Center has seen an increase in patients since the storm.

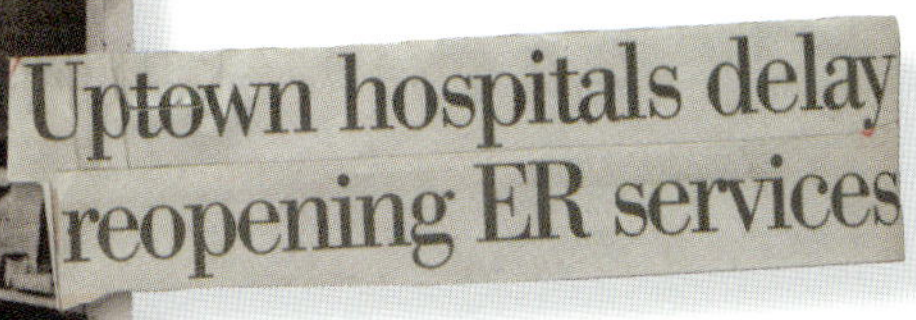

Uptown hospitals delay reopening ER services

Times-Picayune, *September 18, 2005*

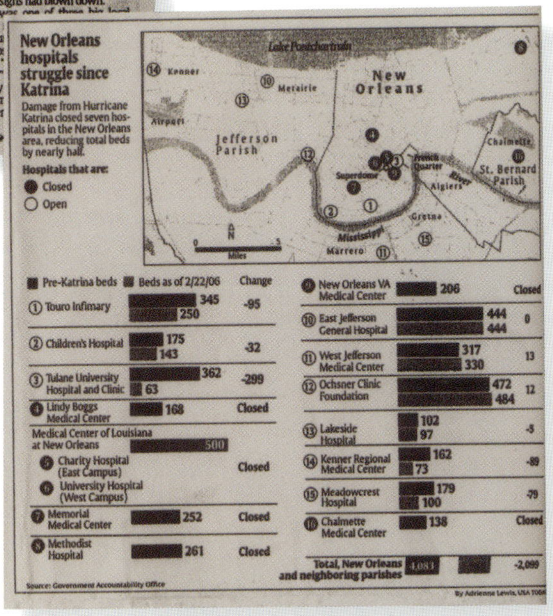

Despite significant damage, Ochsner was one of the few healthcare facilities in New Orleans able to remain open throughout the storm and its aftermath. USA Today, *April 26, 2006*

ammunition for the National Guard personnel. Ironically, the biggest call for security during the three weeks of getting back to normal after Katrina came from truckers who were delivering supplies to the Hospital and Ochsner neighborhood health centers.

A Team security members took pains to track down every rumor. When a New Orleans Special Weapons And Tactics (SWAT) team member called his mother, an Ochsner employee, to tell her to evacuate because a well-known local mall was under siege from armed gunmen, Grant Walker got on his cell phone to a police officer at the mall—some 15 miles away—and confirmed that two small fires had caused minor damage at the mall, and an inebriated resident with a .22 rifle was arrested for shooting at tin cans in the mall's parking lot.[5] The case was typical of the way the media and the rumor mill blew events out of all proportion.

"From then on," Walker said, "all reports were sent to the security director and were considered rumor unless verified, which ended up being the case in all accounts."[6]

Personnel from the Federal Emergency Management Agency (FEMA) began arriving in New Orleans mid-week following the hurricane's landfall, and A Team members spent a fair amount of time devising methods to get supplies to Ochsner without having them commandeered by FEMA. Support from city, state and parish officials was virtually non-existent during the first chaotic weeks after the storm.[7] Ochsner had to go it alone.

• WHAT OCHSNER MEANS TO ME •

"Everyday I get the opportunity to work with physicians, peers, nurses and employees to provide new services, help bring state-of-the-art technologies and new clinic services to improve and raise the QUALITY of care for our region."

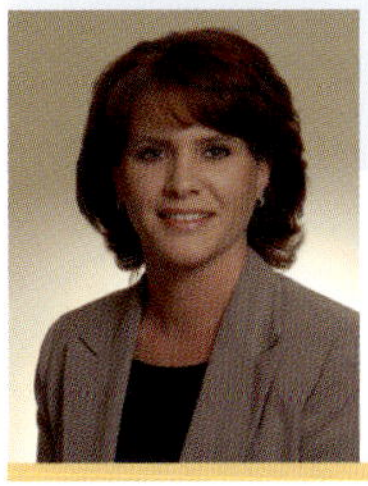

Nicole Gonzales, Assistant Vice President of Clinic Operations, Ochsner Health Center – Covington

To watch the full interview with Nicole Gonzales, visit **ochsner.org/history**.

REACHING OUT TO THE COMMUNITY

National media reports didn't obscure the fact that many New Orleans residents who had not evacuated ahead of the storm were in deep trouble. On September 1 and 2, A Team members loaded up a truck with food and water and began driving up and down the streets surrounding the Hospital passing out supplies to Ochsner's neighbors. CEO Patrick Quinlan rode shotgun in a van loaded with food and water that visited a low-income housing complex just down the street from the Jefferson Highway campus. Ochsner staff went where many feared to tread and helped hand out a four-day supply of food to the residents, many of whom had eaten nothing since Monday morning.[8]

Late that week after landfall, recovery teams visited most of Ochsner's neighborhood health centers. They reported back that three health centers were still under water and one was a total loss after the roof blew off. The other neighborhood health centers, however, could easily be repaired and reopened.

Meanwhile, Emergency Department physicians, nurses and support staff set up a MASH (Mobile Army Surgical Hospital) unit at the intersection of Interstate 10 and Causeway Boulevard, just north of the Hospital. Military units and FEMA were using the exit as a staging area for residents plucked from roofs in the city's flooded areas.[9] Ochsner ER personnel helped treat those who were injured or sick.

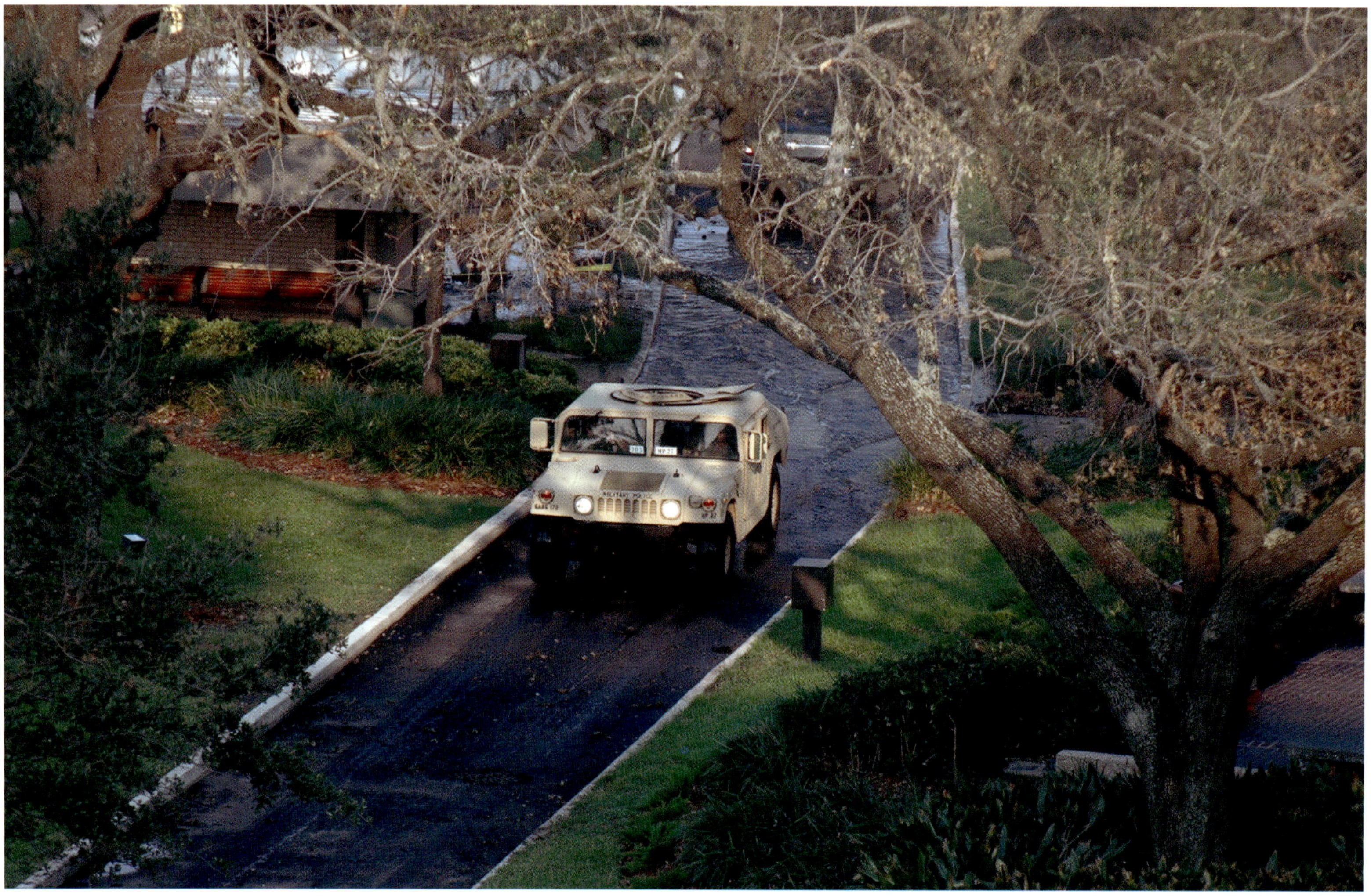

A National Guard HumVee patrols the front driveway of Ochsner Medical Center in New Orleans during the days following Katrina.

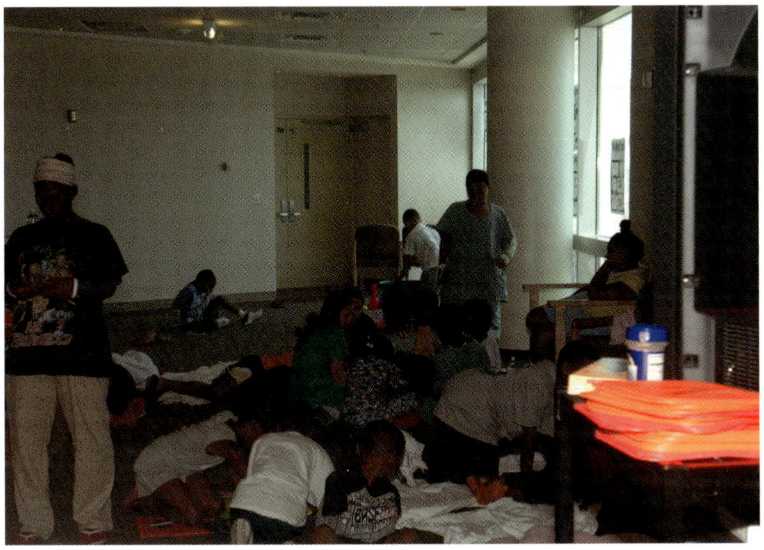

To care for the children of visitors and employees during Katrina, the Volunteer Services Department at Ochsner Medical Center set up a child care area in a hospital waiting room.

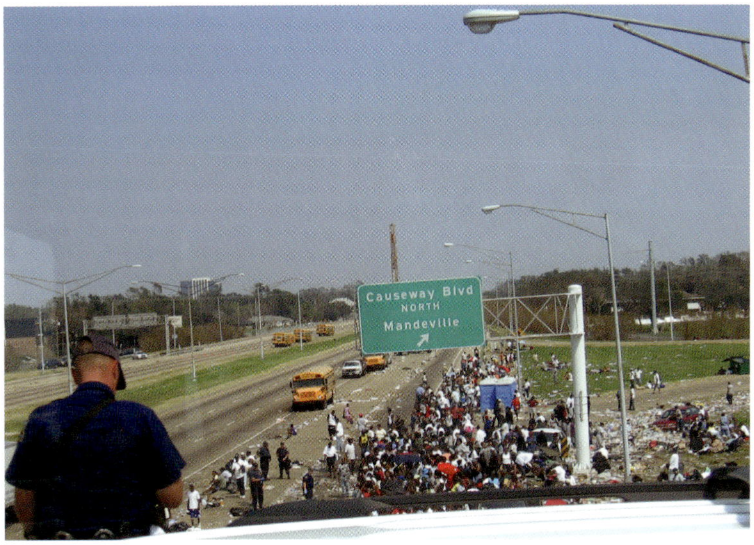

Ochsner set up a MASH hospital and staged supplies for transport to the Hospital at the FEMA staging area at the intersection of Interstate 10 and Causeway Boulevard.

OPEN FOR BUSINESS

While the nation's attention was focused on the devastation wrought by Katrina, Ochsner leadership was laying the groundwork for reopening the System facilities and accepting new patients. On Friday, September 2, patients on the 11th floor were moved to the 3rd floor, where air conditioning was more reliable. A 50-man damage recovery team was busy preparing the 10th and 11th floors of the Hospital for occupancy and would be assigned to rehabilitate the Rothschild and Metairie Clinics before the weekend was over. Roofing crews began tackling the repair and replacement of damaged roofs at Ochsner facilities across the metropolitan area.

That Friday night, Entergy, the electric utility company serving Louisiana, restored electric power to the Jefferson Highway campus. A Team members had climbed up on to the Hospital roof each night since the hurricane passed over, watching the inexorable march of lights coming from Kenner as power was restored. Restoration of electric power was a signal to the world that Ochsner was well on its way to recovery.

On Saturday, September 3, team members taped the word "OPEN" in 20-foot letters made of red garbage bags to the concrete top deck of the facility's parking garage. Patrick Quinlan went on national television to proclaim that Ochsner was, in fact, open for business and accepting new patients.[10]

The word was circulating throughout the community. On Labor Day weekend, Jefferson Parish officials asked Ochsner to open its Kenner and Lapalco Clinics because hospitals in those areas had evacuated. Ochsner was able to quickly get standby generators to both clinics in preparation for reopening. By the second week of September, Quinlan and Warner Thomas were making the rounds of local government offices asking what Ochsner could do in the way of support. New Orleans residents would not soon forget that Ochsner put a key element of the city's healthcare infrastructure back into operation and then went out into the community seeking to help wherever needed.

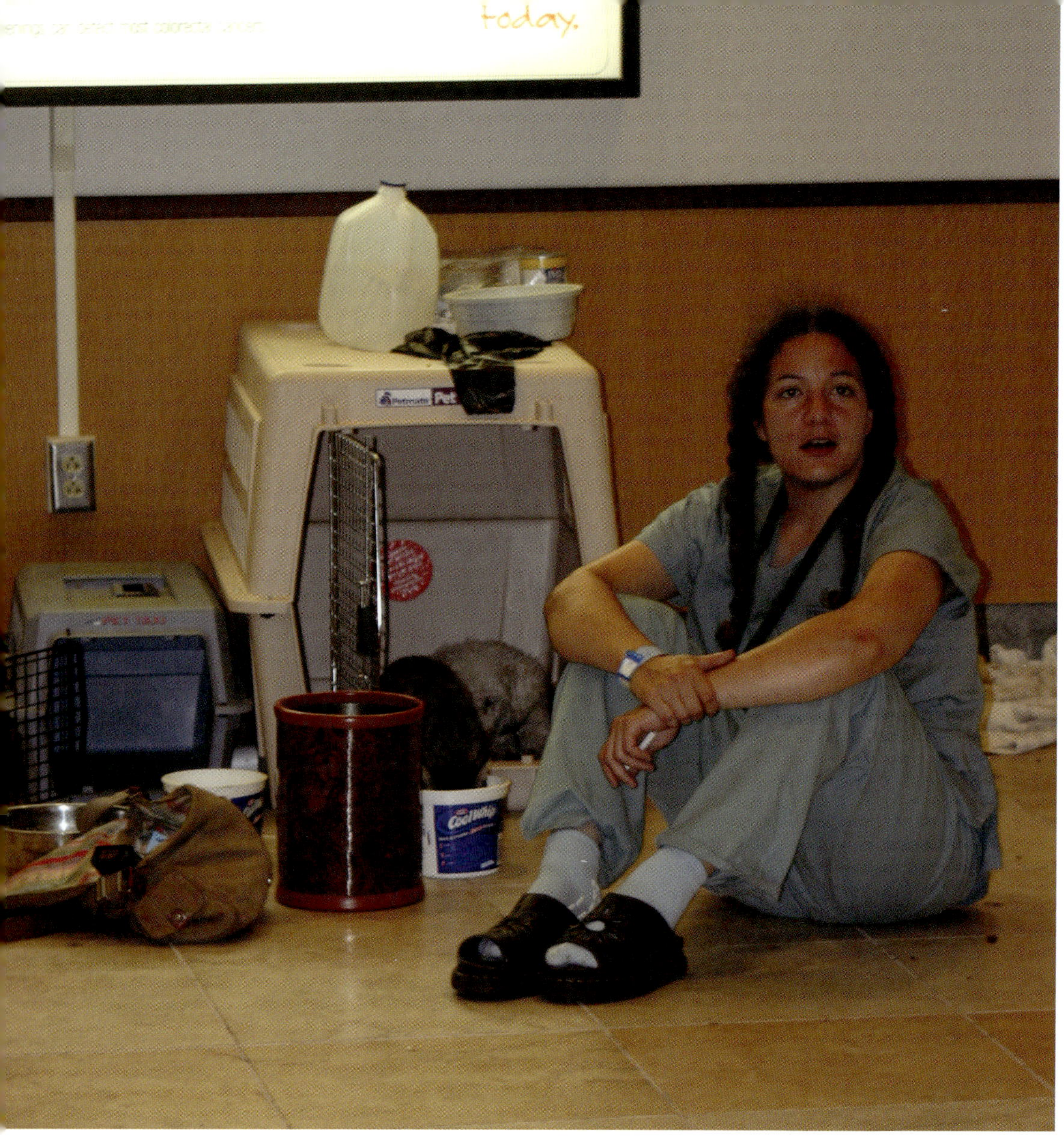

Ochsner's commitment to employees and their families even extends to family pets, as reflected in the fact that employees who stayed at the Hospital during Hurricane Katrina were allowed to bring their pets and house them in the parking garage elevator lobbies.

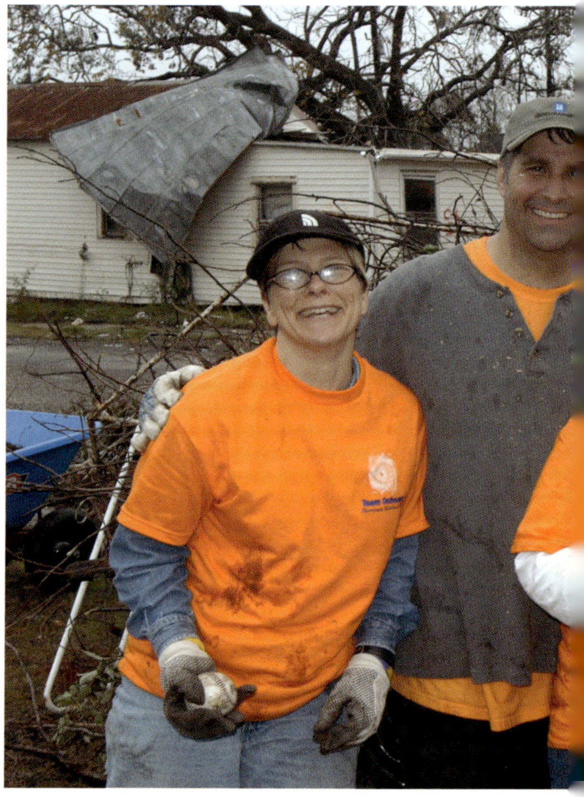

HELPING TEAM MEMBERS

Patrick Quinlan likes to point out that Ochsner's employees are what make the institution so special. And many of Ochsner's physicians, nurses, administrators and employees were personally hurting following the hurricane's passage.

"We are all about trusting people," Quinlan said, "but if you want loyalty, you have to give it in return. It takes trust. There was real-time decision making. There was problem solving as a group."[11] That willingness to give loyalty was tested dozens of times every day during the days, weeks and months following Katrina.

Hundreds of Ochsner employees lost everything they had in the wind and water of the storm. Quinlan remembered one case in particular when a nurse looked up at a television monitor on her ward to see an aerial view of her flooded house with a dog on the roof. She continued to work, knowing there wasn't anything she could do about the house.[12]

Grant Walker finally made it to his home Labor Day weekend to discover that "we only got seven feet of water in the house. My second floor is high and dry. We will be able to rebuild."[13] Walker, who lived near the 17th Street Canal off of Veterans Memorial Boulevard, was one of the flood victims. Walker returned to his home by boat a week after the storm to rescue his cats and the valuables he forgot to take with him. Ten days later, after pumps had finally drained the floodwaters, he returned to the neighborhood and began gutting the house so he could dry it out and begin rebuilding. Three years later, only 50 percent of the people in Walker's neighborhood had returned.[14]

Thousands of Ochsner employees sustained flood or storm damage during Katrina. Ochsner did everything it could to help. "Some people lost everything," said Grant Walker. "We gave free meals in the cafeteria to every employee for nine months. We had a helping hands program that gutted 55 employee homes."[15] Ochsner knew early on which of its employees were flooded out. The Ochsner Relief Fund, set up shortly after the floodwaters had receded, raised more than $3 million. One hundred percent of the fund went to employees in need.[16]

Charles Heim, Ochsner's Vice President of Philanthropy who was displaced to Houston and then to Connecticut for more than a

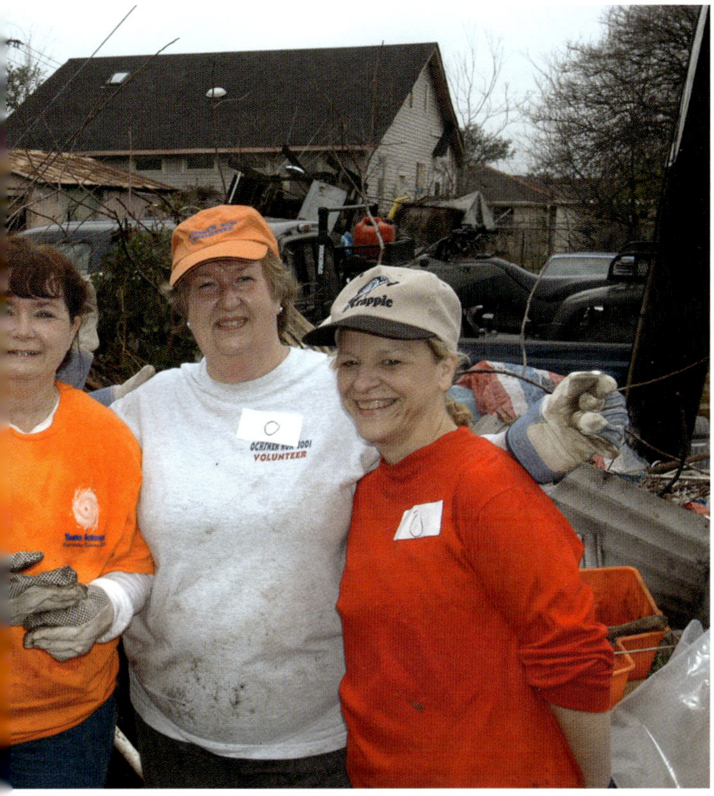

Ochsner's Employee Relief Fund provided housing assistance for the thousands of employees who sustained damage to their homes.

month, helped raise money for the Ochsner Relief Fund on the Internet. "There are only two occasions when the American public responded to e-philanthropy initiatives," Heim said, "for 9/11 and Katrina."[17]

Employees whose homes were relatively unaffected by the storm joined teams to help rehabilitate the employee homes that had sustained major flood damage. Betty Wells from Environmental Services had closed on a house in New Orleans in early June, less than three months before Katrina came ashore. Wells, who was at Ochsner for nearly a month following the storm, didn't know how she would ever clean the mud and silt out of her home.

"I will forever be eternally grateful to my co-workers," she said. "They gutted my house so we could rebuild. Ochsner is such a loving environment. They alleviated so many of my hardships."[18]

HELPING TO SAVE THE SAINTS

One of the enduring images of New Orleans in the days following Katrina was the chaos at the Louisiana Superdome. Originally designated as an evacuation point, the Superdome became a symbol of everything that had gone wrong in one of the worst natural disasters to strike the United States in decades. Thousands of local residents waited in vain for rescue or supplies. Gaping holes in the roof allowed the rain to pour in on the green artificial turf that was home to the New Orleans Saints, the city's representative in the National Football League (NFL).

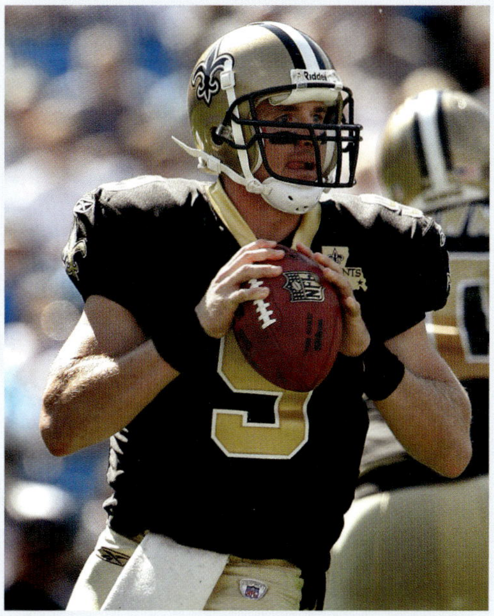

Ochsner's partnership with the New Orleans Saints helped bring the professional football team back to New Orleans for the 2006 season. Image courtesy of the New Orleans Saints.

By the time a week had passed, most of the evacuees had been bussed to better-equipped evacuation centers. The Saints were left with a home stadium that was all but destroyed. Working with the NFL, the team agreed to play its home games in San Antonio for the 2005 season, which started 10 days after Katrina roared through Louisiana.

Following that 2005 season, an increasing number of people questioned whether the Saints would return to New Orleans for the 2006 season opener. The Louisiana Superdome was on schedule to reopen for the Saints' first home game in September, but loss of population led many to wonder if the Saints would, in fact, return.

Once again, Ochsner stepped up to help the community. Ochsner's CEO and the Ochsner Clinic Foundation Board saw the Saints as an essential part of the fabric of the community and an organization that affected the morale of the city. As a result, Ochsner came on board as a major team sponsor as the "Official Healthcare Provider of the New Orleans Saints," a move that helped ensure the return of the team to New Orleans and helped lift the morale of employees and the community. What seemed to be a major risk turned into a community celebration when the Saints, behind Quarterback Drew Brees, won the NFC South division title and made it all the way to the NFC championship game against the Chicago Bears. Three years later, following the 2009 season, the Saints beat the Indianapolis Colts 31-17 to capture the Lombardi Trophy at Super Bowl XLIV.

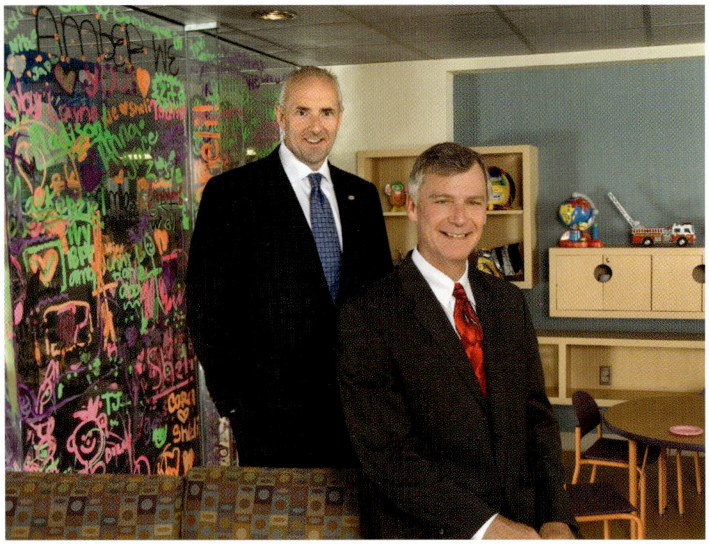

Warner Thomas and Patrick Quinlan arrived at Ochsner within months of each other in 1999. They formed a leadership team that consolidated the Clinic and Foundation, re-established Ochsner as one of America's best hospitals and transformed healthcare in New Orleans in the wake of Hurricane Katrina.

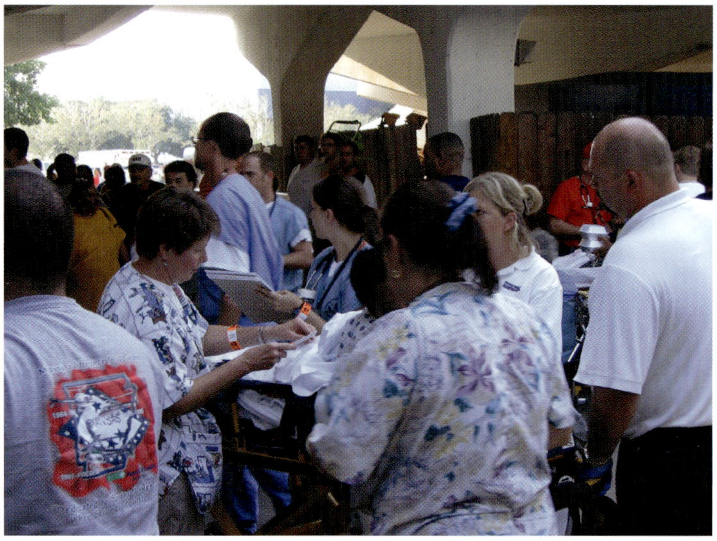

One of the busiest places in Baton Rouge in the days after Katrina passed was the LSU Assembly Center triage area for patients who were transferred from New Orleans.

'THERE WOULDN'T BE A NEW ORLEANS'

A month into the post-Katrina era, it was evident that Ochsner had emerged as a leader of the future of healthcare in Louisiana and adjacent areas of Mississippi and Alabama. The organization had been tested in a way previous Ochsner generations might have found inconceivable, but it had not been found wanting. Katrina had forged a bond among those who survived her fury that few would ever forget. Three weeks after the passage of the storm, homeless employees were still living in the Merrill Hines Surgery Center, and only 20 percent of the Hospital's food and housekeeping personnel were back to work.

Even with the shortfalls of personnel, morale at Ochsner remained high, and everyone pitched in to get the job done. Physicians volunteered every day to serve food in the cafeteria, washing dishes and cooking food in a 110-degree kitchen so the overworked dietary staffers could take breaks. Nursing staff helped to clean the units, and one patient, the wife of a non-Ochsner physician, had refused to be admitted to another New Orleans hospital because it was so dirty. She commented that the shiny floors at Ochsner meant that the hospital's patient care must be outstanding.[19]

A month after the storm, Ochsner staff reserved 750 hotel rooms for employees, many of whom had been sleeping on air mattresses in the Hospital. Ochsner arranged for buses to transport employees back and forth from the Jefferson Highway campus to the hotels.[20] For Ochsner, it was a simple matter of doing the right thing.

There was no thought given to the cost of housing, feeding and helping employees. In the first month after Katrina, Ochsner lost $30 million. Quinlan and the leadership team refused to let the organization get distracted. Ochsner was in it for the long haul, and the long haul involved continuing to provide quality healthcare for the people of Louisiana. Before that first month was over, Ochsner teams were back to performing kidney transplants at the Jefferson Highway campus.

"We were focused on fundamentals," Quinlan said, explaining that Ochsner kept its eye on a very important goal. "We were getting hospitals and clinics back up and running. If there were no medical care to come home to, there wouldn't be a New Orleans. Public safety and public education and public health—those were our focus."[21]

On October 1, Ochsner's New Orleans inpatient census stood at 276 patients, roughly half of pre-storm volume. Clinic visits were up to 40 percent of pre-storm volume. Ochsner Clinic of Baton Rouge was approaching 200 percent of capacity. "Every day," one staffer commented, "things get better."

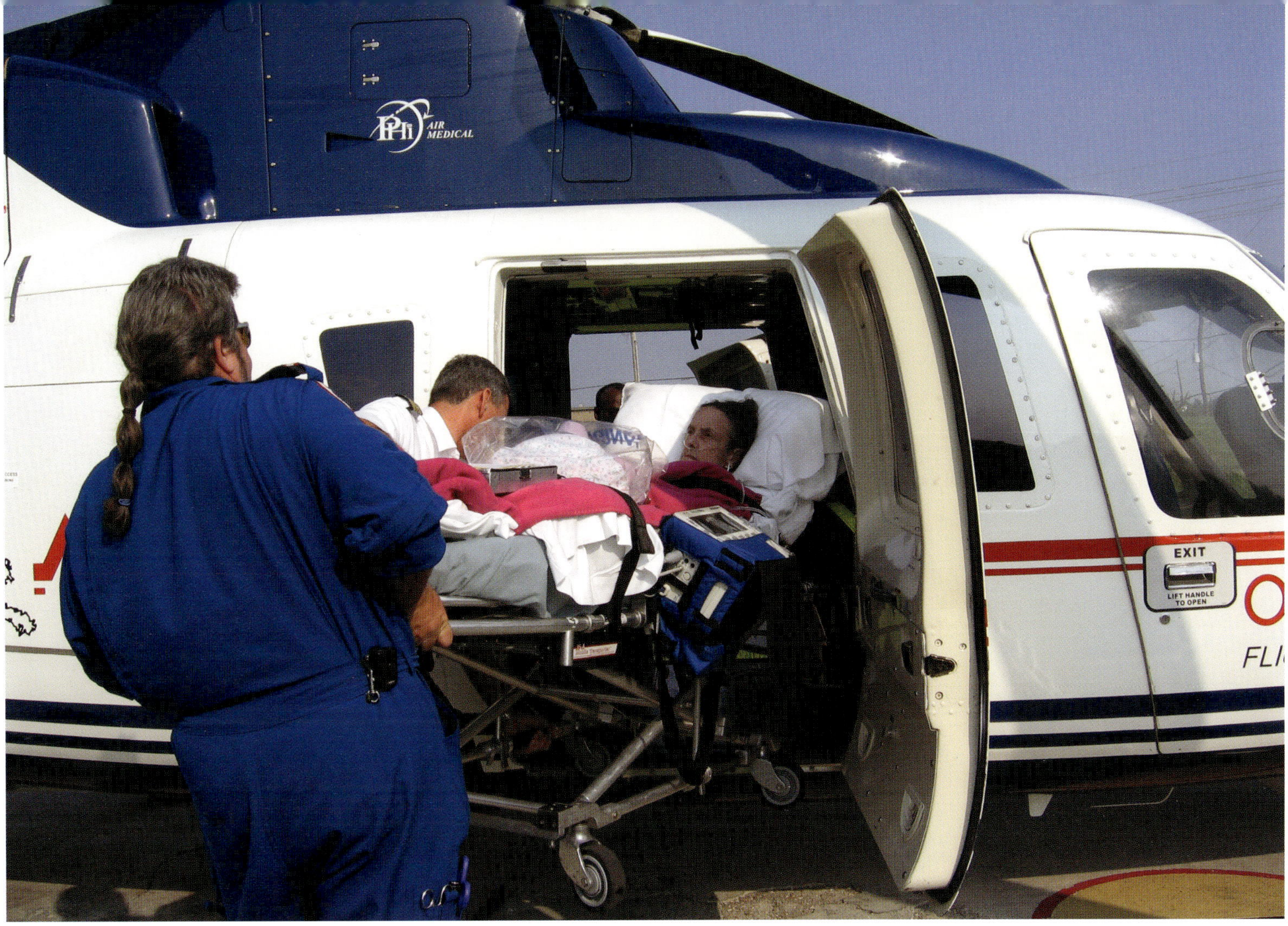

The original decision in 1954 to build a helipad definitely paid off during Katrina as the Ochsner Flight Care team worked to transfer patients to and from the Hospital.

UPROOTED

The aftermath of the Category 4 hurricane uprooted thousands of Ochsner physicians, nurses and employees. When New Orleans Mayor Ray Nagin issued a mandatory evacuation order on Saturday morning, August 27, many Ochsner personnel not assigned to either the A or B Teams evacuated all over the country, literally dispersed across the nation.

Perhaps the most wrenching decision for Ochsner employees displaced by Katrina was whether or not to return to New Orleans. Some who came back had to bow to the inevitable when spouses could not commit to rebuilding lives in a city that had nearly been destroyed. Others took their insurance money and rebuilt elsewhere. All told, several hundred physicians, nurses and employees who had been a part of the Ochsner family in the summer of 2005 were no longer there two years later.

Others did come back. John Lockwood "Lock" Ochsner evacuated his family to his wife's hometown of Chattanooga, Tennessee, the weekend before Katrina came ashore. The family was in the mountains of Tennessee for most of the fall of 2005, but there was no question they would eventually come home to New Orleans.

"Some people are never going to leave the institution," Ochsner said. "They're just not going to leave New Orleans. They are the people who have adapted to New Orleans and its environment."[22]

For Lock Ochsner, it was simply a matter of wanting to practice at a place named for his grandfather. "I don't think I could do as good a job someplace else," he said. "I wouldn't have the same staff commitment everywhere down the line as I do here."[23]

One year later, Ochsner continued to lead in the rebuilding of healthcare in New Orleans. Normalcy came back in incremental stages. Ochsner was at 100 percent of pre-storm volume by the spring and early summer of 2006. The Hospital's Emergency Department was at 140 percent of pre-storm volume; some patients had to wait up to 48 hours to be admitted because all of the beds were full.

As New Orleans marked the first anniversary of the storm that would forever be linked with the city's past and future, Ochsner was preparing a major initiative that would propel it to the forefront of New Orleans' healthcare infrastructure.

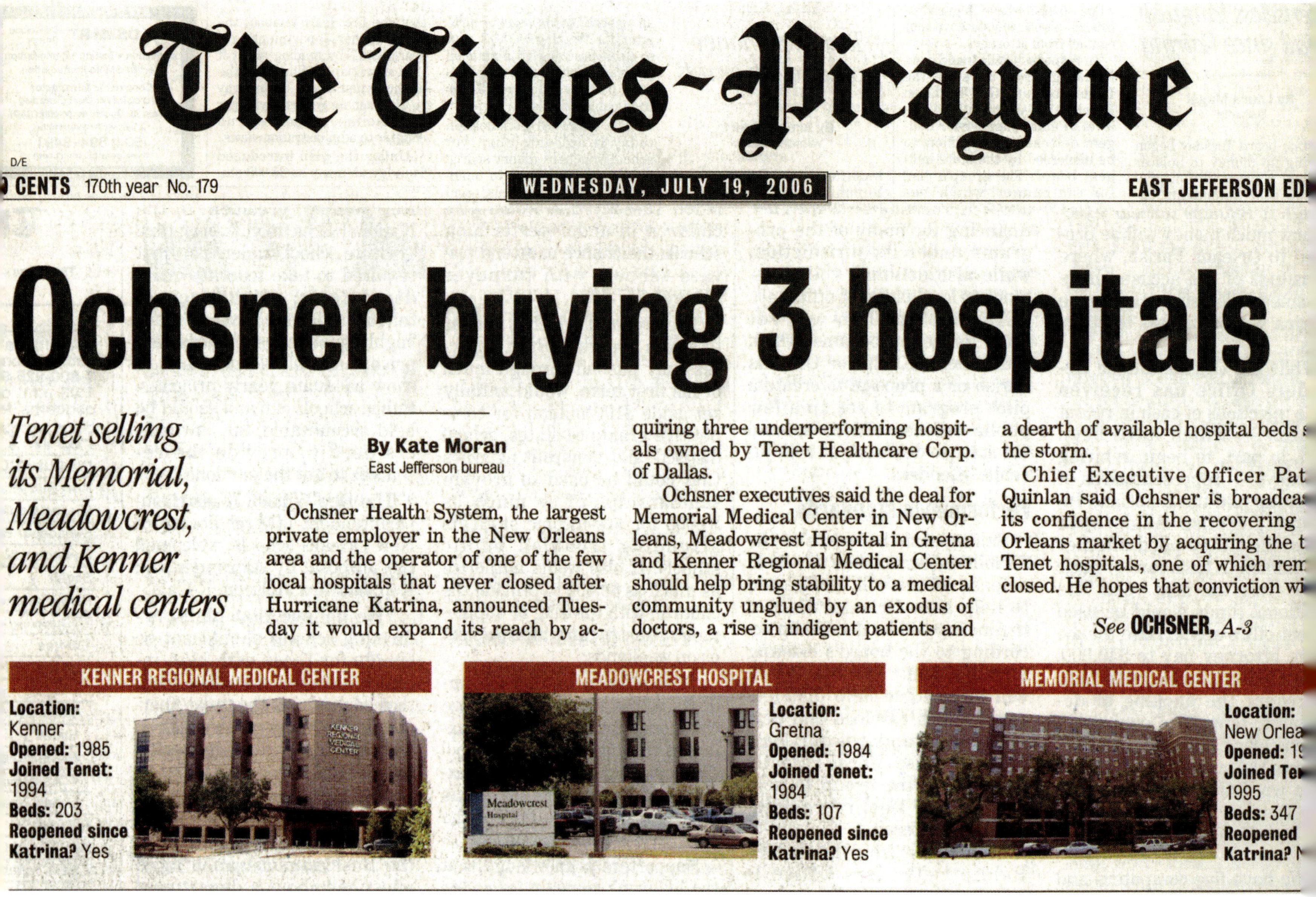

The Times-Picayune

D/E

CENTS 170th year No. 179 | WEDNESDAY, JULY 19, 2006 | EAST JEFFERSON ED

Ochsner buying 3 hospitals

Tenet selling its Memorial, Meadowcrest, and Kenner medical centers

By Kate Moran
East Jefferson bureau

Ochsner Health System, the largest private employer in the New Orleans area and the operator of one of the few local hospitals that never closed after Hurricane Katrina, announced Tuesday it would expand its reach by acquiring three underperforming hospitals owned by Tenet Healthcare Corp. of Dallas.

Ochsner executives said the deal for Memorial Medical Center in New Orleans, Meadowcrest Hospital in Gretna and Kenner Regional Medical Center should help bring stability to a medical community unglued by an exodus of doctors, a rise in indigent patients and a dearth of available hospital beds s the storm.

Chief Executive Officer Pat Quinlan said Ochsner is broadcas its confidence in the recovering Orleans market by acquiring the t Tenet hospitals, one of which rem closed. He hopes that conviction wi

See **OCHSNER,** *A-3*

KENNER REGIONAL MEDICAL CENTER

Location: Kenner
Opened: 1985
Joined Tenet: 1994
Beds: 203
Reopened since Katrina? Yes

MEADOWCREST HOSPITAL

Location: Gretna
Opened: 1984
Joined Tenet: 1984
Beds: 107
Reopened since Katrina? Yes

MEMORIAL MEDICAL CENTER

Location: New Orlea
Opened: 1
Joined Te 1995
Beds: 347
Reopened Katrina?

Ochsner's decision to buy the three Tenet hospitals in New Orleans was rooted in the institution's focus on doing what was right for the community.

CHAPTER 12:

BUILDING STRENGTH THROUGH CONSOLIDATION

OCHSNER LED THE RESURGENCE OF HEALTHCARE in southeast Louisiana in the wake of Hurricane Katrina. Through a combination of preparedness and luck, Ochsner maintained service throughout the hurricane and the aftermath of flooding and chaos.

"The heroism, the generosity, the selflessness and the sense of teamwork that was presented by everyone inside and outside this organization dwarfs anything negative that I have seen or heard," Dr. Patrick Quinlan told Ochsner employees two weeks after Katrina hit.[1]

While Ochsner was providing assistance and help to the thousands of employees who had sustained damage or lost their homes, other New Orleans healthcare institutions were struggling just to survive. Seven hospitals in the New Orleans metropolitan area remained closed eight months after Katrina's passage. All told, nearly 2,100 hospital beds in Orleans, Jefferson and St. Bernard Parishes were lost to Katrina.[2]

Ochsner might well have thanked its lucky stars, looked inward and gone about its business of providing outstanding patient care without giving thought to the unfortunate institutions that were not as lucky or as prepared. That, however, is not the Ochsner way.

"In August and September of 2005, the whole city became an emergency room," Quinlan said. "Ochsner rose to the challenge. We stepped up, not back."

Stepping up and not back became Ochsner's post-Katrina mantra. In 2006, stepping up meant taking some of the biggest risks in Ochsner's history, including purchasing, reopening and expanding three Tenet hospitals, one of which remained closed after the storm.

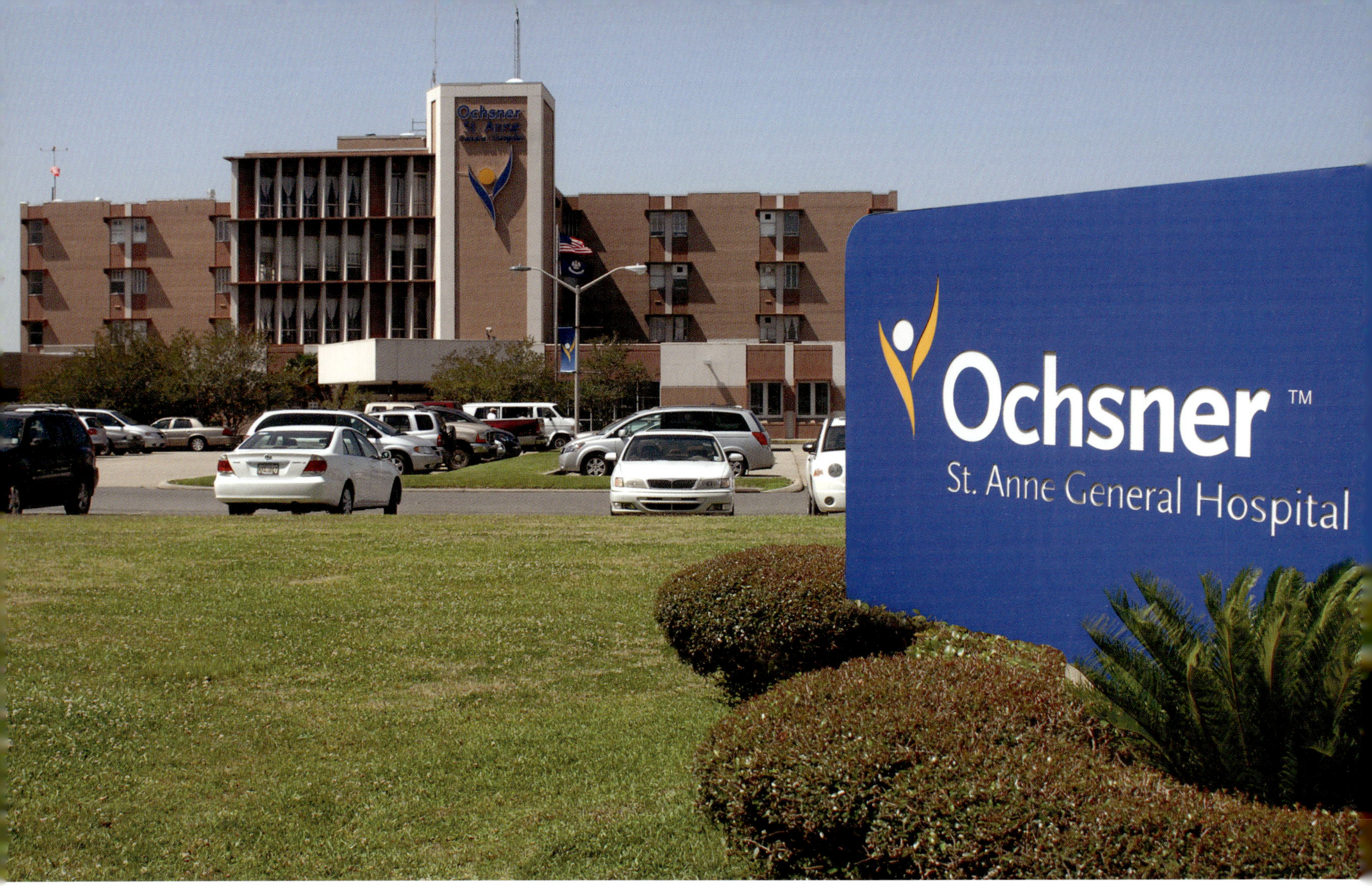

Ochsner St. Anne General Hospital in Raceland brings a wide range of healthcare services to the residents of Lafourche Parish.

'TOGETHER, WE MADE IT WORK'

The closure of Charity Hospital of New Orleans in the wake of Katrina left a gaping hole in the local healthcare safety net. LSU had operated the only Level I Trauma Center in southeast Louisiana at Charity Hospital. When Katrina devastated that hospital, the Level I Trauma Center was relocated to LSU Medical Center in Shreveport.

LSU Health Care Services Division CEO Donald Smithburg contacted Ochsner for the solution. New Orleans simply could not go without Level I Trauma Care for any length of time, he said.[3] Ochsner agreed and quickly stepped up, offering to lease space to LSU at Ochsner Hospital – Elmwood. Ochsner had unused capacity at the Elmwood facility, which it had purchased in 2002. FEMA spent $3 million to renovate the space, which included two surgery suites, a recovery room, a radiology suite and a number of inpatient beds on the facility's third floor.[4]

"We were all in this together," Ochsner leaders told the community. "Together, we made it work."[5]

Ochsner began the difficult task of consolidating healthcare in southeast Louisiana in April 2006 when it formed a partnership with St. Anne General Hospital in Raceland. "We have a very loyal patient following in the bayou region," Warner Thomas explained to *Louisiana Medical News,* "and have had a relationship dating back to the late 1990s. We are bringing in more physicians and more medical technology."[6]

In 2006, about the same time it formed its partnership with St. Anne General Hospital, Ochsner changed its formal name from Ochsner Clinic Foundation to Ochsner Health System. The name change was symbolic of what Ochsner had become in the wake of Katrina: a health system serving the needs of residents of a broad swath of southeast Louisiana and adjacent Gulf Coast Mississippi.

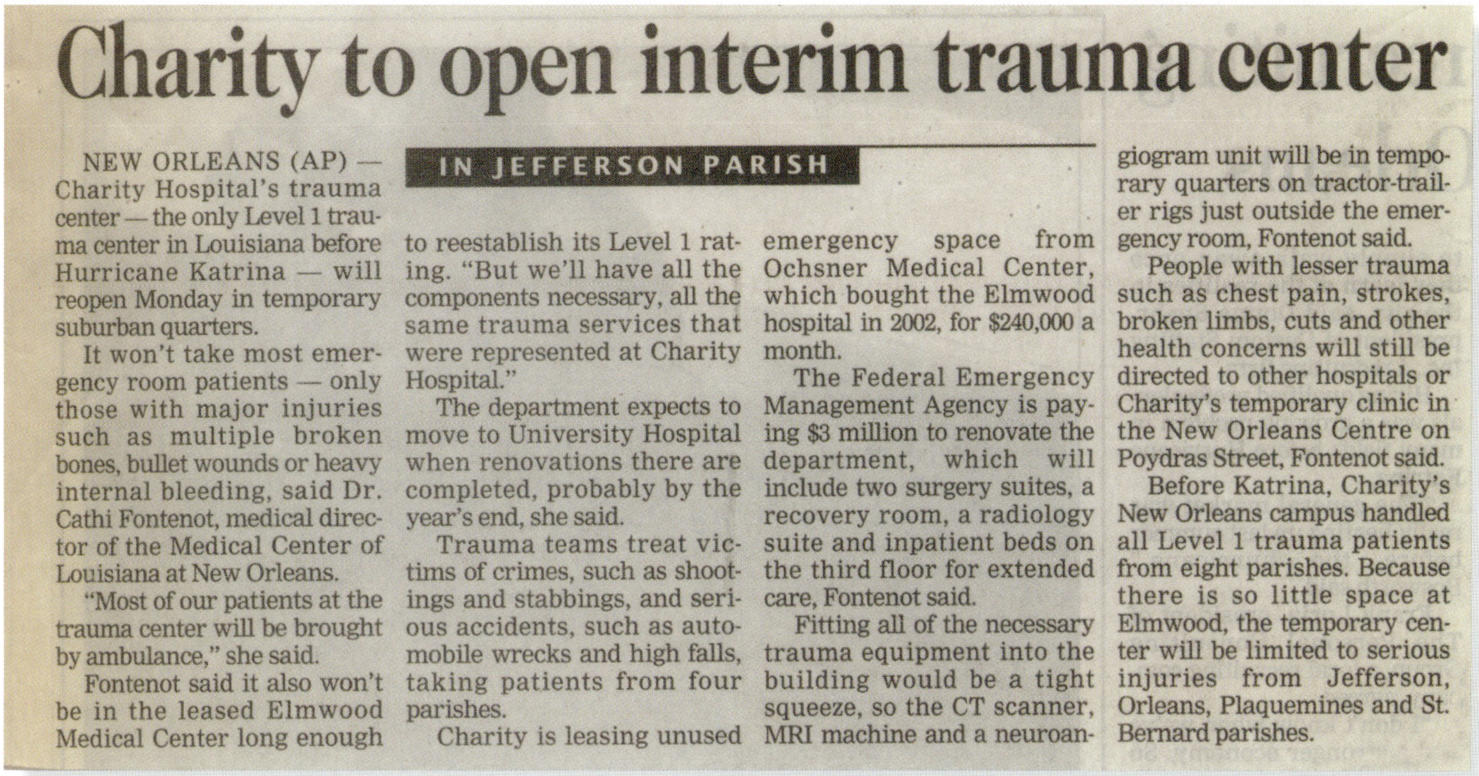

Charity to open interim trauma center

IN JEFFERSON PARISH

NEW ORLEANS (AP) — Charity Hospital's trauma center — the only Level 1 trauma center in Louisiana before Hurricane Katrina — will reopen Monday in temporary suburban quarters.

It won't take most emergency room patients — only those with major injuries such as multiple broken bones, bullet wounds or heavy internal bleeding, said Dr. Cathi Fontenot, medical director of the Medical Center of Louisiana at New Orleans.

"Most of our patients at the trauma center will be brought by ambulance," she said.

Fontenot said it also won't be in the leased Elmwood Medical Center long enough to reestablish its Level 1 rating. "But we'll have all the components necessary, all the same trauma services that were represented at Charity Hospital."

The department expects to move to University Hospital when renovations there are completed, probably by the year's end, she said.

Trauma teams treat victims of crimes, such as shootings and stabbings, and serious accidents, such as automobile wrecks and high falls, taking patients from four parishes.

Charity is leasing unused emergency space from Ochsner Medical Center, which bought the Elmwood hospital in 2002, for $240,000 a month.

The Federal Emergency Management Agency is paying $3 million to renovate the department, which will include two surgery suites, a recovery room, a radiology suite and inpatient beds on the third floor for extended care, Fontenot said.

Fitting all of the necessary trauma equipment into the building would be a tight squeeze, so the CT scanner, MRI machine and a neuroangiogram unit will be in temporary quarters on tractor-trailer rigs just outside the emergency room, Fontenot said.

People with lesser trauma such as chest pain, strokes, broken limbs, cuts and other health concerns will still be directed to other hospitals or Charity's temporary clinic in the New Orleans Centre on Poydras Street, Fontenot said.

Before Katrina, Charity's New Orleans campus handled all Level 1 trauma patients from eight parishes. Because there is so little space at Elmwood, the temporary center will be limited to serious injuries from Jefferson, Orleans, Plaquemines and St. Bernard parishes.

Ochsner offered LSU Medical Center of Louisiana, New Orleans space at its Elmwood facility for a Level 1 Trauma Center because New Orleans simply could not be without Level 1 trauma care in the wake of Katrina. American Press, *April 24, 2006*

'A MAJOR POSITIVE STEP'

The April 2006 lease of space at Ochsner Hospital – Elmwood to LSU and Charity Hospital was simply the precursor to a much more significant Ochsner commitment to the community to follow in July. With the city's healthcare system crippled by Katrina, it became apparent that many of the hospitals closed in the wake of the hurricane might never reopen. Those fears might well have become reality without Ochsner.

However, Ochsner stepped up. On July 19, 2006, Ochsner announced it was purchasing three New Orleans-area hospitals from Tenet Healthcare Corporation of Dallas, Texas, as Tenet had decided to leave the New Orleans market. Memorial Medical Center was still closed, nearly a year after the hurricane. Kenner Regional Medical Center was operating with a little over 40 percent of its 163 pre-Katrina beds, while Meadowcrest Hospital on the West Bank was operating at about 60 percent capacity.[7]

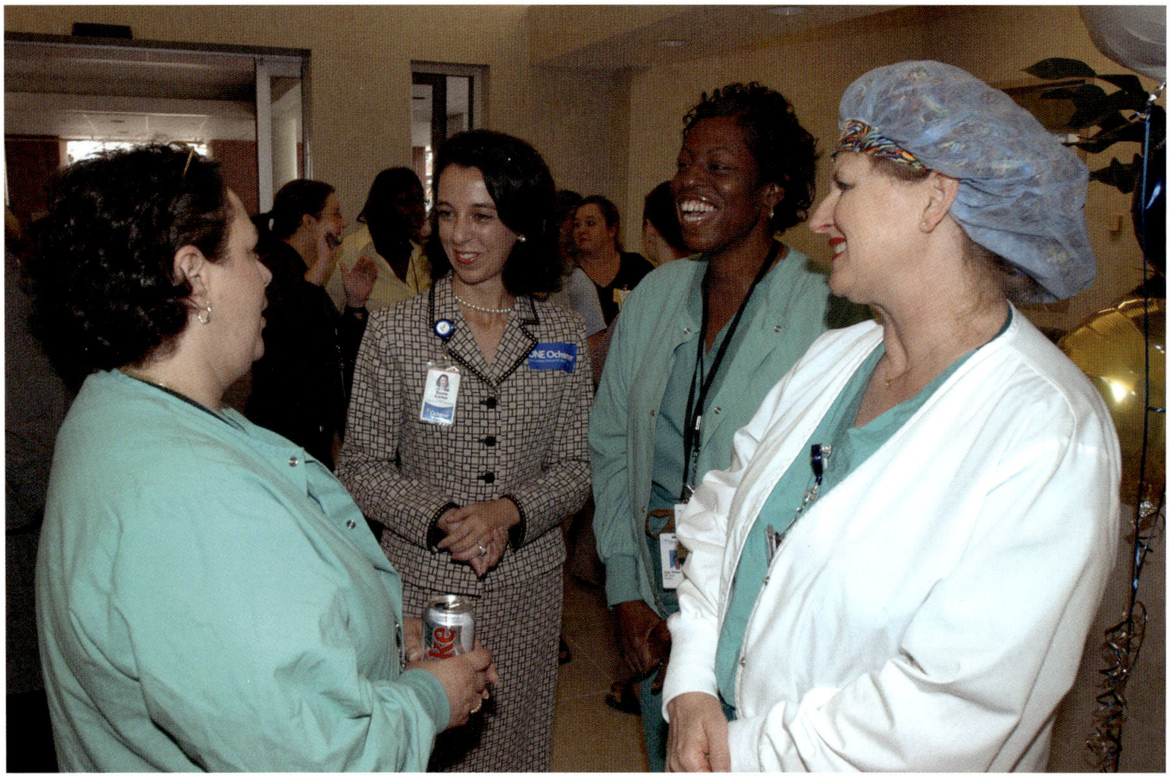

Sonia Carter and Patient Relations staff celebrate the grand reopening of Ochsner Baptist Medical Center.

A REFUGE FROM THE STORM

Built in 1926 as Southern Baptist Hospital, Memorial Medical Center—as it was known in 2005—was perhaps one of the chief victims of Hurricane Katrina. Located a couple of miles south of the French Quarter, the hospital occupied one of the lowest points of New Orleans, three feet below sea level. Local residents had gotten in the habit of seeking refuge at the hospital in time of storms.

When Katrina passed over that Monday morning, nearly 2,000 people had taken shelter in the hospital, more than half of them residents from the Uptown community surrounding Memorial. The winds blew, the tide surged and the walls withstood the gusts. Electric power was out just before 5 a.m. Monday, but the hospital's emergency generators cycled on flawlessly and lit emergency lights and needed equipment. The air conditioning was out, but with the exception of Ochsner, that was the condition of most hospitals in the path of the storm.[8]

What the staff at Memorial did not know at the time was that the surge of floodwater had breached industrial canals in the city. On Tuesday morning, August 30, administrators, physicians and employees watched helplessly as a wall of dirty brown water lazily made its way down Napoleon Avenue. By noon, Memorial Medical Center was effectively cut off from the outside world; early that afternoon, administrators began making plans to evacuate the more than 180 patients. The hospital's doctors and nurses quickly agreed that infants in the NICU, pregnant mothers and adult ICU patients should have priority in evacuating the hospital.[9]

Memorial spent the next three days evacuating patients and refugees from the hospital. Staff struggled against what sometimes seemed to be insurmountable problems, but with the use of a fleet of sport fishing boats organized by hospital employees, they began evacuating patients. Tenet Healthcare had chartered private helicopters to evacuate the hospital. All day on Thursday, September 1, helicopters descended on the parking garage roof in a steady stream. By 9 p.m., Memorial Medical Center had been evacuated.

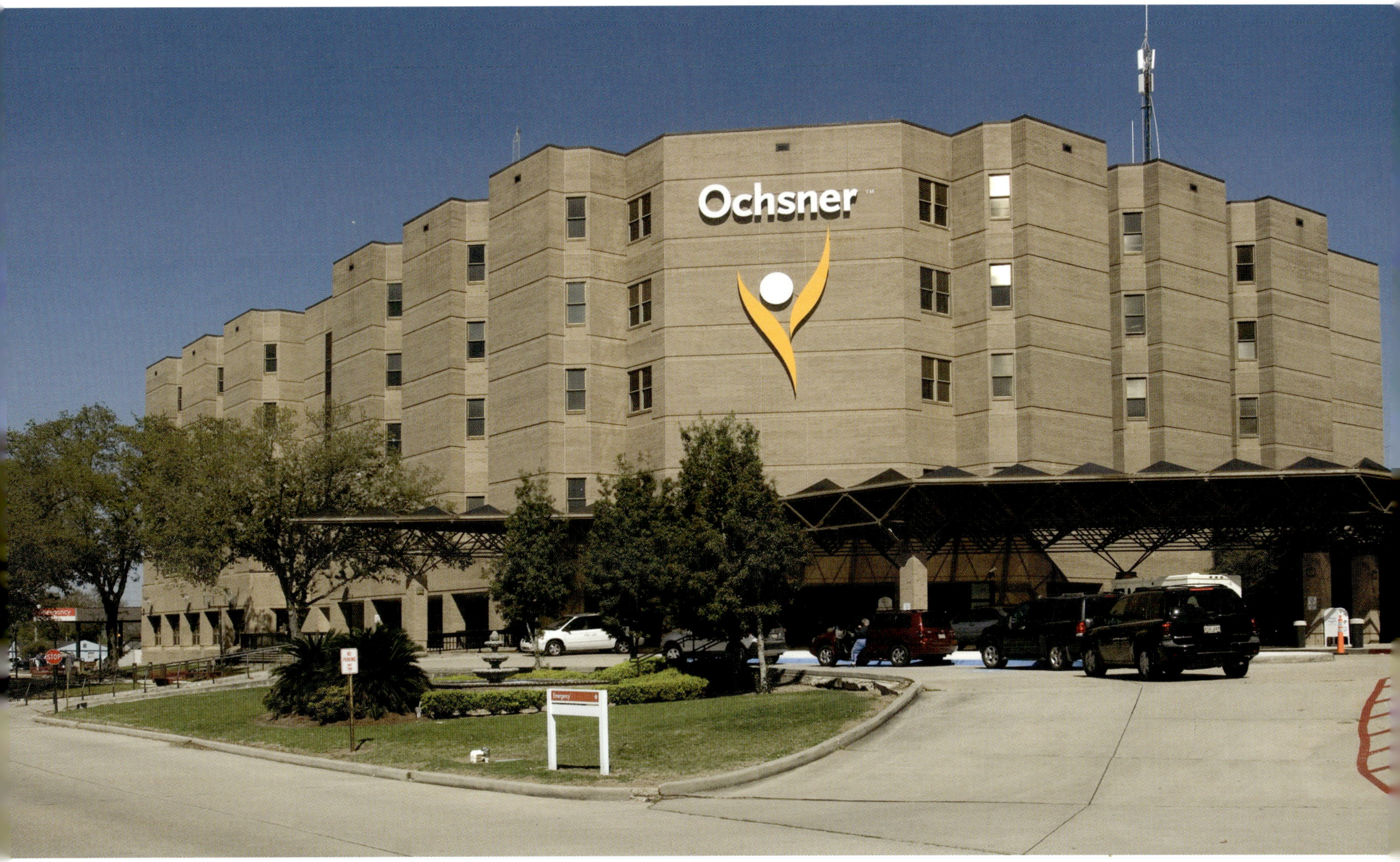

Kenner Regional Medical Center became Ochsner Medical Center – Kenner in July 2006.

• WHAT OCHSNER MEANS TO ME •

"Ochsner is about hope. Ochsner is about giving back to the community and being there for the community. Ochsner is about EXCELLENCE in everything we do. That is evident in the positive outcomes for our patients, and in our constant striving to be better."

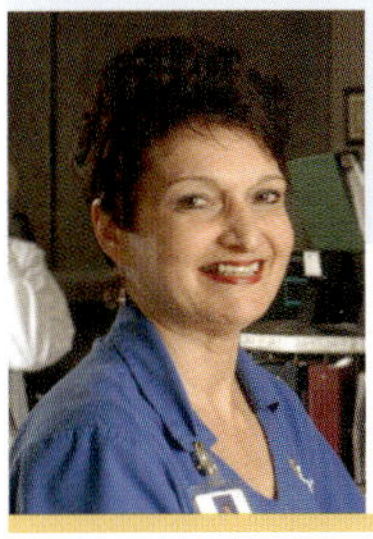

Joan Rooney, Assistant Vice President of Women's, Neonatal and Primary Care Services, Ochsner Medical Center – West Bank Campus

To watch the full interview with Joan Rooney, visit **ochsner.org/history**.

LEADING THE RECOVERY OF HEALTHCARE

Given the severe structural damage from the effects of Katrina to Memorial Medical Center, it would have been understandable if Ochsner had elected not to consider the acquisition of the Uptown hospital. Ochsner would have received more than enough kudos from the community for taking responsibility for Tenet's other New Orleans-area hospitals, Kenner Regional and Meadowcrest.

Ochsner had originally approached Tenet in October 2005 with the suggestion the two institutions partner in restoring quality healthcare to the community. Within a month, Tenet suggested to Ochsner that its three hospitals were for sale. Ochsner didn't hesitate. Ochsner and Tenet announced the transaction on October 1, 2006. Soon after, Ochsner announced plans to double the staffed beds of Ochsner Medical Center – Kenner and Ochsner Medical Center – West Bank Campus in order to bring more healthcare services to those areas. Plans also called to re-open medical surgery beds at Memorial—renamed Ochsner Baptist Medical Center—by late 2007. The Tenet purchase was the best example of Ochsner's commitment to lead the recovery of healthcare in New Orleans.

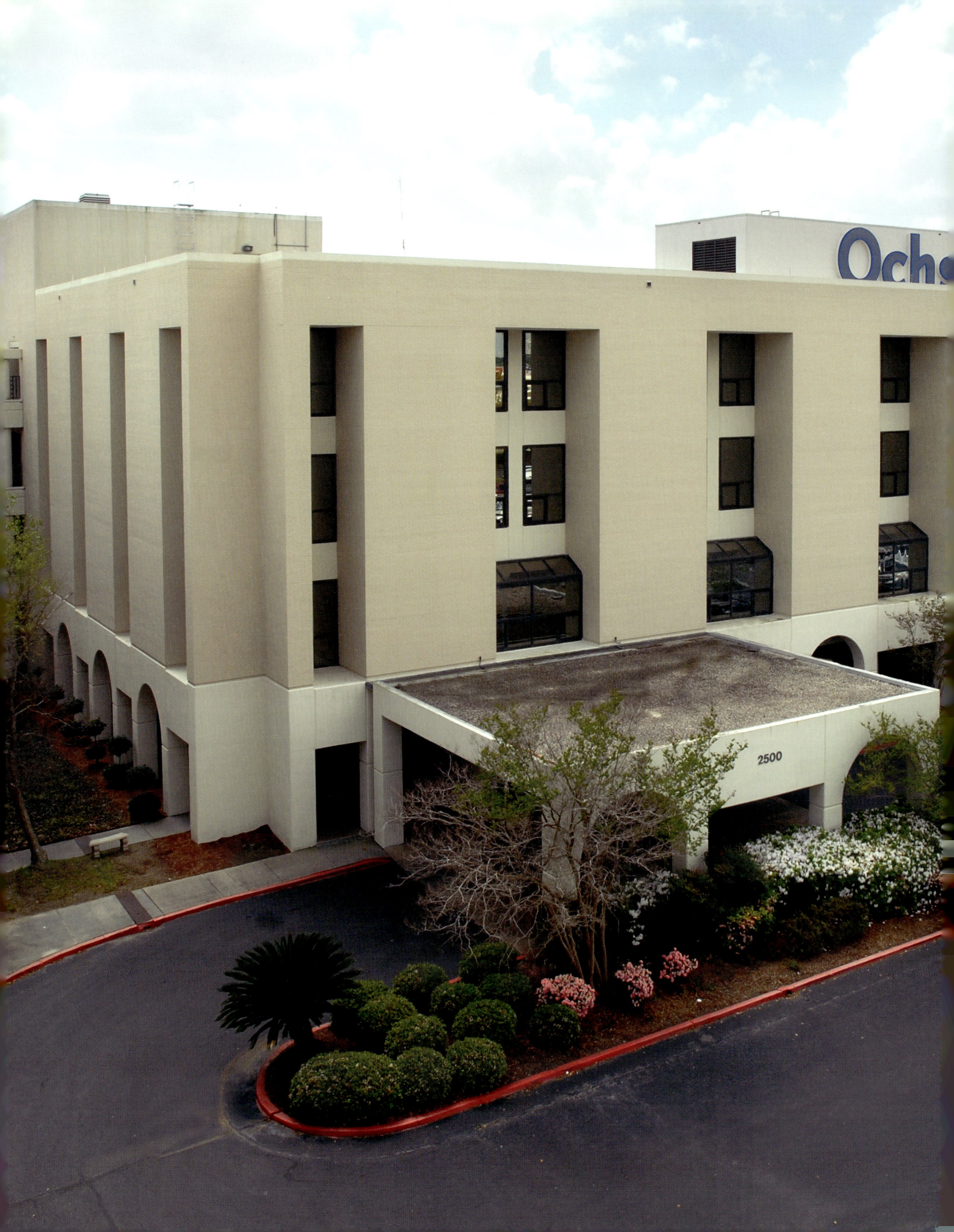
Ochs
2500

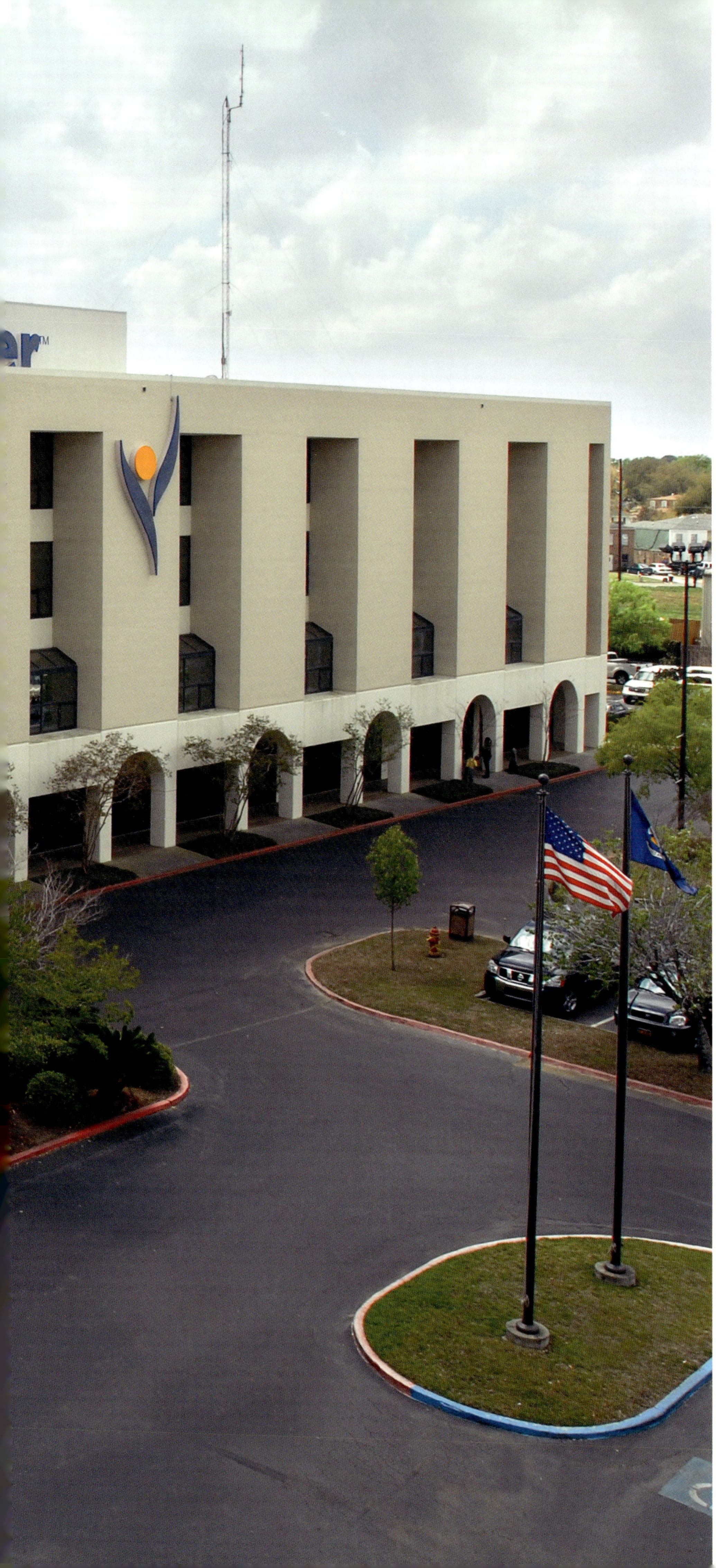

Ochsner Medical Center – West Bank Campus was known as Meadowcrest Hospital in Gretna before Ochsner purchased it in 2006.

'THE FOUNDERS OF OCHSNER WOULD HAVE DONE THE SAME'

Patrick Quinlan told New Orleans media in July 2006 that Ochsner's purchase of the three hospitals should help convince other businesses of the viability of New Orleans and should assure doctors, nurses and hospital workers that they had a future in the rebirth of the community.[10]

Quinlan went on to tell reporters that Ochsner would no longer be a "quiet company" content to step away from the glare of publicity and hide the work it does to better the community. "This can be a major positive step in changing the national perception of healthcare in New Orleans," he noted.[11] He added it was essential to stop the large and growing "brain drain" that occurred following Katrina.[12]

Rejoicing from the community greeted the news that Ochsner had upped the ante in its bid to help New Orleans recover from Katrina. Jack Finn, President of the Metropolitan Hospital Council of New Orleans, hailed the fact that "decisions will be made in our community rather than 1,000 miles away. That is the core of this transaction. Our community is going to have these facilities."[13]

The Tenet purchase represented an enormous financial risk for Ochsner, but one the organization was willing to take. Treasurer Bobby Brannon reported that Ochsner took out a $100 million bridge loan from Lehman Brothers to buy the hospitals. "That was part of $483 million in bonds," Brannon said. "Dr. Quinlan, the board, the management team—they all said, 'We need to do this now. Let's do it.'"[14]

OCHSNER HEALTH PLAN

One key financial milestone that paved the way for the acquisition of the three hospitals occurred before Katrina hit. The Ochsner Health Plan (OHP) had recouped much of its losses following the unification of the Clinic and Foundation. Terry Shilling, the Atlanta-based consultant who joined the Ochsner Health Plan full time in 2000, explained that the Foundation had made a capital infusion of $25 million into OHP, a factor that ultimately made the 2001 unification work.

"They gave them breathing room," Shilling described the Foundation's decision to invest in OHP. "They gave OHP management time to right the ship. It was merely a question of becoming more effective, more efficient. The organization already had a wonderful brand name."[15]

By 2003, the Plan had paid back $20 million of the $25 million in seed capital. Ochsner began to seriously investigate the feasibility of selling OHP. "They made the initial strategic decision in the spring of 2003," Shilling said. "The bottom line was that the capital deployed in the Health Plan, along with the capital derived from the sale of OHP, was better deployed in patient care and research. It was an $800 million entity. It was a huge risk profile."[16]

It was a decision Ochsner deemed worth making. Scott Posecai, Ochsner's CFO, and Executive Vice President and Director of Finance Bobby Brannon headed a team that investigated the potential sale of OHP. "We looked at potential buyers through CitiGroup," Posecai said. "We worked on that deal for quite some time. Eventually, we identified Humana as the best buyer."[17]

Negotiations with the Louisville, Kentucky-based health insurance giant continued throughout late 2003 into early 2004. In April, Ochsner and Humana announced an agreement in principle concerning the sale of OHP. What had been a liability turned into a multi-million dollar asset overnight. Without the financial boost to Ochsner's bottom line provided by the 2004 sale of OHP, Ochsner might never have been able to take a leadership role in acquiring the Tenet hospitals in 2006. Ochsner was able to leverage its OHP asset into an audacious plan that helped transform healthcare in New Orleans in the wake of Katrina.

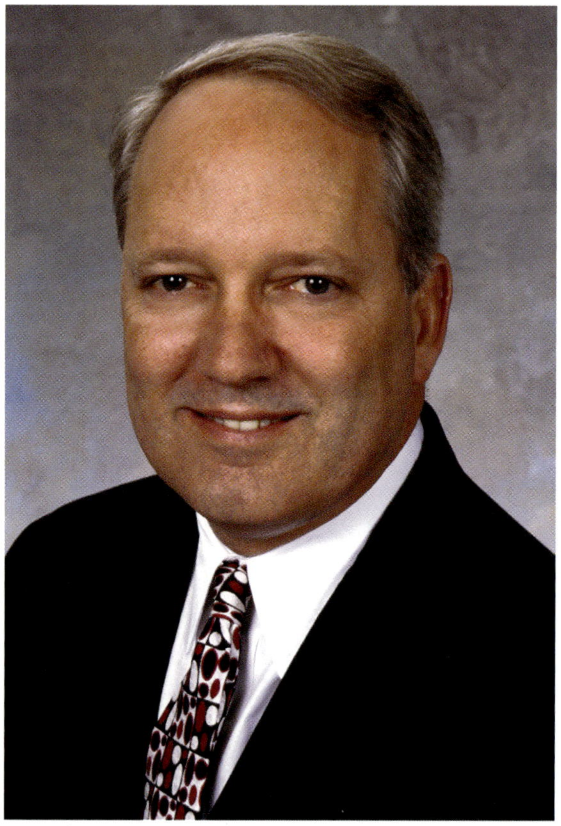

Terry Shilling was CEO of the Ochsner Health Plan and helped Ochsner turn around the ailing managed care plan.

The acquisition also was an immense cultural challenge for the organization as well as a financial risk. Ochsner had just unified five years before in 2001, integrating the staff and physicians of the Clinic and Hospital into Ochsner Health System. Now, Ochsner was preparing to integrate non-Ochsner physicians and staff into the system framework it had worked so strenuously to construct. It was one of the gutsiest moves in Ochsner's long history.

Skeptics said Ochsner might never get Memorial Medical Center reopened. Ochsner publicly pledged to reopen the hospital by the following year. It was renamed Ochsner Baptist Medical Center in honor of the facility's original name and 80-year New Orleans roots. In October 2006 the 10-bed New Orleans Surgery and Heart Institute on the Baptist campus reopened.[18] By the fall of 2007, Ochsner had invested $50 million in Ochsner Baptist and was completing the second part of a four-phase reopening and expansion plan for the hospital located at 2700 Napoleon Avenue in Uptown New Orleans.[19]

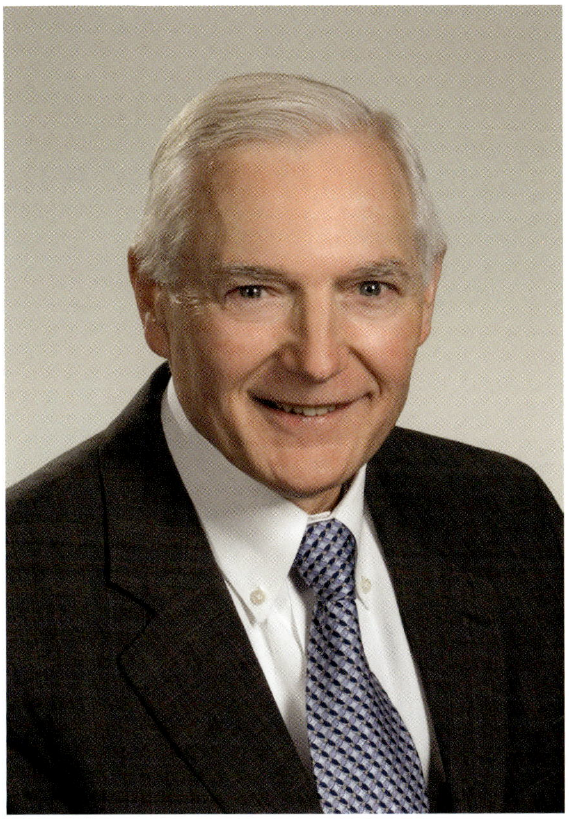

Bobby Brannon, Executive Vice President and Director of Finance, provided long-term financial leadership and secured the funding for the 2006 purchase of the Tenet hospitals.

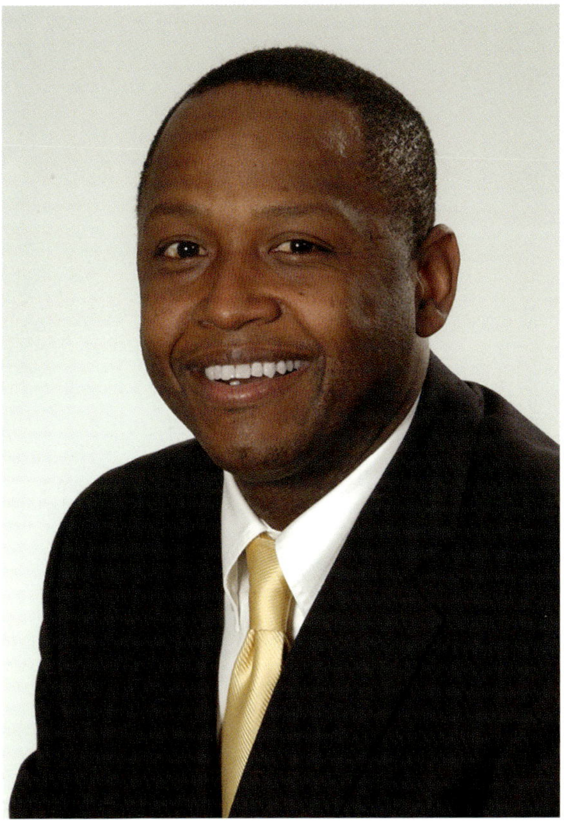

Yvens Laborde, M.D., is the Medical Director for West Bank Region.

Less than two years later, Ochsner Baptist was helping to spearhead the redevelopment of the nearby Freret Street business corridor recovery zone. Ochsner reclaimed part of the Clara Wing and reopened the two medical office buildings as well as the surgical hospital. The reopening of a brand new Ochsner Baptist Emergency Room in January 2009 gave further evidence that the Ochsner strategy of using healthcare investments to jumpstart economic development in New Orleans was working.[20]

The reopening and expansion of Ochsner Baptist Medical Center, Ochsner Medical Center – Kenner and Ochsner Medical Center – West Bank Campus was a shining example of the Ochsner Mission Warner Thomas called "doing great things for the community." For Ochsner, reopening and expanding the hospitals was the right thing to do, in spite of the financial risks involved. "We believe the founders of Ochsner would have done the same," the organization told stakeholders in its annual report.[21]

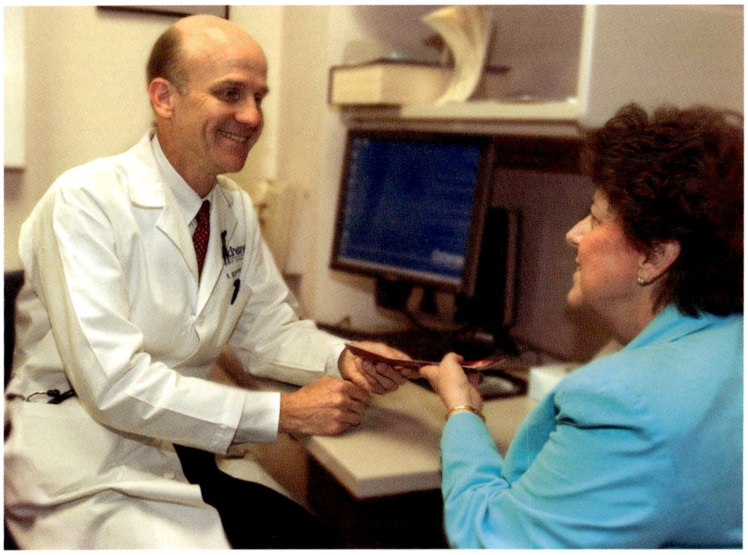

Richard E. Deichmann Jr., M.D., was Chair of Internal Medicine at the hospital that became Ochsner Baptist after Hurricane Katrina and joined the Ochsner staff after the storm.

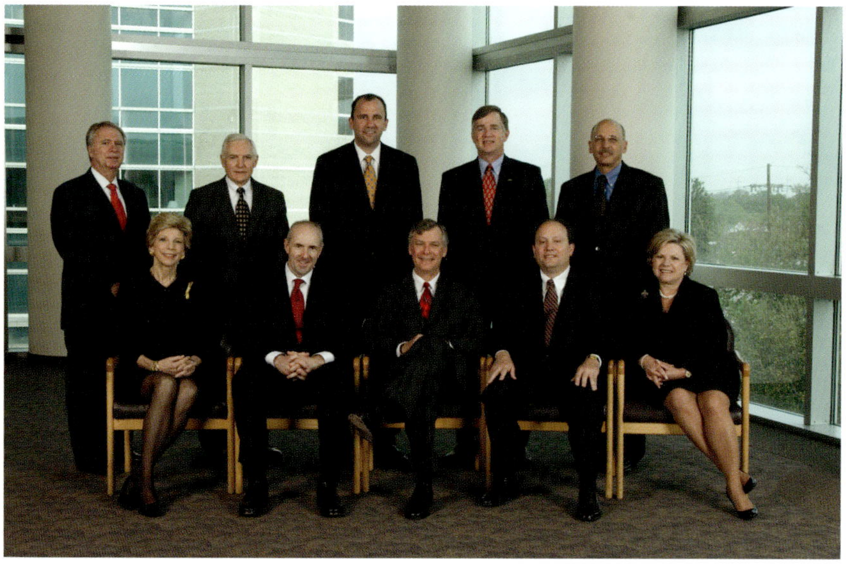

The Executive Operating Committee is responsible for the strategic direction Ochsner takes in the twenty-first century.

'A LOCALLY BASED HEALTHCARE SYSTEM'

Ochsner's commitment to "doing great things for the community" was exemplified by the ribbon-cutting ceremony for the Ochsner Baptist Imaging Center on November 14, 2007. The opening of the 22,000-square-foot facility on the Ochsner Baptist campus marked the completion of Phase 4 of Ochsner's overall plan to revitalize the Uptown facility. The new Imaging Center offered the latest state-of-the-art equipment and sophisticated medical imaging. Ochsner leadership also announced the Ochsner Baptist Imaging Center would begin offering radiation therapy services in January 2008.

Warner Thomas told attendees at the Imaging Center ribbon-cutting that "just two months ago, we unveiled this campus' two-year plan—and we're right on track. We are already moving forward with Phase 5: the renovation of the Clara Wing."[22]

Thomas went on to say that "Ochsner has grown tremendously in the past year, and I want to assure you that we are first and foremost a locally based healthcare system that supports our local physicians as well as Ochsner physicians. We are excited about the momentum and positive physician and patient response to our Baptist campus. We'll continue to expand the services on this campus and bring more services back to the residents of the Uptown area and Orleans Parish."[23]

Patrick Quinlan told the ribbon-cutting crowd that Ochsner viewed the revitalization of Baptist as a catalyst for future growth in New Orleans. He pledged Ochsner's commitment to the city's future and rededicated Ochsner's efforts to continue to expand medical services in Orleans and surrounding parishes.

"Ochsner was founded on the mission to provide quality healthcare to the communities we serve, and for the Baptist campus our community includes all of the Uptown neighborhoods," he said. "Ochsner Baptist is here to serve the needs of the community, physicians and their patients."[24]

Curtis Dosch, Chief Executive Officer of Ochsner Baptist Medical Center at the time, reported the hospital was undergoing a literal rebirth, with more than 170 active physicians on staff. By the time the new Imaging Center opened, Ochsner Baptist was performing more than 220 surgical procedures a month.

Dosch paid special compliments to Ochsner Baptist's facilities and information technology teams for making the new Imaging Center possible. "Getting this campus in shape is an ongoing joint effort," he said, adding that "hundreds of people have been working night and day for months."[25]

Dosch told the crowd that Ochsner's commitment to Baptist was contagious and none of the improvements would have happened without the direction and support of Baptist's new owners. "I am proud of this facility," he said, "and I'm proud of Ochsner's commitment and dedication to rebuild it for the community."[26]

New Orleans City Councilman Arnie Fielkow summed up the feelings of Uptown residents when he paid tribute to Ochsner for all it had done and was doing to bring Baptist back. "Ochsner has proven to this community that it is committed to bringing back the Baptist campus for Uptown residents," Fielkow said. "Today's opening is one more example of Ochsner's promise to revitalize this campus and to help rebuild healthcare in the region."[27]

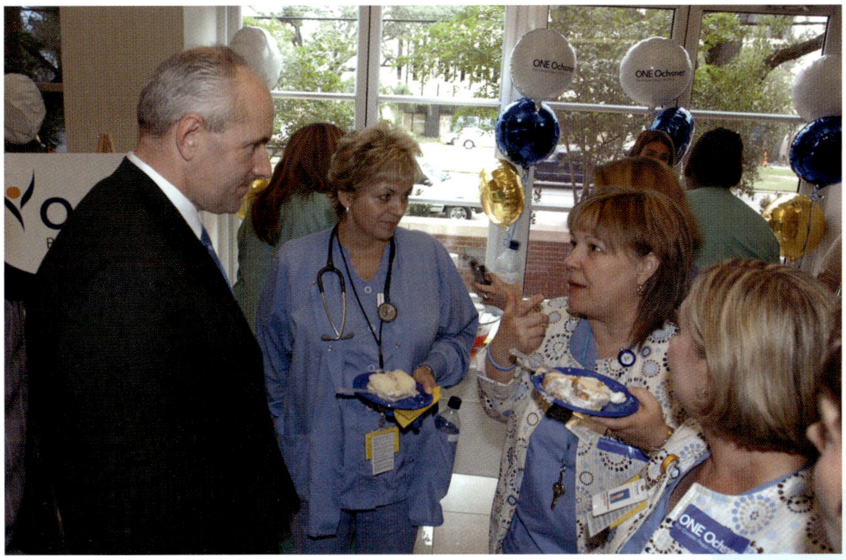

President and COO Warner Thomas welcomes Memorial Medical Center employees to Ochsner at a celebration and open house held immediately following the 2006 acquisition.

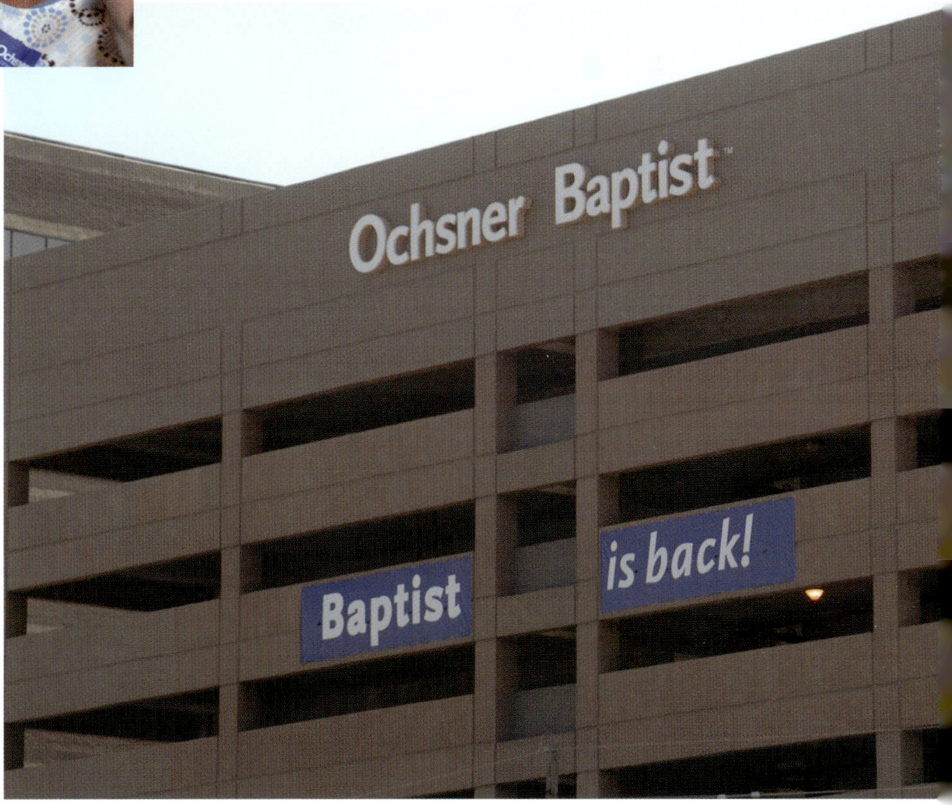

The "Baptist is Back" sign on the Ochsner Baptist parking garage announced to the world that a longtime member of the New Orleans healthcare community was once again open for business.

COMMITTED TO BRINGING BAPTIST BACK

Ochsner's decision to acquire the three Tenet hospitals gave a new lease on life to the thousands of employees of the three facilities who feared their jobs and livelihood were in jeopardy.

JoAnn Cardaro, Unit Director of the ICU at Ochsner Baptist, was operating a 10-bed surgical unit when Ochsner acquired Baptist in 2006. In short order, Ochsner expanded the unit from 10 beds to 36 beds. "That changed a lot of my role," Cardaro said, "going from 10 beds to 36. We hired more staff, and pretty soon, we were planning and organizing for the move into the new wing in January 2009."[28]

Cardaro gave credit to Ochsner's decision to restore Baptist. "Ochsner was committed to bringing Baptist back to the Uptown community," Cardaro said. "Knowing we were able to bring Baptist back was truly inspirational to me."[29]

Since joining the Ochsner team, Cardaro said she could feel the commitment to the patient, excellence and quality medicine in a way she never experienced in her healthcare career before. It was a feeling that was shared by most of the staff of the Tenet hospitals. "I can really take pride in that," Cardaro said. "What I believe, they focus on."[30]

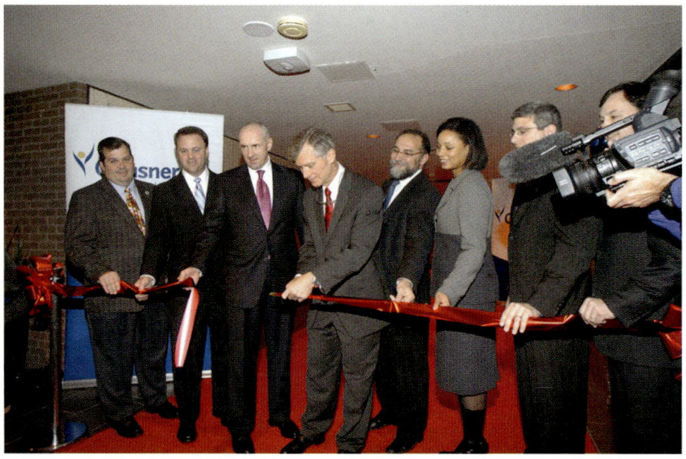

Ochsner renamed Memorial Medical Center as Ochsner Baptist Medical Center, bringing back a name familiar to generations of local residents.

'WE'VE COME A LONG WAY'

Just 14 months after opening the new Imaging Center at Ochsner Baptist Medical Center, Ochsner hosted a second ribbon cutting to commemorate the opening of the new Baptist Emergency Room and Clara Wing. The January 12, 2009, dedication ceremony celebrated the opening of a full-service Emergency Room, a 43-private bed Clara Hospital Wing and an expanded Intensive Care Unit.

Ochsner had completed the Phase 5 rebuilding of Baptist in the teeth of the worst recession to hit the United States since the Great Depression. Ochsner ignored the financial conditions and forged ahead with Phase 5 because it fostered the system's goal of doing great things for the community. Patrick Quinlan explained the new community resources at Baptist would help ease Emergency Room crowding, bring medical care closer to the hospital's Uptown community home and provide local physicians with a facility that met their patients' needs.

James Maurin, a well-known local developer and 2009 Chair of the Ochsner Health System Board of Directors, pointed out Ochsner's investment in rebuilding Baptist was a sign of its strong conviction to always do what's best for patients. "The fact that Ochsner is willing to invest over $30 million to revitalize a single facility should serve as a symbol of hope for our region and a sign that this organization is willing to go the extra mile for the citizens of New Orleans and the patients and physicians of Baptist," Maurin said.[31]

Rob Wolterman, who was named Chief Executive Officer of Ochsner Baptist in 2008, noted another addition to the Baptist campus being initiated that winter was Ochsner's electronic medical records system. "Beyond all the technology," Wolterman said, "was the work of Baptist's employees. This campus has an extraordinarily committed staff that believes in this facility, its history and its name, and they have worked tirelessly to bring this campus back."[32]

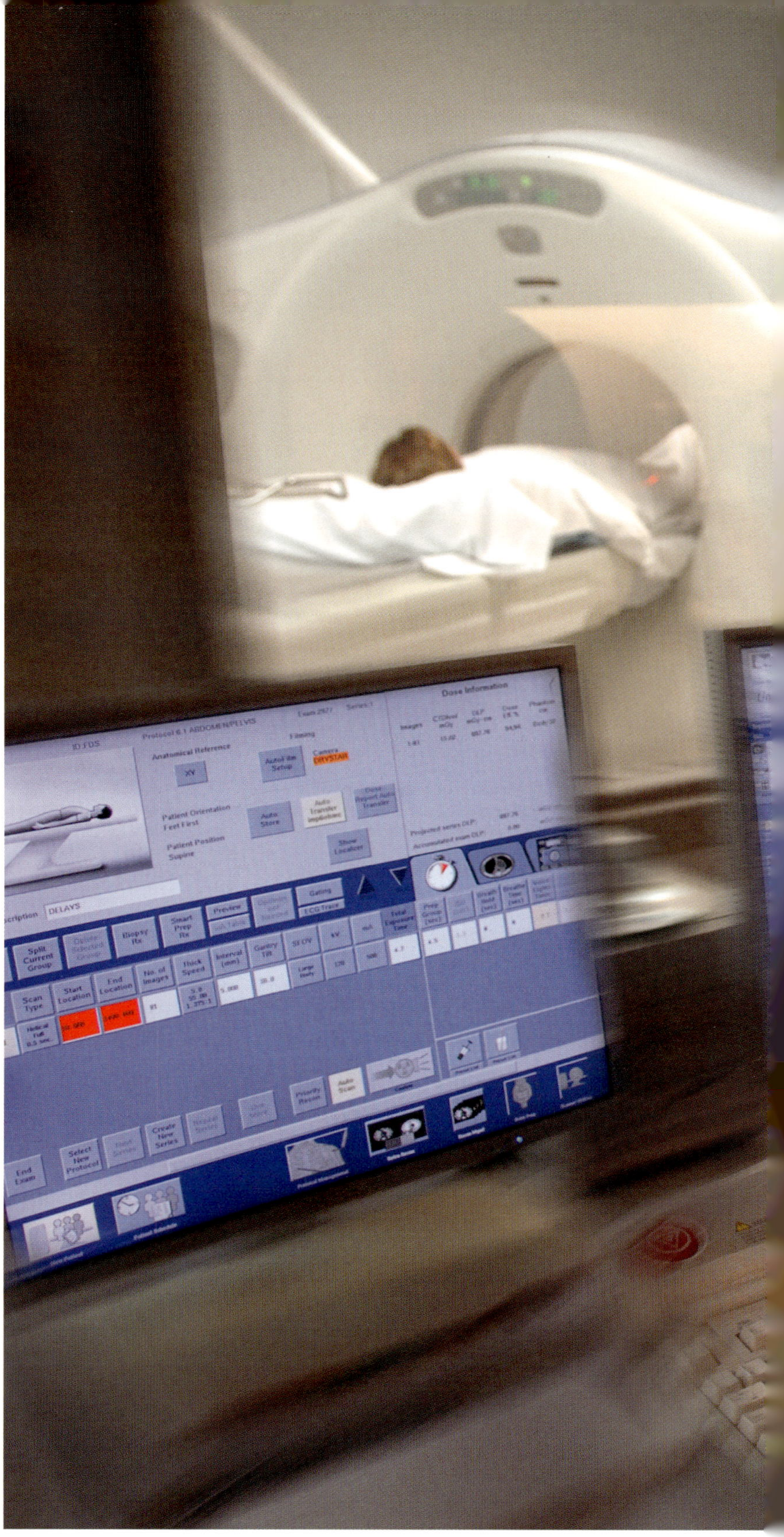

Seconding those sentiments was Patrick Quinlan. "Three years ago, we assumed ownership of this campus and New Orleans was struggling," he said. "After watching construction at Ochsner Baptist for the past three years, I'm proud of what our city has accomplished, of Ochsner's contribution and of the people who've helped rebuild and revitalize our city. We've come a long way!"[33]

He wasn't the only one feeling a sense of pride. The day Ochsner Baptist opened its new Emergency Room was a source of immense pride to JoAnn Cardaro and her co-workers. "That day," she said, "I was truly proud. It

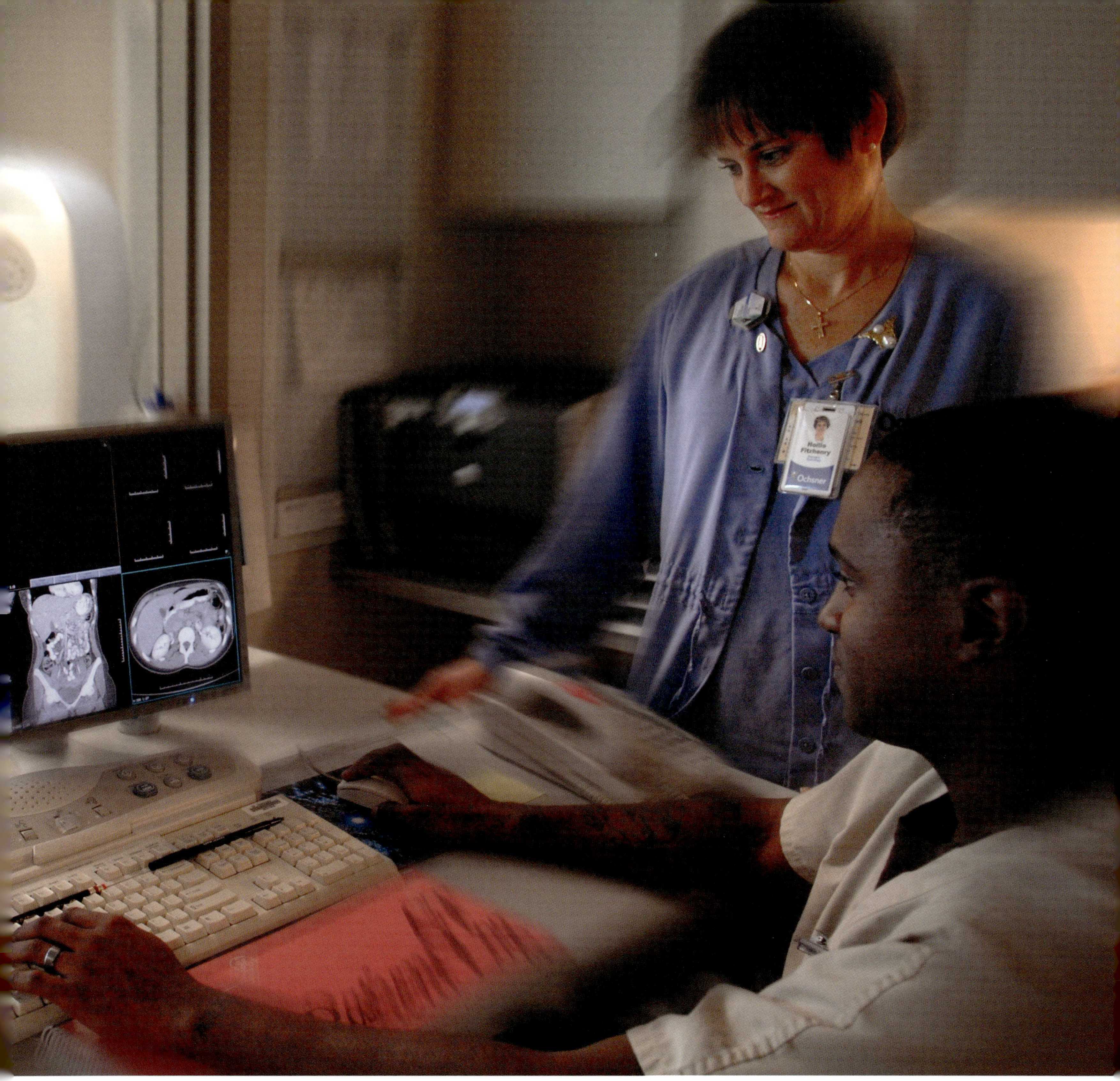

would not have happened without the leadership of Ochsner. We worked together as a team."[34]

Quinlan viewed Ochsner's support of the new Emergency Room and Clara Wing at Baptist as a continuation of the legacy handed down to Ochsner and its employees by Alton Ochsner and the other founders. "As stewards of the community, Ochsner is committed to improving our neighbors' health through education, medical care and community involvement," he said. "This is part of our mission, and one we will continue to build upon."[35]

The Ochsner Baptist Imaging Center on Napoleon Avenue in New Orleans was part of the $30 million in investments that Ochsner has made since 2006 to make Ochsner Baptist a leader in state-of-the-art healthcare.

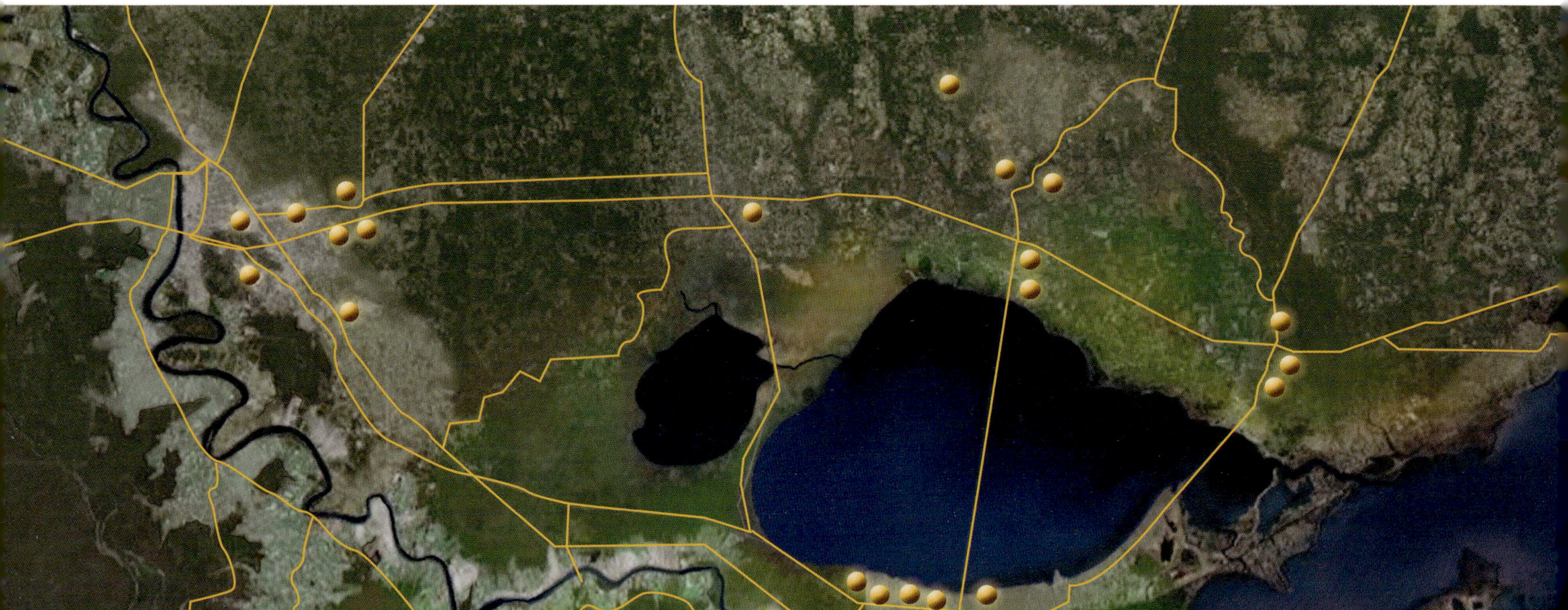
Ochsner™
Healthcare With Peace Of Min

CHAPTER 13:

EXERCISING HEALTHCARE LEADERSHIP

IN JANUARY 2008, OCHSNER HEALTH SYSTEM and the Louisiana Organ Procurement Association (LOPA) held a joint press conference to announce they were joining together to issue a challenge to Louisiana residents and businesses to consider the life-saving benefits of organ donation. The two institutions called their new program "Make Life Happen."[1]

LOPA Executive Director Kelly Ranum was at the press conference at the Brent House Hotel Conference Center to present the Number One Donor Award to Ochsner and to stress the importance of organ donation. Dr. Patrick Quinlan accepted the award on behalf of Ochsner and announced that the entire Health System had become a LOPA "Workplace Partner," pledging to inform its more than 10,000 employees about the benefits of donating life. Ochsner's support of the innovative program was further evidence of the healthcare system's emergence as a community leader in medicine.

Quinlan said he was proud "to announce that Ochsner has reached several major medical milestones; this year we are celebrating our 1000th liver, 1000th kidney and 700th heart transplant. That's 2,700 lives saved thanks to our physicians, nurses, anesthesiologists, transplant coordinators, social workers and entire medical, surgical, administrative and clerical staff who work daily with transplant patients. That's 2,700 lives that were saved by organ donors—people who made the decision, and their wishes known, while they were alive and healthy."[2]

Ochsner is the largest private, not-for-profit healthcare system in southeast Louisiana.

Quinlan challenged peers and business colleagues to become LOPA "Workplace Partners" and educate employees on organ donation and how the decisions they make today can save lives tomorrow. "Ochsner's 1,000 livers, 1,000 kidneys and 700 hearts demonstrate that organ donation does save lives," Quinlan told the press conference, which was beamed via video conference to a number of Ochsner facilities, including Ochsner North Shore, Ochsner St. Anne and Ochsner Baton Rouge.[3]

Hector Ventura, M.D., a cardiologist associated with Ochsner for more than a quarter-century, told the conference he had recently treated a Baton Rouge man for three years "fighting to save his heart and his life. In the end, he needed a heart transplant and thanks to someone like you, who signed up to be an organ donor, we were able to save his life and mark our 700th heart transplant."[4]

Ventura went on to say that organ transplantation is "truly a team effort to save a life and Ochsner has a great team. Only a handful of hospitals around the world can say they've saved over 2,700 lives in transplant operations, and I'm proud to be part of this team."[5]

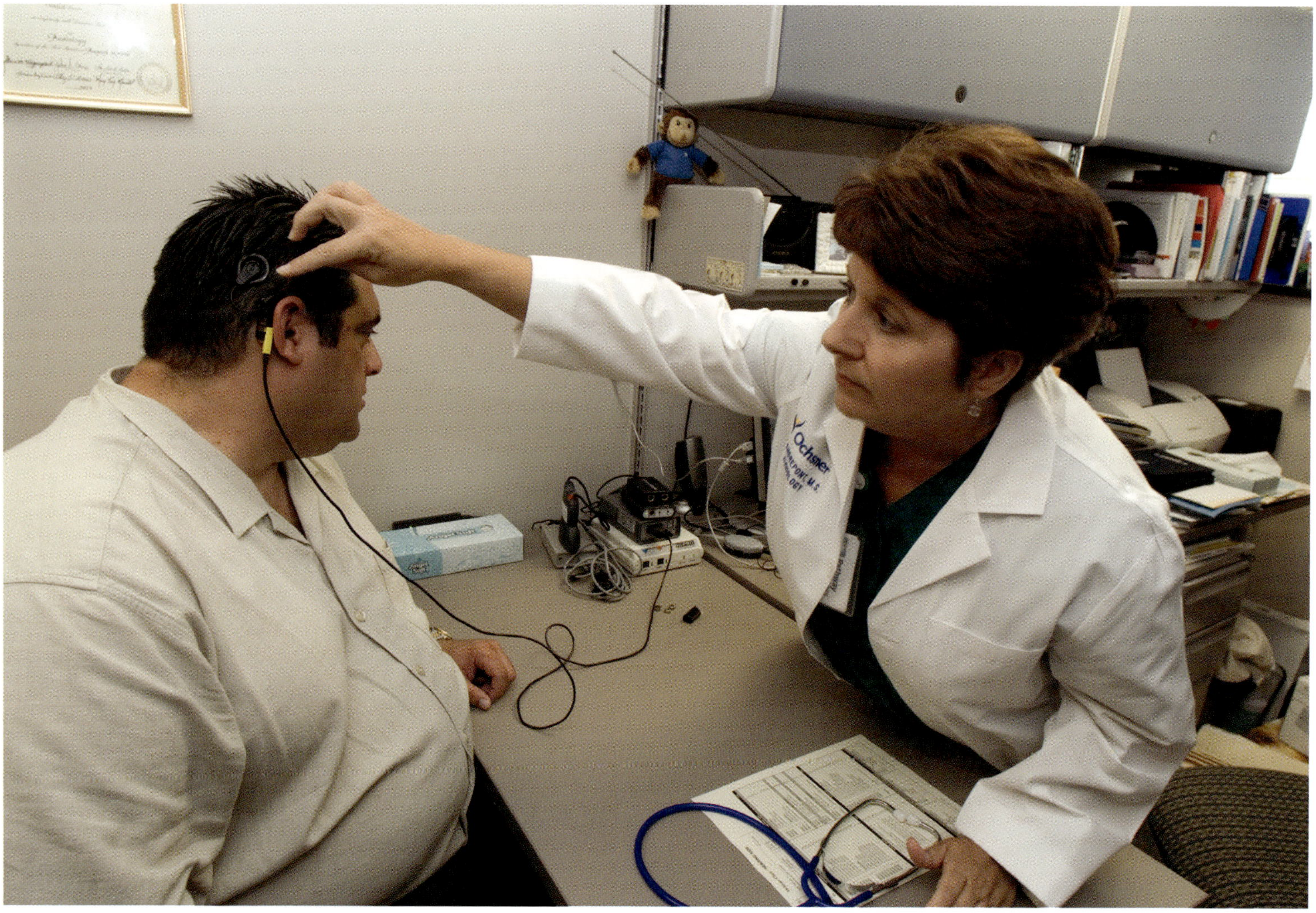

Since 1990, more than 300 people have been helped by cochlear implants performed by surgeons at Ochsner Medical Center. The implants, which stimulate the hearing nerve in the inner ear, help both adults and juveniles afflicted with profound hearing loss to regain much of their hearing.

• WHAT OCHSNER MEANS TO ME •

"It's really about the people here. We have a lot of great buildings and a lot of great technology, but frankly so do a lot of other places. The difference is our PEOPLE. I think we have some of the best physicians, the best surgeons, the best nurses and the best staff in the country. They are a cut above the rest."

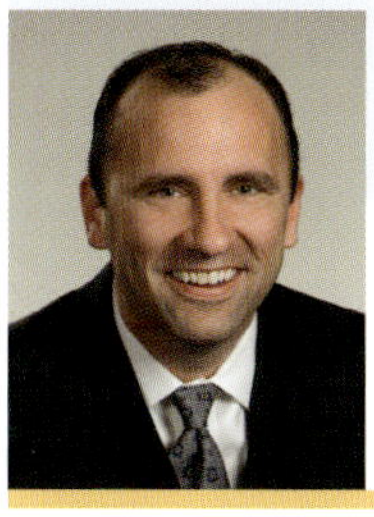

Mike Hulefeld, Chief Executive Officer, Ochsner Medical Center

To watch the full interview with Mike Hulefeld, visit **ochsner.org/history**.

THE BEST MEDICAL RESULTS

The transplant conference of early 2008 served as a reminder that even after undergoing one of the worst natural disasters in American history, Ochsner Health System had firmly fixed its sights on delivering the best medical results it possibly could. The pursuit of excellence continued to drive everything Ochsner did in the wake of Katrina.

Warner Thomas has operational responsibility for Ochsner's hospital locations, regional neighborhood health center locations and all corporate functions. Establishing Ochsner as a healthcare institution that exemplifies the best medical results in the United States is a passion he shares with Patrick Quinlan and the other members of the Ochsner leadership team.

"According to HealthGrades®, Ochsner is in the top 5 percent of hospitals in the United States in clinical outcomes," Thomas said. "We are a diamond here in New Orleans that is continuing to get better. It is such a treasure to have in the area. And we have always had a patient focus."[6]

Over the years, Ochsner has been ranked many times by *U.S. News & World Report* and the July 15, 2009, issue named them one of "America's Best Hospitals" in three categories: Heart and Heart Surgery, Ear Nose and Throat and Urology.[7] "There are many 'best lists,'" Quinlan noted in an August 2009 press conference, "but *U.S. News'* rankings are recognized by the medical community as one of the most commercially unbiased. It's a comprehensive representation of hospitals with ranking quality care, quality staff, academic prominence and cutting-edge technology. This annual list reflects the top one percent of all hospitals in the nation."[8] Ochsner was the only hospital in Louisiana and Mississippi to be listed in the prestigious survey.

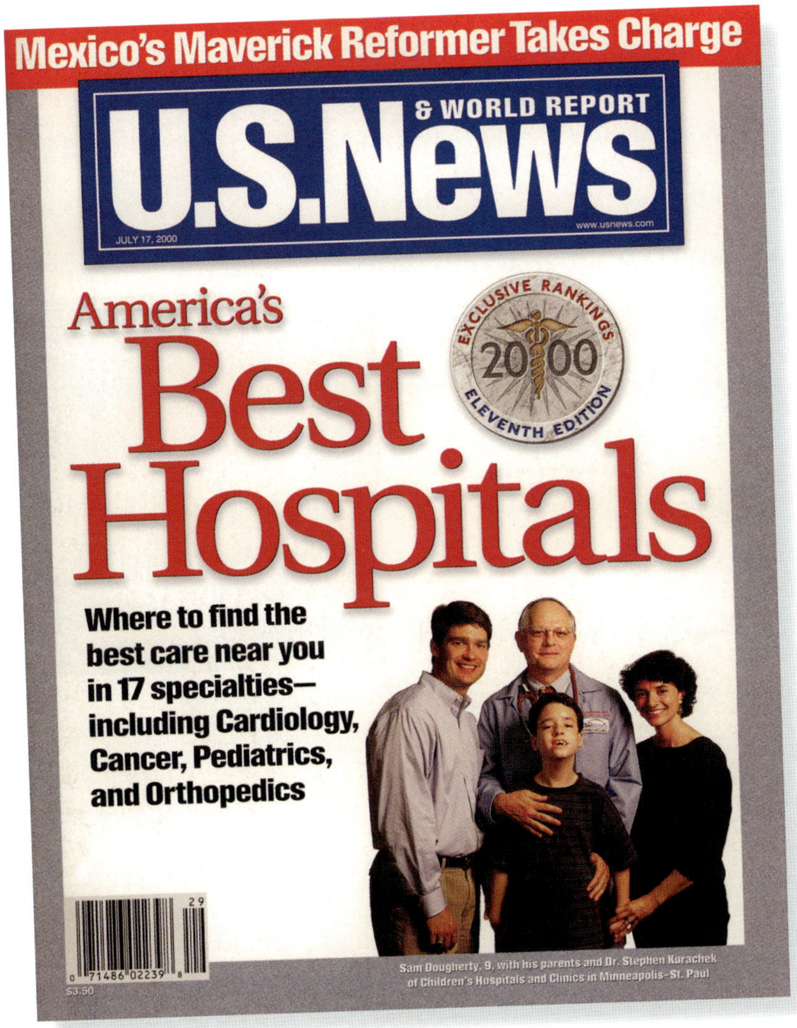

Ochsner remains the only New Orleans-area hospital honored as one of "America's Best Hospitals" by U.S. News & World Report.

Ochsner received further confirmation of its status as one of the nation's elite hospitals early in 2010 when HealthGrades, the nation's leading independent healthcare ratings organization, singled out Ochsner Medical Center as the only Louisiana hospital ranked in the top 5 percent in the U.S. The ratings organization's *8th Annual Hospital Quality and Clinical Excellence Study* identified Ochsner as one of 269 of more than 5,000 U.S. hospitals that received HealthGrades' *Distinguished Hospitals for Clinical Excellence* Award.[9] The study pointed out that "patients who choose to receive their care at a *Distinguished Hospital for Clinical Excellence* will have a lower risk for an adverse clinical outcome relative to all other hospitals."[10]

Ochsner patients, many of them the second or third generation of their families to seek treatment at Ochsner, didn't need to be told that Ochsner was a Distinguished Hospital for Clinical Excellence. They knew clinical excellence when they walked through the doors at Ochsner.

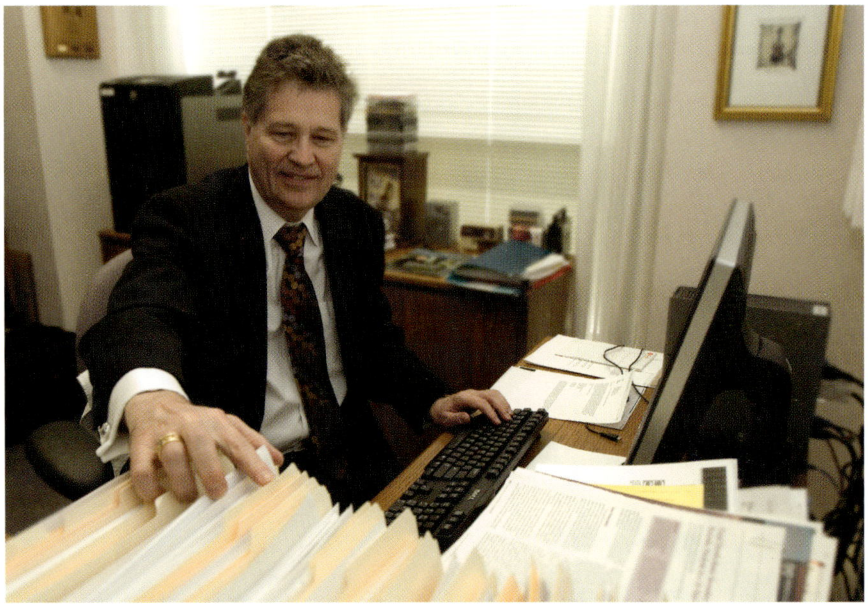

Lynn Witherspoon, M.D. serves as Ochsner's System Vice President, Chief Medical Information Officer. He was critical in guiding the organization in its adaptation of electronic medical records and planned the expansion of the organization's information technology.

A HEALTHCARE MODEL

Beyond being an honor for the Ochsner team and promising news for Louisiana residents, the HealthGrades rankings were a reaffirmation of the fact that Ochsner Health System was leading a revitalization of healthcare in New Orleans and surrounding Louisiana parishes, just four years after Katrina came ashore with such devastating consequences.

Ochsner correctly noted that the HealthGrades rankings were driven by hard data that included reputation, death rates, patient safety and care-related factors such as nursing and patient services. The reality was that because of Ochsner, New Orleans residents four years after the hurricane were receiving healthcare equal to or better than the healthcare offered in other areas of the country.

"We began working with HealthGrades in 2005 to improve our patient outcomes, lower complication rates and decrease mortality rates in cardiovascular diseases, pulmonary disorders, sepsis, stroke, and most recently, orthopedics," explained Dr. Sandra Kemmerly, Ochsner Medical Director for Clinical Practice Improvement. As a result, Ochsner concentrated its efforts on delivering reliable, standardized care, based on scientific evidence. "As we've expanded these processes throughout our hospital," Kemmerly said, "we're seeing improvements in all the patients we serve."[11]

Patrick Quinlan and the leadership team took great pride in the HealthGrades rankings. "This award is a reflection of our mission and the promise we make to our patients every day: to serve, heal, lead, educate and innovate," he said."[12]

Warner Thomas added that Ochsner could become a living model for healthcare in the twenty-first century. "President Obama appeared at the Cleveland Clinic earlier this year and talked about the fact that the Cleveland Clinic is the model everybody in the healthcare community should emulate," Thomas said in 2010. "Ochsner is an integrated system that fits that model. There is a team of practitioners. The clinical team coordinates the care of patients."[13]

For Thomas and the Ochsner leadership team, the larger challenge resides in the general healthcare community, where there is a lack of coordination and outright fragmentation. "Ochsner is further integrating hospitals into its system," he explained. "That's our role, and definitely the right model. So how can we be the integrator of healthcare in the region? How do we spread the model to others?"[14]

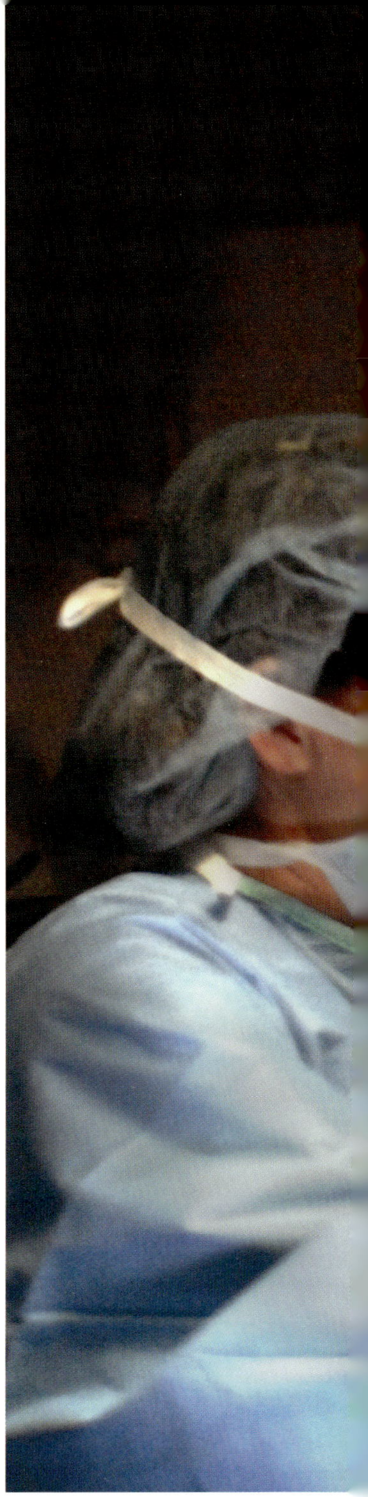

John Bolton, M.D., shown here during a surgical procedure, is the Chairman of Ochsner's Department of Surgery. Bolton is a Surgical Oncologist as well as an accomplished General Surgeon.

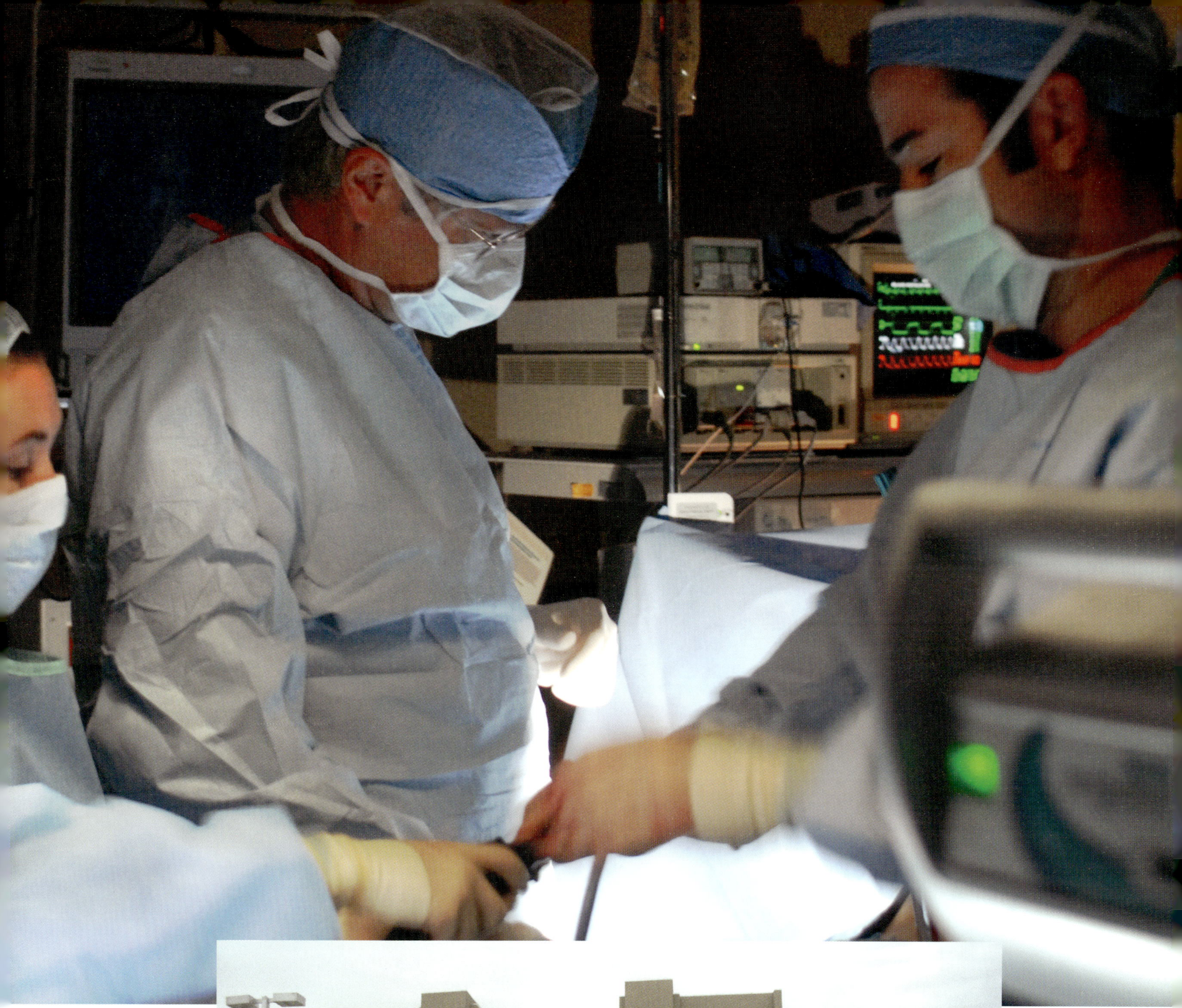

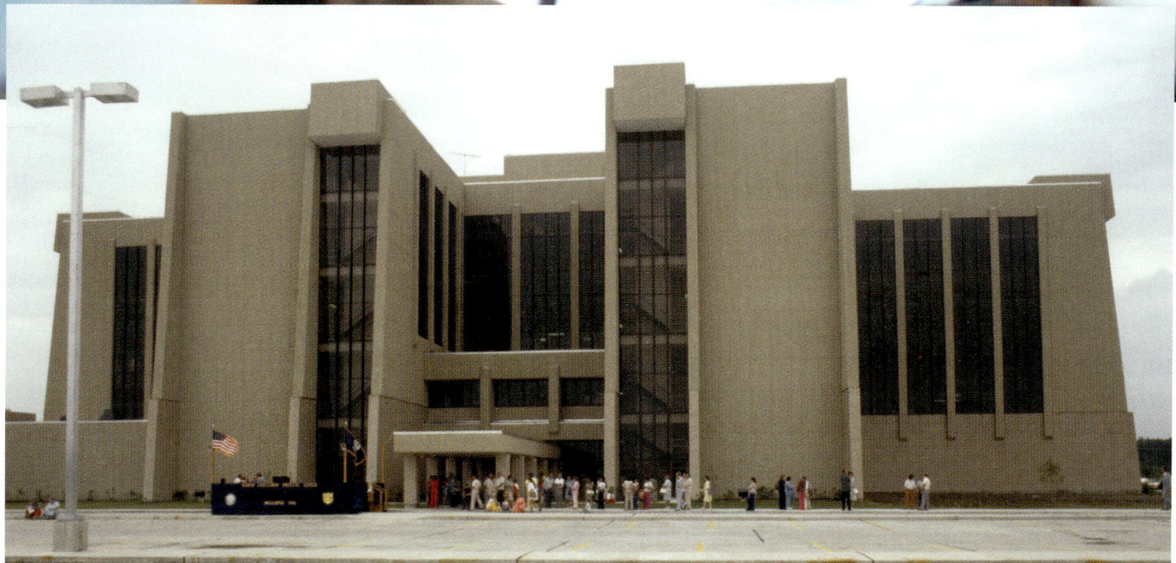

Since the mid-1970s, Ochsner has enjoyed an effective, mutually beneficial relationship with Leonard J. Chabert Memorial Hospital in Houma, 75 miles southwest of New Orleans. For much of that period, Ochsner residents in several specialties have received education and training at the Houma hospital.

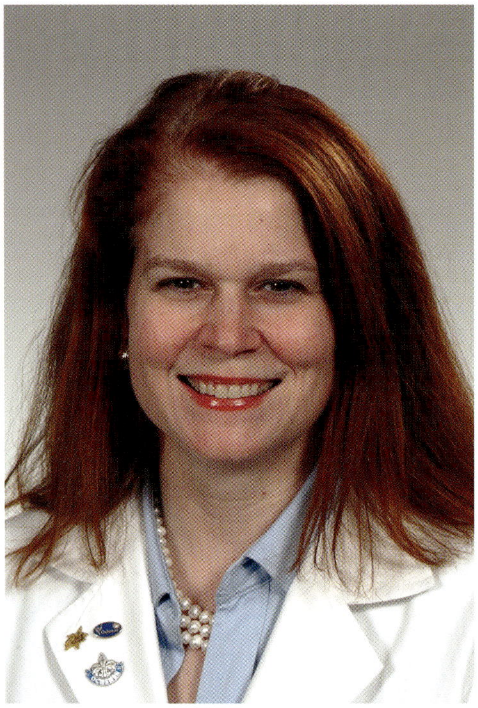

A Radiologist at Lieselotte Tansey Breast Center and Section Head for Breast Imaging, Dana Smetherman, M.D. helped bring digital mammography to Ochsner.

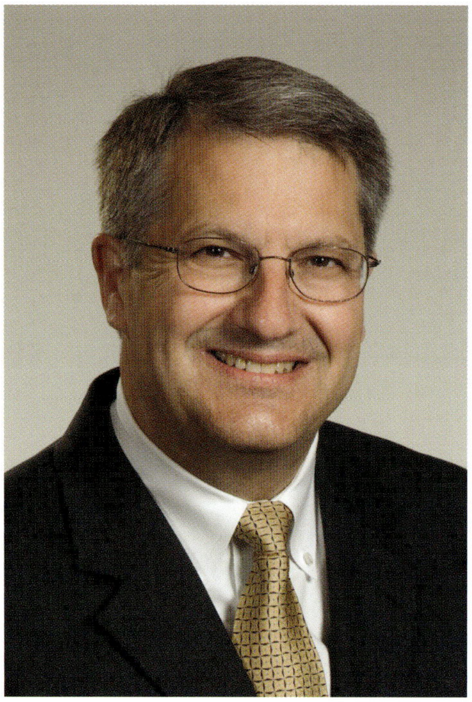

Edward Martin Jr., M.D., a Family Medicine physician, is the Medical Director for the North Shore Region.

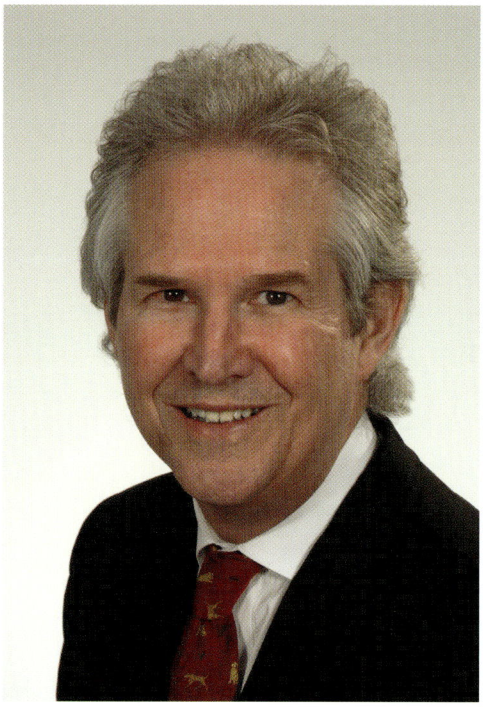

Alfred Robichaux III, M.D., Chairman of the Department of Obstetrics and Gynecology and Section Head of Maternal-Fetal Medicine, led the significant expansion of the OB/GYN Department at Ochsner Medical Center to medical centers across the System.

MEDICAL EDUCATION

The answer to that question lies in Ochsner's efforts to attract physicians to New Orleans and surrounding Louisiana parishes. The area lost hundreds of physicians and medical personnel in the wake of Katrina, and Ochsner has been doing everything it could since then to reverse that healthcare "brain drain." Medical education, one of the three pillars of the Clinic when it was founded in 1942, has never been so important to New Orleans and Louisiana as it is today.

Ochsner's educational programs have been affiliated with Leonard J. Chabert Medical Center, a 250-bed member of Louisiana's Charity Hospital System, located in Houma, Louisiana, 75 miles to the southwest, since its opening in 1977. The affiliation enables Ochsner's various residencies in the surgical disciplines to provide the required hands-on operating experience as a leader of the surgical management team. In exchange for the opportunity, Ochsner is expected to arrange senior staff physician coverage at the hospital.

Ochsner addressed the problem by creating a separate professional corporation, South Louisiana Medical Associates (SLMA), linked to leadership of Ochsner, but largely composed of newly recruited physicians employed by SLMA, supported by Ochsner consultants. SLMA contracted with the state to oversee resident education, to provide patient care services and to direct clinical hospital service departments. Based on the group practice model, SLMA is funded by hospital contracts and by patient care revenues. The business models introduced by Ochsner to conduct the affairs of SLMA were of significant benefit to the hospital as well, and later emulated by other hospitals in the Charity System.

There has been an effective, mutually beneficial relationship between Ochsner, SLMA and Chabert for over 30 years, which has produced excellence in Ochsner's residency education and in patient care to the medically underserved at Chabert. SLMA has a medical staff of 45 physicians and 20 to 30 surgical and medical Ochsner residents are assigned to Chabert at any given time. Ochsner leaders involved were Drs. Frank Riddick, J. Byron Gathright, Donald Erwin, John Bowen and clinic administrator Francis F. "Mel" Manning. SLMA stalwarts over the years include Drs. Tom Ferguson, Alvin Lassen, John Dampeer and Michael Garcia.

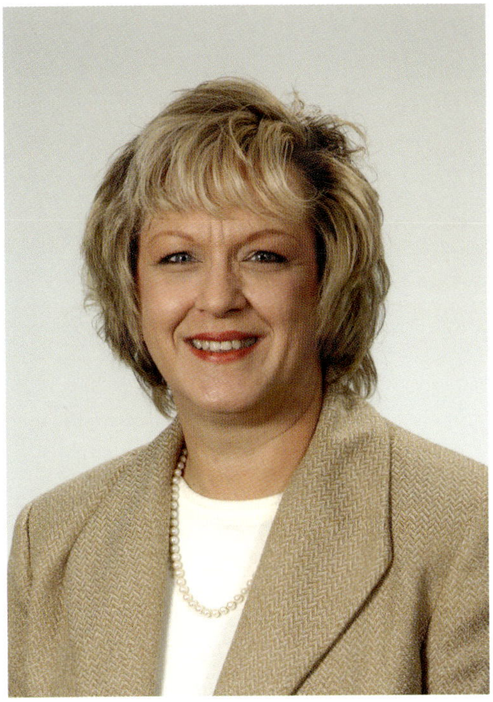

Karen Rice, an Adult Nurse Practitioner and Clinical Nurse Specialist, is the Program Director of the Ochsner Center for Nursing Research.

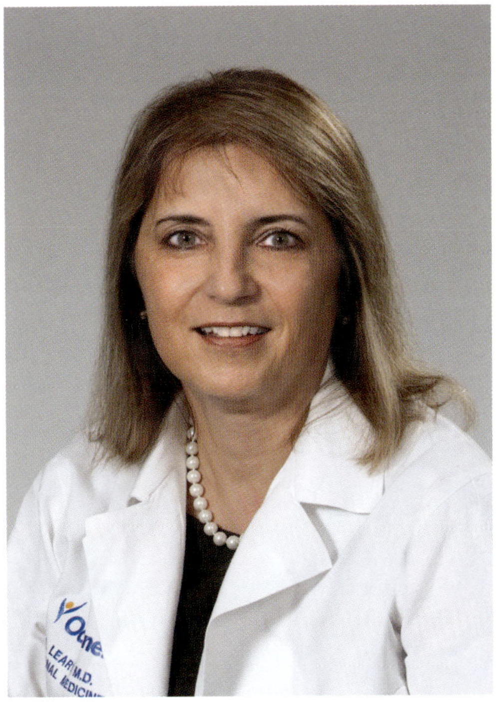

Ochsner's former Head of the Section of General Internal Medicine, Gloria Leary, M.D., is in great demand for her diagnostic and medical skills.

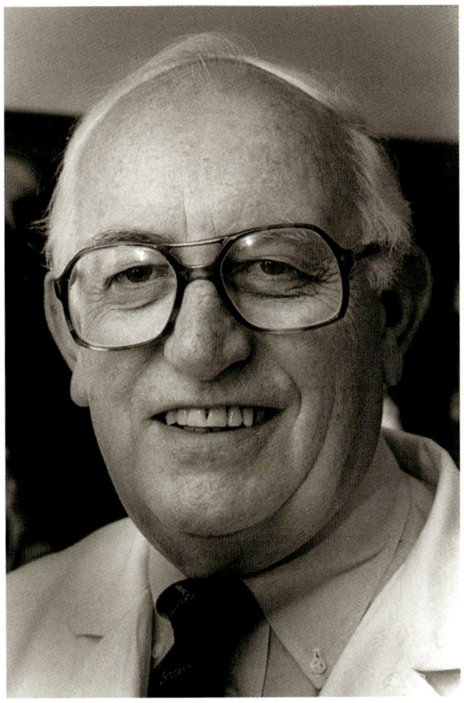

John Ray, M.D. was the longtime Chair of Ochsner's internationally renowned Department of Colon and Rectal Surgery and led several of the professional organizations in that discipline.

Education continues to be a critical part of Ochsner's Mission, a legacy left to future generations by the founders in 1942. Ochsner operates one of the nation's largest independently accredited medical education programs, annually training more than 300 house staff, 450 allied health students, 800 nursing students and 400 medical students. The medical students traditionally rotate to Ochsner for medical training.

As part of the leadership component of its medical education mission, Ochsner moved to fill a void that had been created by the passage of Hurricane Katrina. Much of the knowledge stored in the region's medical libraries had been lost or damaged in the storm. The Ochsner Medical Library and Archive was the first medical library to reopen in the New Orleans area in the wake of Katrina. In September 2005, Ochsner Library staff teamed up with the National Library of Medicine (NLM), librarians at Southeastern Louisiana Area Health Education Center in Hammond and the Leonard J. Chabert Medical Center in Houma to establish the Medical Library Recovery for Southeast Louisiana Project. As part of the innovative education initiative, Ochsner Librarians placed 35 computers, dubbed Library e-stations, at various Ochsner regional and neighborhood health centers. The NLM approved the placement of additional Library e-stations at non-affiliated Ochsner sites in St. Tammany and Terrebone Parishes.

"The Ochsner Medical Library welcomes ALL healthcare professionals, students and community members to use its information services," the Library noted in a 2006 report. "We recognize that access to medical information is more critical than ever as physicians and patients face new health and environmental issues."[15]

THE QUEENSLAND ALLIANCE

Ochsner further enhanced its well-deserved reputation for educating physicians when it established an alliance with the University of Queensland in 2009. One of the three founding principles of Ochsner, medical education has enjoyed a resurgence at Ochsner Clinic Foundation in the twenty-first century. Under the direction of Dr. William Pinsky, education has made great strides in standardization, curriculum and the quality of the Ochsner faculty since Pinsky's arrival.

"We established accountability in our graduate medical education program," Pinsky said. "We have done very well in recruiting students into residency programs, even through the aftermath of Katrina."[16]

Patrick Quinlan explained the quiet leadership Ochsner showed in the wake of Katrina to reestablish quality medical education in New Orleans "can't be glossed over. It's a very complex story. We were helping Tulane and LSU get back on their feet. We were keeping medical students in the city. They helped start the revival of New Orleans."[17]

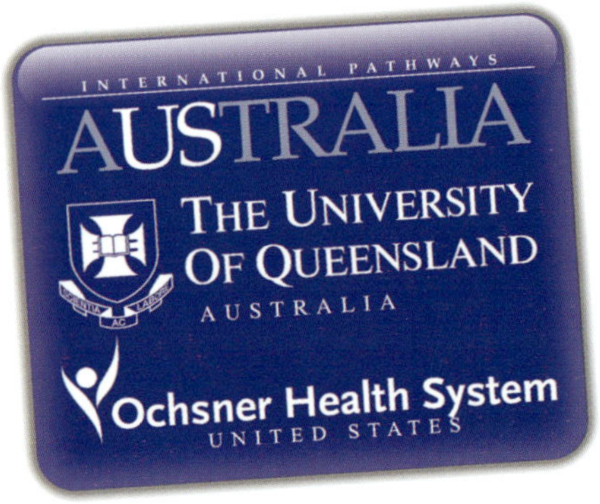

The alliance with the University of Queensland will help alleviate the growing shortage of physicians in Louisiana.

Ochsner's alliance with the University of Queensland in Brisbane, Australia, trains medical students for two years in Brisbane before they arrive in New Orleans to spend two years in clinical training at Ochsner. "It provides the opportunity to train doctors in areas that are important to them, such as multi-specialty practices," Pinsky explained. "It will also help in terms of workforce generation."[18]

Quinlan called the alliance an exclusive agreement with a leading institution to give students a chance to become physicians while expanding the pool of physicians in Louisiana. The potential of 125 graduates per year is almost equal to the number of graduates of a mid-sized medical school.

For Ochsner, the alliance with the University of Queensland will pay huge dividends. "If we can do this successfully," Pinsky noted, "we will increase the number of doctors in the state, increase the quality of training programs and increase the presence of Ochsner in academia globally. The end result is that we want Ochsner to be a medical degree-granting institution."[19]

Pinsky noted the goals of the partnership between Ochsner and the University of Queensland are three-fold. First and foremost, he said, the partnership will open more medical school positions providing local and Australian students with a truly unique medical education. Secondly, the partnership will regenerate Louisiana's physician workforce by educating more physicians and encouraging them to practice in our communities. Finally, the partnership will increase patient accessibility to healthcare by increasing the number of physicians.

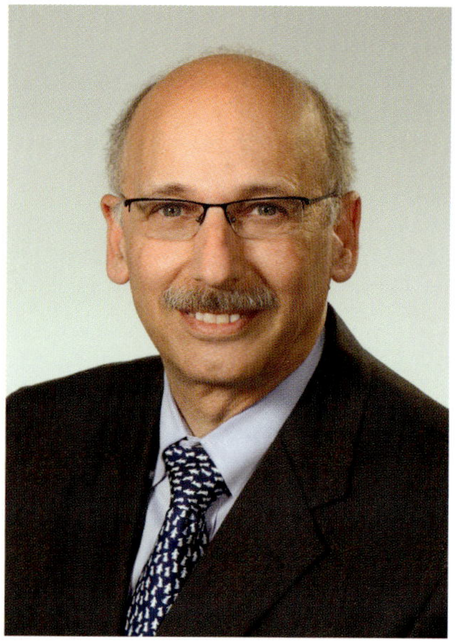

William Pinsky, M.D., Executive Vice President and Chief Academic Officer, helped engineer an alliance with Australia's University of Queensland.

"Ochsner is a seven-hospital system," Pinsky pointed out. "Therefore, we have the capacity to grow our medical education outreach. The breadth and depth of our organization enables us to provide our Australian students, as well as our current LSU and Tulane students, with rural hospital experience, involvement in research programs and core and sub-specialty rotations."[20]

The alliance, however, is bigger than Ochsner or the University of Queensland. In an era of twenty-first century globalization, Ochsner is taking the lead in the creation of the world's first bi-continental medical school.

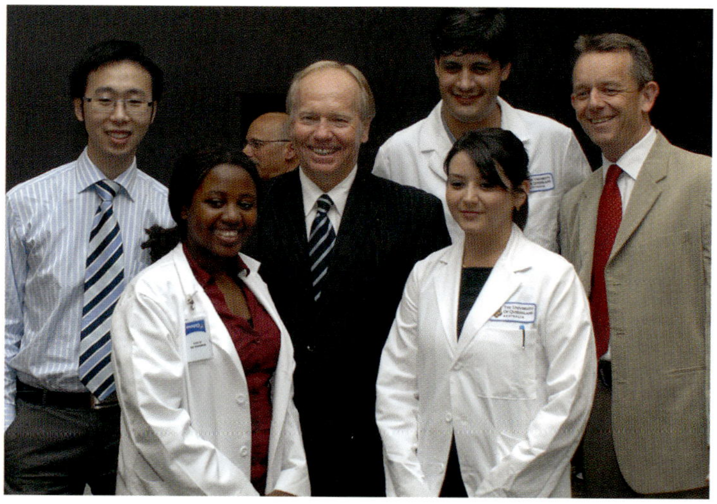

Former Queensland Premier and North American Trade Commissioner, Peter Beattie (standing third from left) and Professor David Wilkinson, BSc(H), MBBS, MSc, MD, PhD, DSc, MFPHM (UK), FACRRM, FRACGP, FAFPHM, FRCP (London), Dean of Medicine and Head of The University of Queensland School of Medicine (standing far right) with the first four University of Queensland students training at Ochsner in the innovative medical education program sponsored by Ochsner and The University of Queensland.

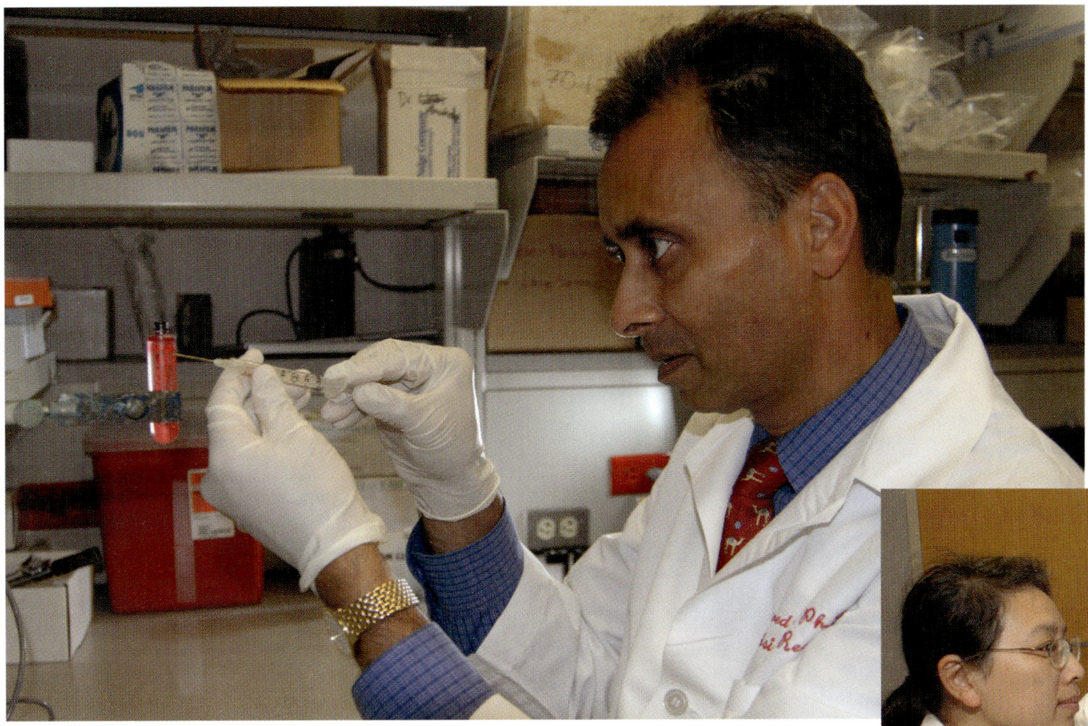

At any given time, more than 300 physicians and scientists, including Li Li, M.D. and Ph.D., Yong Sung Choi, M.D. and Ph.D. (below right and left, respectively) and Jawad Alam Ph.D. (pictured at left) are engaged in research at Ochsner.

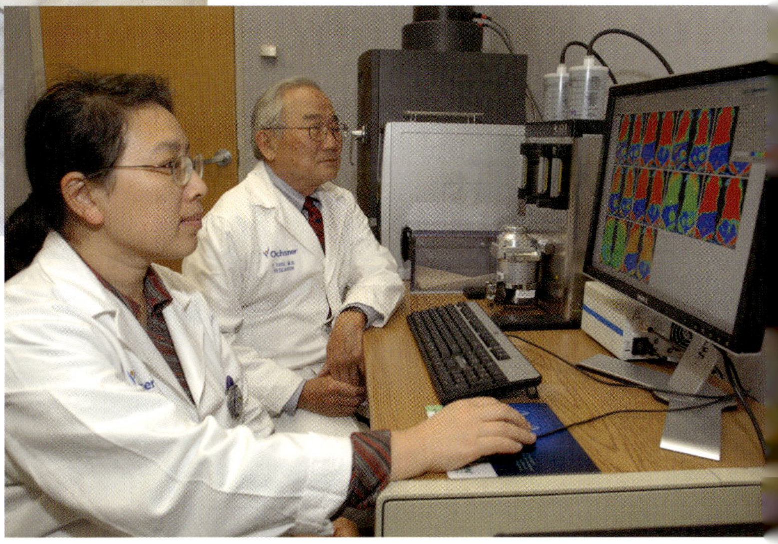

RESEARCH STRIDES

Ochsner continues to make strides in research, another of the pillars of the organization's foundation. Research efforts date from Dr. Alton Ochsner's pioneering work in tying cigarette smoking to lung cancer.

Ochsner researchers were able to resume their projects almost immediately following Katrina. The effective execution of Ochsner's disaster plan meant there was no loss of laboratory animals, research cell lines or tissues. In another example of the community outreach for which Ochsner has become so well known, scientists at the institution threw open their laboratories to researchers from Tulane and LSU until colleagues from other institutions were able to return to their home laboratories.

Today, more than 300 Ochsner physicians and scientists are involved in research at Ochsner's Basic Science Laboratories. Pinsky pointed out that Ochsner physicians and scientists have more than 500 clinical protocols in place, ranging from Molecular Genetics and Cellular Immunology to Transplantation, Pediatric Endocrinology and Hypertension. Nearly 75 percent of research projects are funded outside Ochsner.[21]

In recent years, Ochsner researchers have used some of that funding to support cutting-edge research projects, including cellular research into leukemia, pediatric nutrition and vitamin research.

Julia Cook, Ph.D., one of the talented research scientists at Ochsner, has seen major changes in the research infrastructure during her years at the laboratory. Dr. Richard Ré recruited Cook, Director of Ochsner's Laboratory of Molecular Genetics, to Ochsner from an LSU post-doctoral program in 1989. She helped Ochsner set up a diagnostic laboratory and worked closely with Ochsner endocrinologists and cardiovascular and infectious disease specialists during the 1990s.[22]

Cook said the emphasis on cost and competition has been "a good thing. It has made us a better research department."[23] What it hasn't done is obscure the traditional mission of Ochsner research. "All of the research we do affects patients in the end," she said. "It is invaluable to patients, and it affects the community as well."[24]

ELMWOOD FITNESS CENTER

When *Gambit Weekly* released its 2010 list of the best the Big Easy has to offer, it was no surprise that Elmwood Fitness Center, a service of Ochsner, was listed as Best Health Club in the city.

With locations downtown, in Metairie, Kenner and Harahan, Elmwood Fitness Center offers the largest variety of fitness programming in the New Orleans area. At the club's flagship facility in Harahan, weight rooms house six lines of weight equipment, and each of more than 80 pieces of cardio equipment has a built-in television screen. Elmwood Fitness Center offers more than 100 fitness classes each week. Those interested in sharpening their fitness in the water have access to pools with 20 lap lanes, and members can take advantage of everything from adult swim lessons to water aerobics classes to arthritis aquatics for seniors.[25]

Elmwood Fitness Center believes in helping its members balance physical activity, emotional well-being, proper nutrition and time for fun and relaxation. The Center offers members and non-members nutrition and massage services, private yoga and Pilates training, a fully stocked Pro Shop and the opportunity to consult Dr. Matthew McQueen's Family Practice once a week. Instruction and certification in Basic CPR, Healthcare Provider CPR and Automatic External Defibrilator (AED) are offered on an on-going basis.[26]

Personal Training and Weight Loss is a specialty at Elmwood Fitness Center. The Center offers one-on-one and small group training to help members of all different fitness levels take their workouts to the next level. A fully equipped Applied Physiology Laboratory helps members and their trainers maximize workout efficiency and keep an accurate track of progress.

Those who have resolved unsuccessfully in the past to lose weight need look no further than the multitude of weight-loss programs at Elmwood. The Weight No More, Power of 3 and Biggest Loser programs have helped members and non-members to lose weight, keep weight off, reach an optimal level of physical fitness and incorporate positive nutritional habits into their daily lifestyles.[27]

Ochsner and Elmwood Fitness Center believe a healthy lifestyle starts at a young age and fitness should involve the entire family. The Center offers a wide variety of programs for the younger set, including children's fitness, aquatics, gymnastics, Kidsports and cheerleading, as well as childcare and birthday parties. The Center's KidSports program offers up to 11 weeks of summer camp for children.[28]

Organized medicine has long known that exercise can be a critical component of preventive medicine programs. Diabetes, blood pressure and obesity can all be controlled if patients engage in a regular program of exercise.

As a service of Ochsner, Elmwood Fitness Center offers medical fitness programs to accommodate all ages and abilities. After receiving approval from an Ochsner physician, Ochsner patients are eligible to enroll in the Medical Fitness Exercise Program that coordinates their fitness needs with their healthcare needs.

"As healthcare costs continue to rise," said Matthew McQueen, M.D., Family Practice, Primary Care Sports Medicine, and Elmwood Fitness Center's Medical Director, "there is a tremendous economic urgency to maximize fitness as an affordable therapeutic measure. Fit people do not need as many medicines and they live stronger, happier lives. These facts are well established by science."[29]

SEEING A NEED

One of Ochsner's greatest strengths is the healthcare system's innate ability to see a need and fill it. When Ochsner physicians began to notice an alarming rise in childhood obesity among their patients, they brought their concerns to Ochsner management.

In August 2010, Ochsner's Elmwood Fitness Center began offering the latest fitness technology designed to get children off the sofa and into physical activity. Called XRKade, the technology was unveiled at Kidsports at Elmwood Fitness Center on August 7, 2010.

XRKade is described as an active gaming system that links video games—suspected as the cause behind many cases of childhood obesity—with exercise equipment that makes working out more like playing an intense, interactive video game that allows children to compete with other children around them in real time.

"With this system," explained Damon Kremer, Assistant General Manager, Director Satellite Facilities and Member Services, "you're not just riding a stationary bike, you're racing other players up a mountain side. This is the next generation of active gaming, and it's so much fun you hardly remember you're exercising."[30]

Kremer added that the XRKade system is a way for children and adults to use their bodies to play engaging, interactive games, but with more physical activity. He noted that the XRKade system is another manifestation of Ochsner's continuing commitment to improving the health of children and adults in southeast Louisiana.

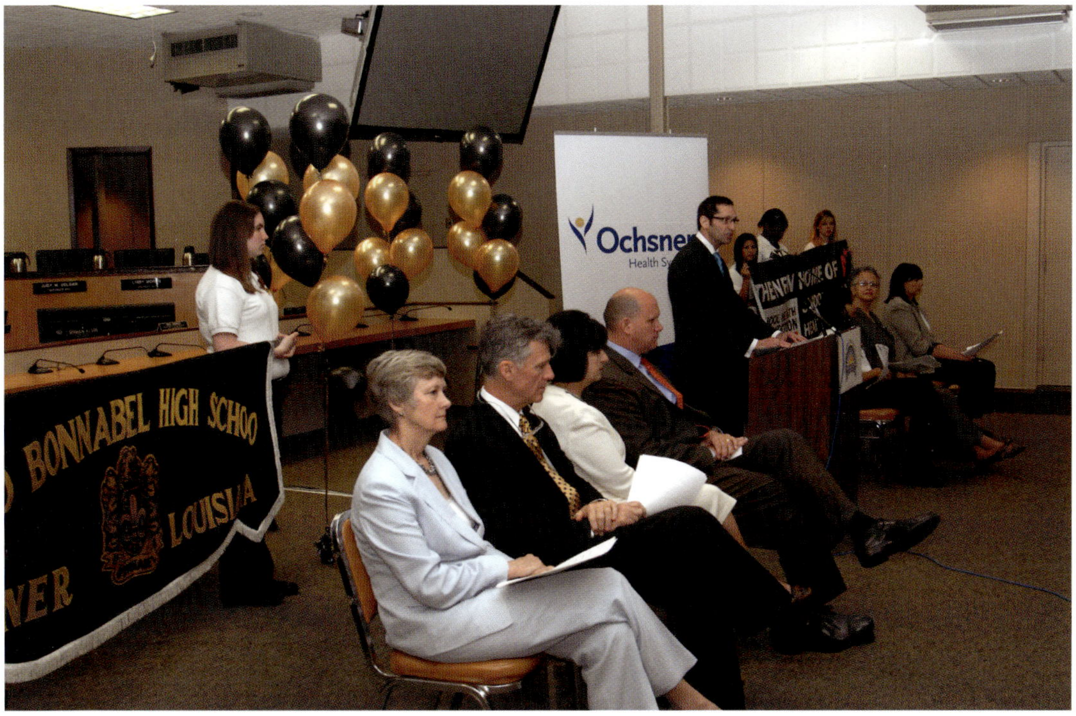

Ochsner and Jefferson Parish Public Schools have partnered to create an on-site clinic for students, teachers, and staff at Bonnabel High School. Ochsner staffs a nurse practitioner at the high school five days a week and a pediatrician four hours a week. The clinic also provides its patients with a full time social worker. As a fully functioning medical office, the clinic is able to see patients who walk in or schedule an appointment for a variety of medical and psychological needs, just another example of how Ochsner reaches out to serve the needs of the community.

BIG ENOUGH TO MATTER

Ochsner's journey has consumed 70 years since Alton Ochsner first began discussing his vision of a multi-specialty clinic with colleagues at Tulane Medical School. Today, that vision is reflected in Ochsner's continuing focus on clinical practice, research and medical education. Patrick Quinlan said Ochsner Health System in the twenty-first century is "standing on the shoulders of those who came before, and it is standing pretty tall. Our legacy is medical excellence. And one thing we do is take excellent care of our patients."[31]

Still, he is convinced Ochsner can get better. "We do things on an immensely different scale than we did in the early days," he said. "Medicine is very complex. We need to learn how to quantify the results to get even better."[32]

Warner Thomas echoed Quinlan's comments. "We do some things very well," he said. "We are certainly not satisfied where we are."[33]

Thomas said Ochsner is pushing its clinical teams internally to seek improvement. Transparency, he said, "is where healthcare needs to go. We have to be more transparent about quality and cost. We can be a leader there."[34]

Thomas ticked off several goals Ochsner is seeking to attain: starting a bone marrow transplant program; tripling the size of the cancer program; and encouraging and growing a global strategic relationship with General Electric concerning business and management practices and imaging developments.

"Our folks are taking delivery of care to a new level," Thomas said. "We want to touch more people, touch more healthcare institutions, to help make them better. It's a challenge, but we can play a huge leadership role in regional healthcare."[35]

For Patrick Quinlan, the hope is that Ochsner Health System never loses its ties to the past or its vision of a better future. "I hope we never depart from that ability to derive our value from service to patients, service to the community," Quinlan said. "It's a place that's known for innovation. It's in our mission statement: to serve, heal, lead, educate and innovate."[36]

As the scale increases, Quinlan added, "it means we can do more and more for more patients. We want to have the best medical outcomes in this country. We work on it continually, and the bar will be raised higher. We want to take what we have and improve on it."[37]

And, he concluded, Ochsner wants to continue, "to be big enough to matter, and small enough to get it done."[38]

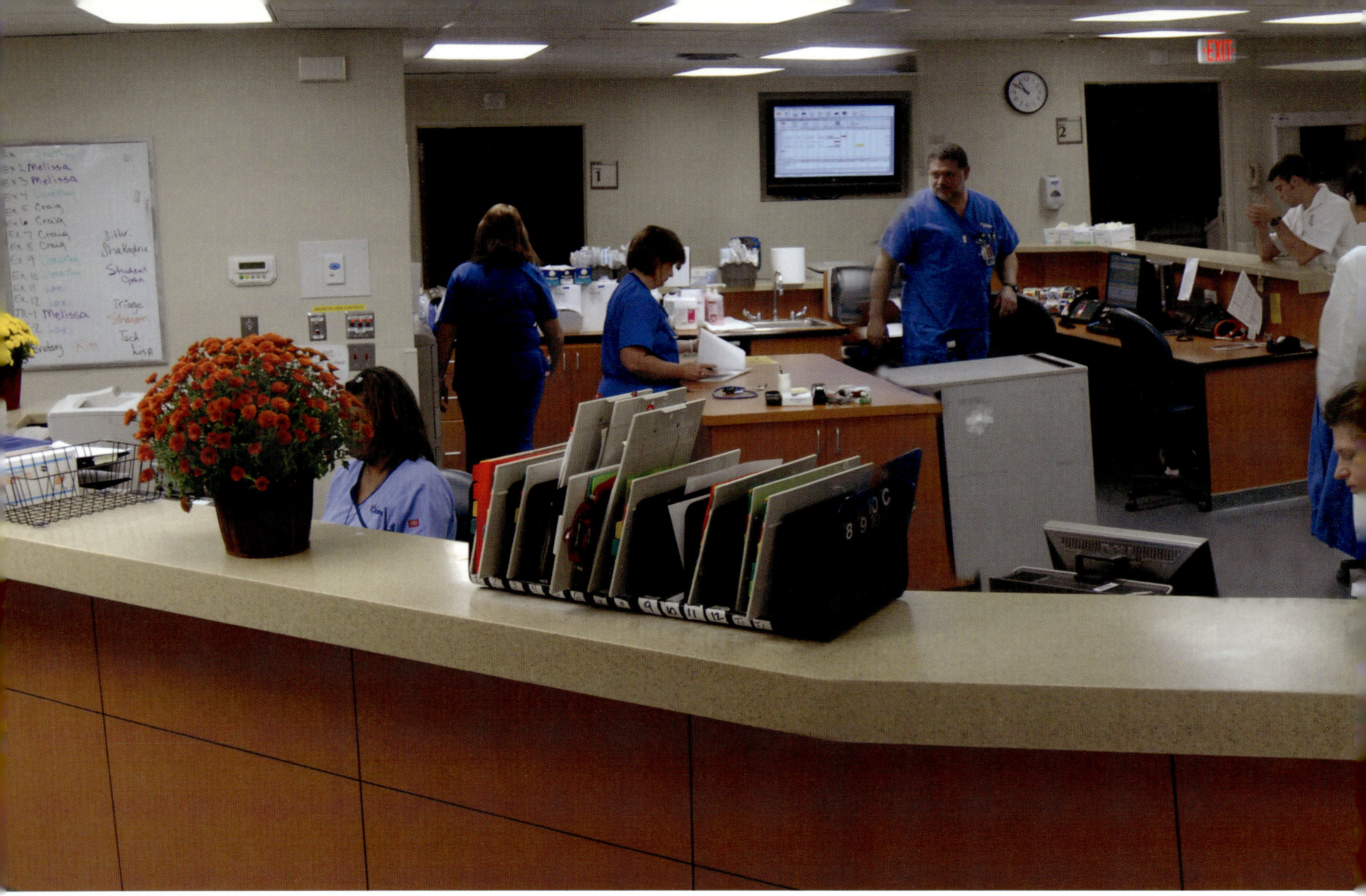

CHAPTER 14:

OCHSNER TODAY... AND TOMORROW

WALK INTO THE ATRIUM in Ochsner's Jefferson Highway campus on any morning of the week and you are likely to see New Orleans residents encountering the face of twenty-first century healthcare. Doctors, nurses, employees and patients are bustling through the brightly lit mall, accompanied by the sound of piano music and the lilt of conversation. Some are stopping in for a bite to eat at the bustling café or grabbing a quick cup of coffee at the popular coffee shop in the center of the Atrium. Others are picking up a greeting card in the gift shop or checking to see if there is a wait for a haircut in the barbershop. A steady stream of people passes down the corridor to and from the adjacent Brent House Hotel.

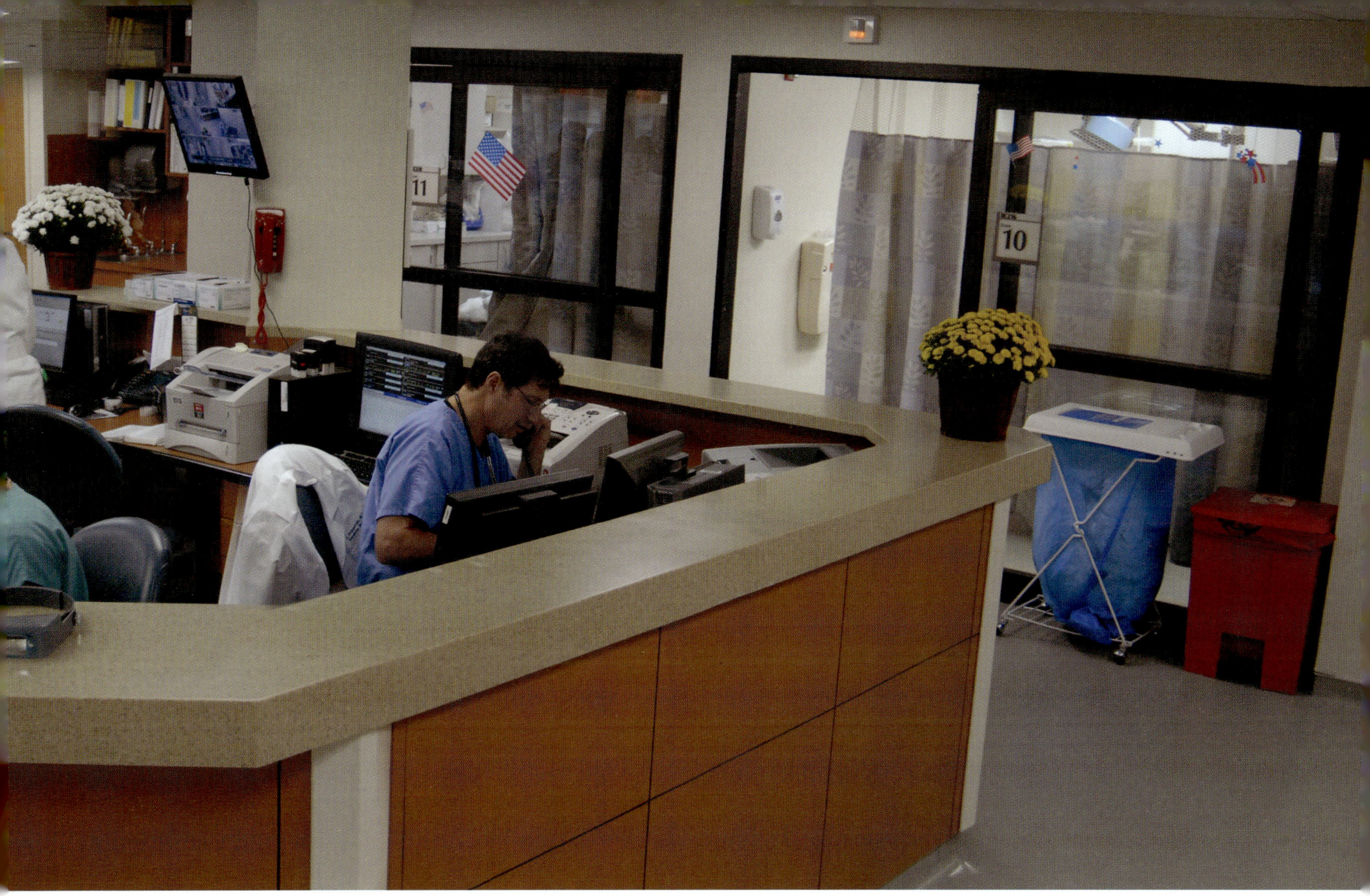

A renovated Emergency Department helped Ochsner Medical Center – Kenner earn the 2008 Louisiana Hospital Quality Award – Gold for its treatment and care of acute myocardial infarction patients.

The scene might be an enclosed shopping mall, for all the hustle and bustle, but in fact it is the hub of the largest private not-for-profit healthcare delivery system in the region, one that includes eight hospitals and more than 38 neighborhood health centers. Many of the people passing through the Atrium on a typical morning are patients utilizing the impressive list of Ochsner healthcare services, including the John Ochsner Heart and Vascular Institute, Primary Care, the Center for Digestive Disorders, Women's Services, the Sleep Disorders Center, the Bone and Joint Center, the Multi-Organ Transplant Institute, Cancer Services, Ochsner for Children, the Sports Medicine Institute, International Health, Spine Services and Surgical Weight Loss.

Ochsner™

Healthcare With Peace Of Mind™

Ochsner Health System is a not-for-profit, academic, multi-specialty healthcare system serving southeast Louisiana.

The patients at the Jefferson Highway campus come from a wide variety of backgrounds and neighborhoods. They might be fourth-generation New Orleans residents who use Ochsner Medical Center as their primary care facility, or they might be suburban residents referred from Ochsner Medical Center – West Bank Campus, Ochsner Medical Center – Kenner or Ochsner St. Anne General Hospital in Raceland. They could be transfers to or from Ochsner Baptist Medical Center, Ochsner Medical Center North Shore, Ochsner Medical Center – Baton Rouge, or other hospitals throughout the region. Other patients passing through the Atrium could be referrals from Ochsner's network of 38 neighborhood health centers or from physicians in Louisiana, Mississippi, Texas, Florida and countries south of the border.

Although Ochsner is as hometown New Orleans as king cakes and po-boys, patients arrive from far beyond the New Orleans – Baton Rouge corridor. Some 2,200 patients last year came to Ochsner for treatment at the Gayle and Tom Benson Cancer Center, which opened in June 2010. The Center provides advanced chemotherapy at 40 infusion stations.[1] Another 2,100 patients with an uncommon type of cancer receive treatment at the Neuroendocrine Tumor Program at Ochsner Medical Center – Kenner, one of only five such units in the United States.[2]

Patients from across the United States as well as from overseas continue to come to Ochsner for life-saving liver, pancreas, kidney, heart and lung transplants. Ochsner's Multi-Organ Transplant Institute is one of the nation's leading transplant centers. At the Institute, the one-year survival rates for Ochsner's kidney and liver transplant programs are consistently higher than the national average, and the wait time for transplants at Ochsner is well below the national average.[3] The John Ochsner Heart and Vascular Institute provides world-class diagnosis and treatment of heart disease for residents of the region, including the Mississippi and Alabama Gulf coasts.

In fact, Ochsner boasts of caring for more than 336,000 patients from 26 countries. As a global leader, Ochsner has been inspired to stretch across continents, countries and boundaries with innovative healthcare services.

In 2009 and 2010, Ochsner expanded its cardiovascular surgical capabilities, restarting pediatric cardiovascular surgery as a regular area of specialty and performing more than 200 surgical cases in the first year. It expanded heart care services through the addition of a new state-of-the-art outpatient catheterization laboratory.[4]

Ochsner opened a new ER and 43-room Clara Wing at Ochsner Baptist Medical Center in 2009 to help fill the crucial needs in the downtown and uptown areas for critical emergency care. At Ochsner Medical Center – West Bank Campus, Ochsner expanded emergency care capabilities so it could serve a patient load more than 20 percent greater than in the past. Ochsner streamlined ER wait times in 2009 when it launched a new service that communicates real-time ER wait times for the four Ochsner New Orleans and Baton Rouge emergency rooms.[5]

• WHAT OCHSNER MEANS TO ME •

"Ochsner's mission is about more than patient care, it's about community service. We want to continue to strive for improvement in disease prevention and education... there's so much more to be done and Ochsner is COMMITTED to providing those services."

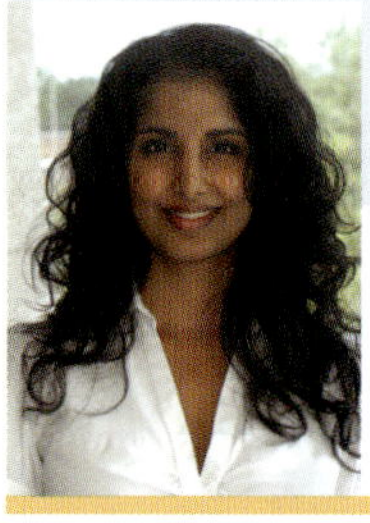

Surveen Klein, Transplant Social Work Supervisor and Kidney/Pancreas Transplant Social Worker, Ochsner Medical Center

To watch the full interview with Surveen Klein, visit **ochsner.org/history**.

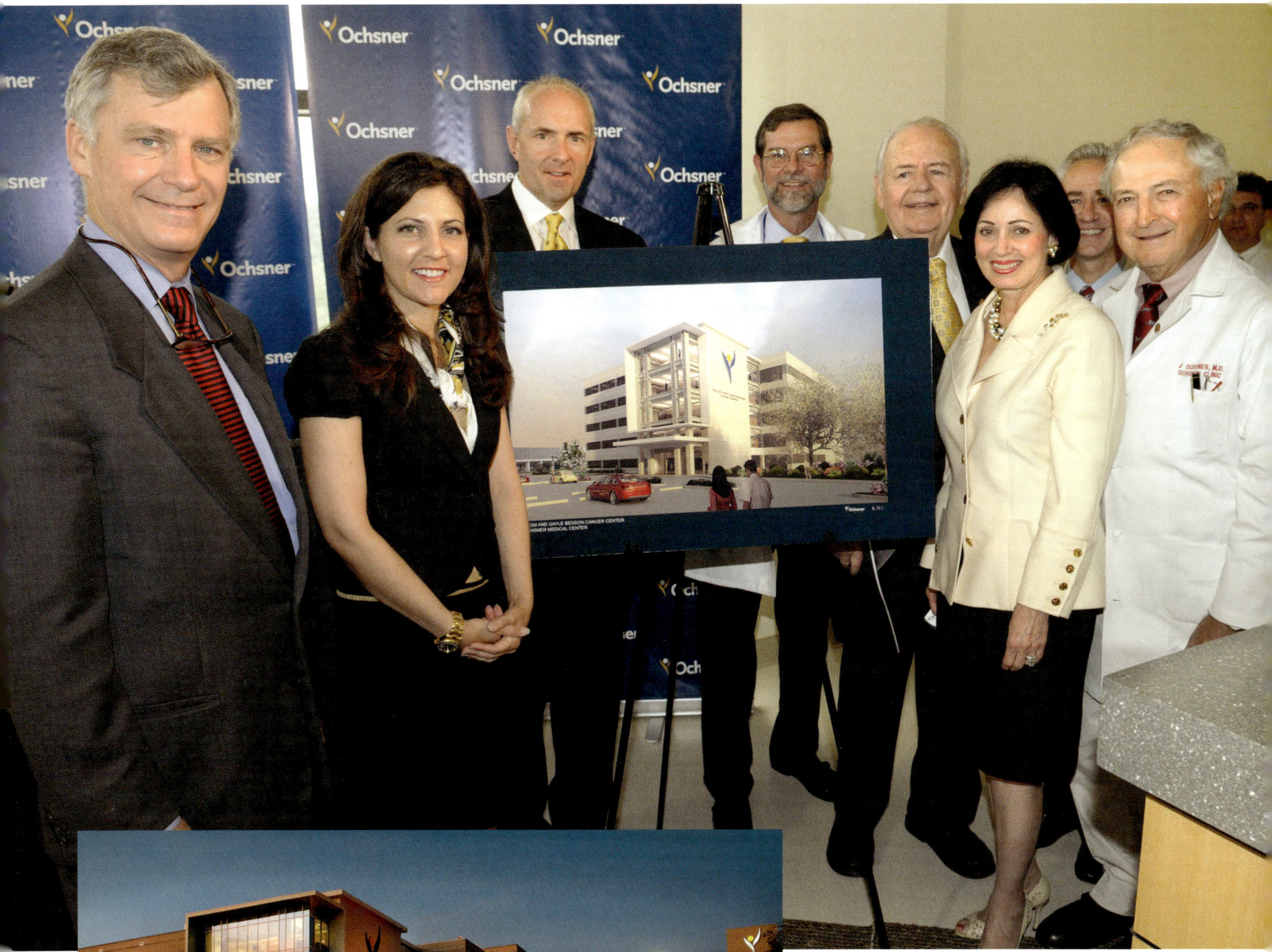

In June 2010, Ochsner unveiled the first phase of the Gayle and Tom Benson Cancer Center at Ochsner Medical Center. The owner of the New Orleans Saints football team, Tom Benson and his wife Gayle, standing fifth and sixth from left, donated $5 million to help fund the Center.

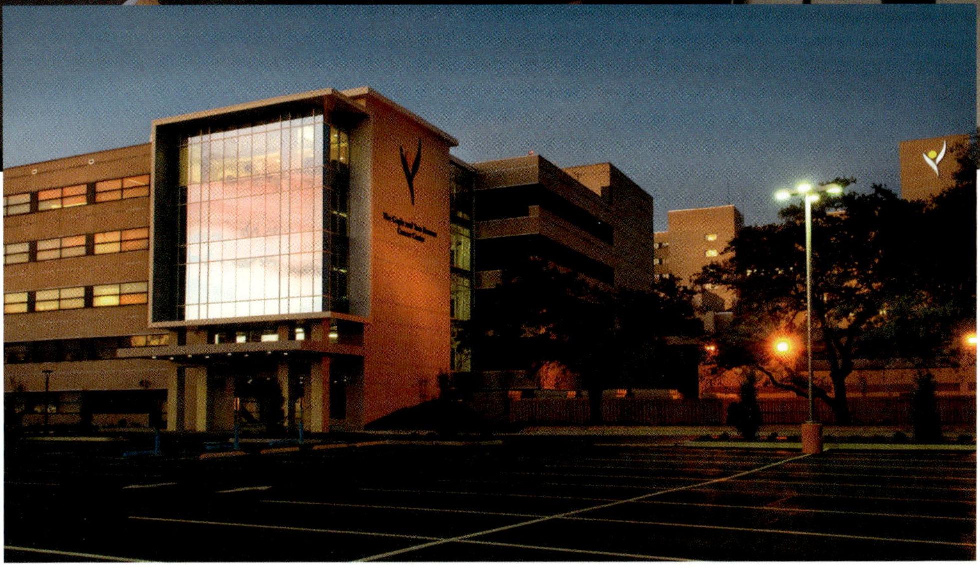

Construction is underway on Phase 2 of the Gayle and Tom Benson Cancer Center, which will house comprehensive cancer treatment services and clinical trials.

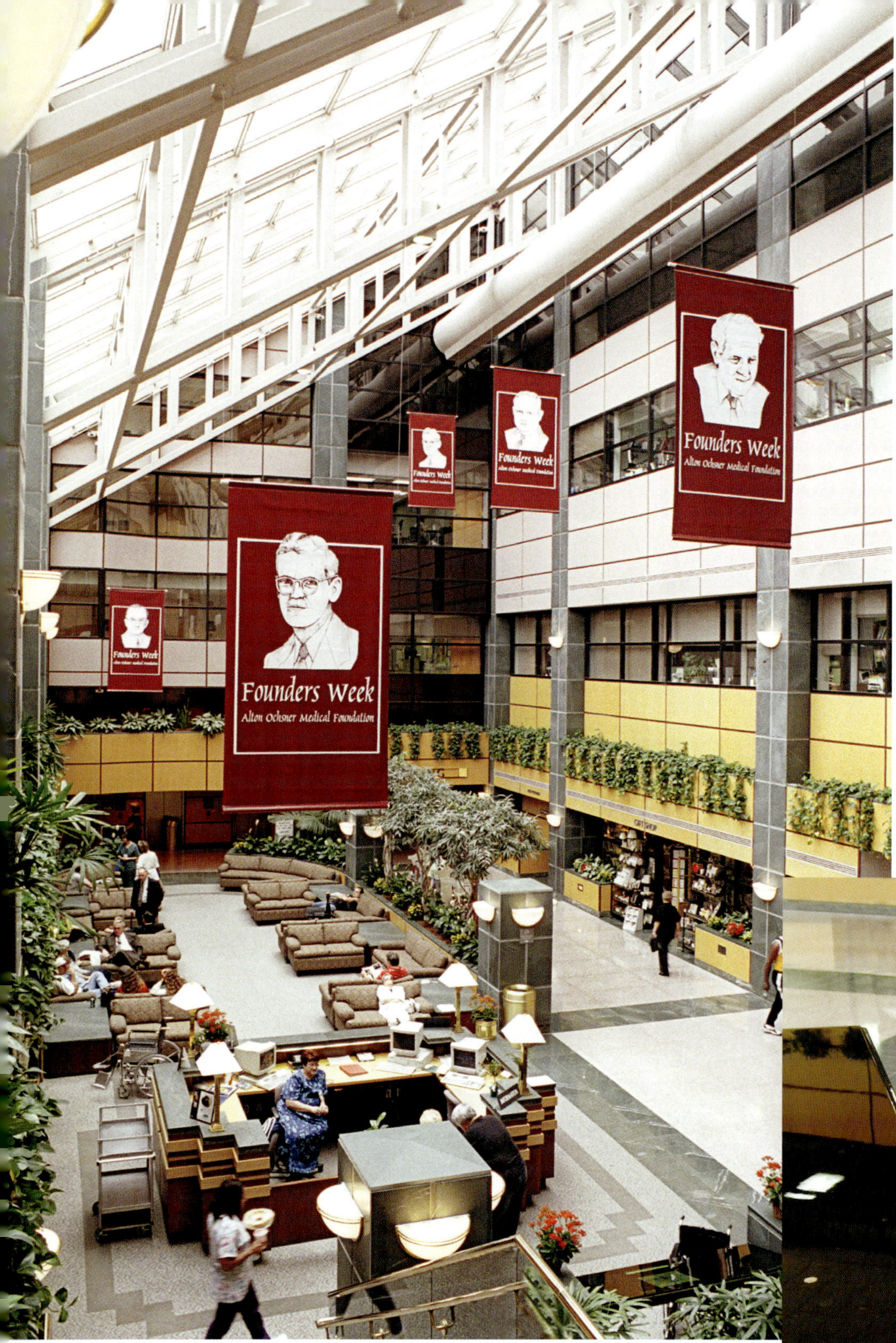

Ochsner annually celebrates its heritage during Founders Week.

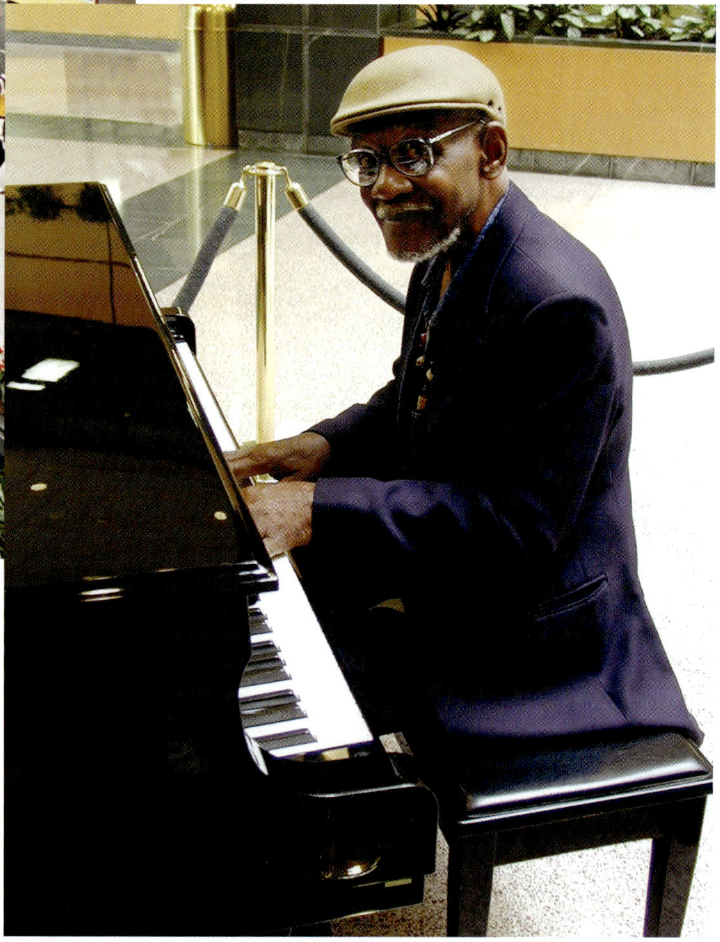

Willy Metcalf plays the piano in the Atrium, providing soothing music for patients, staff and visitors alike.

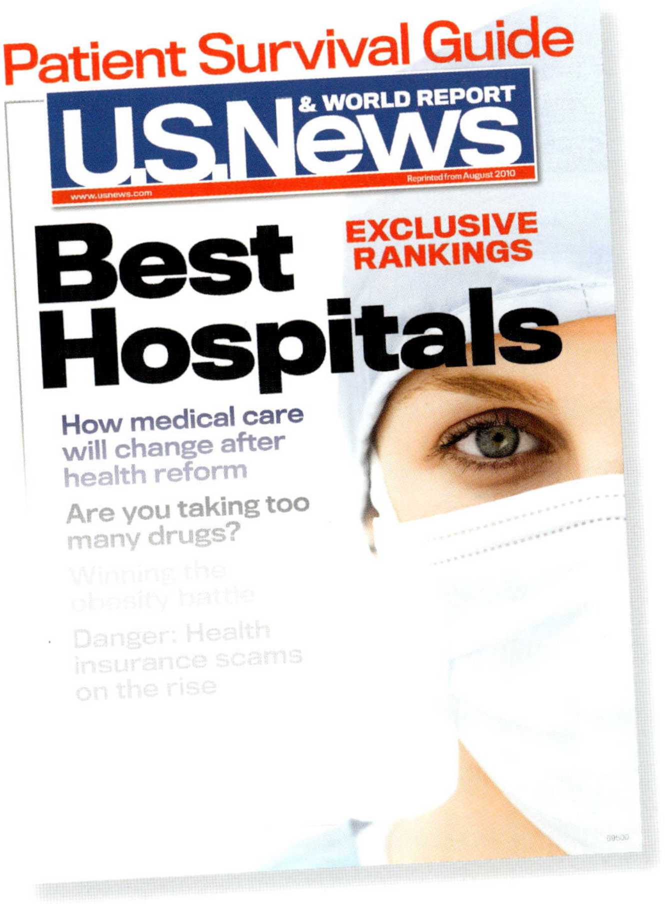

In July 2010, U.S.News & World Report *named Ochsner Medical Center as one of America's Best Hospitals, citing exceptional delivery care across seven categories: Heart and Heart Surgery, Ear, Nose and Throat, Gastroenterology, Orthopedics, Pulmonary, Gynecology, and Geriatrics.*

THE CONSUMER CHOICE FOR HEALTHCARE

With more than 12,500 employees system-wide, Ochsner has consistently been rated as one of the "**Best Places to Work**" **by *New Orleans CityBusiness*.** Ochsner employs more than 850 physicians practicing more than 90 medical specialties and sub-specialties.

Ochsner has been named the **Consumer Choice for Healthcare in New Orleans for 15 consecutive years** and is the **only Louisiana hospital recognized by *U.S. News & World Report* as a "Best Hospital" across seven categories**. In 2010, Ochsner added a new honor when the **Thomson Reuters National Benchmark Study named Ochsner as one of the Top 15 Major Teaching Hospitals** from its annual listing of 100 Top Hospitals.[6]

As a not-for-profit, academic, multi-specialty healthcare delivery system dedicated to patient care, research and education, Ochsner fosters close collaboration between clinicians and scientists that helps bring medical discoveries from the laboratory to the bedside. Each year, Ochsner physicians and scientists are involved in 300 ongoing clinical trials and publish 200 articles in peer-reviewed medical journals.

In 2009, Ochsner Medical Center was the **only healthcare provider in the Gulf South selected to participate as an FDA investigative site in the PARTNER clinical trial**. The PARTNER program (Placement of AoRTic traNscathetER valves) is designed to evaluate the Edwards SAPIEN transcatheter aortic heart valve in patients who are at high risk for open-heart surgery and surgical valve repair.[7]

The clinical and research components of Ochsner are complemented by one of the largest non-university based physician training centers in the nation. In recent years, more than 375 physicians and medical residents have trained at Ochsner each year, along with 800 nursing students and 450 allied health students. The April 2009 opening of the University of Queensland School of Medicine Clinical School at Ochsner creates the opportunity to alleviate physician shortages in Louisiana.

Ochsner's success in integrating clinical practice, research and education has reaped dozens of rewards in recent years. Ochsner **is a recipient of the Consumers Choice Award from the National Research Corporation, which identifies the most preferred hospitals in more than 100 U.S. markets**. It is one of the "**Top 100 Integrated Healthcare Networks" in the nation, according to *Modern Healthcare* magazine**, and AARP calls Ochsner one of the "**Top 50 Best Employers for Workers Over 50." Ochsner continues to be honored by *U.S. News & World Report* as one of "America's Best Hospitals."**

Ochsner now has broader responsibilities. Being the best is no longer good enough. "We have broadened our goal to lift the health status of the community," Quinlan said. "We want to change the kids and change the future."[8]

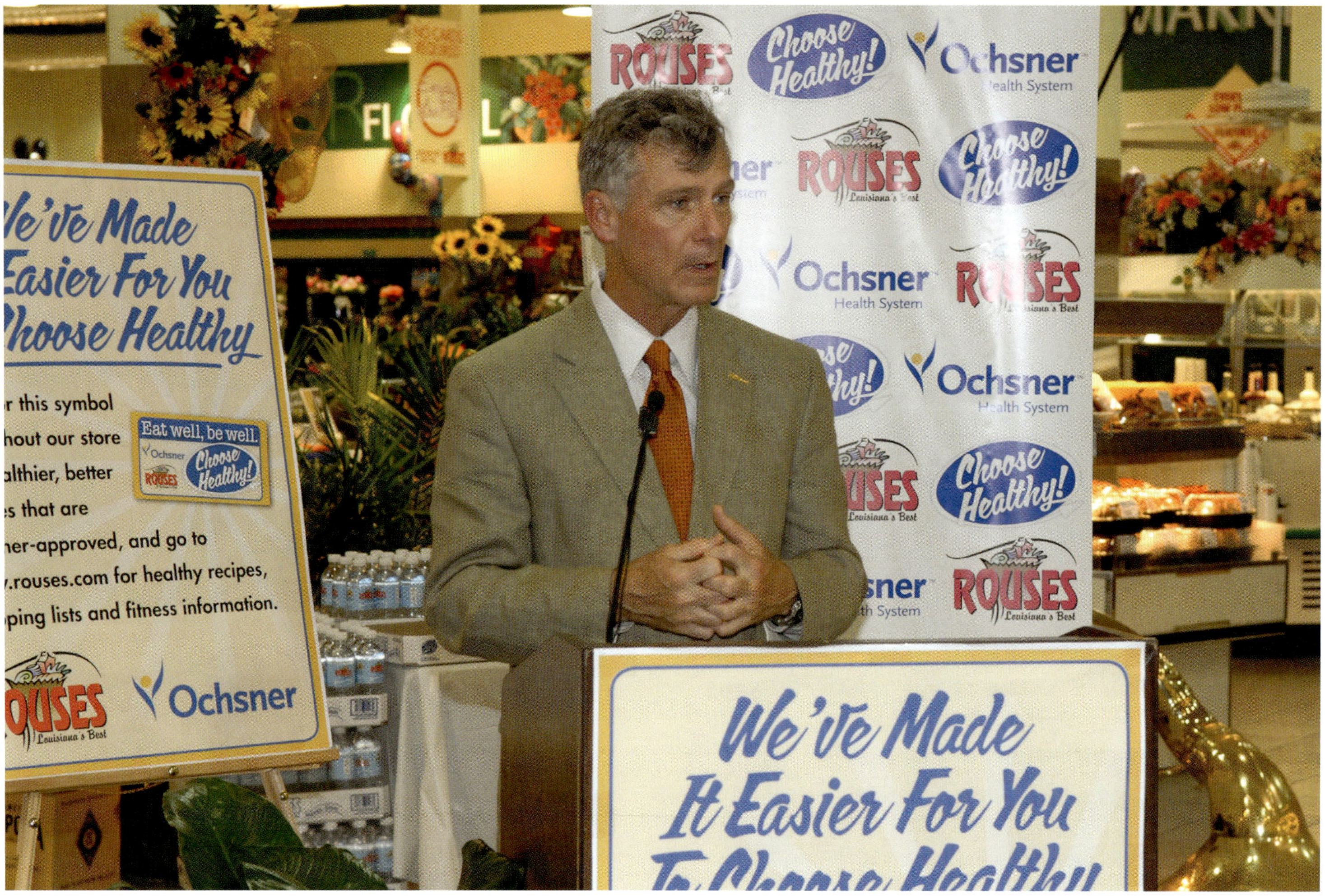

In 2009, Ochsner partnered with Rouses, one of New Orleans' biggest grocery chains, to implement healthy shopping guidelines. At the press conference announcing the innovative partnership, Dr. Patrick Quinlan explained the program would promote locally grown produce, whole grains, lean meat and vitamin-rich seafood in an attempt to stem the epidemic of obesity plaguing Louisiana.

A COMMITMENT TO COMMUNITY PARTNERSHIP

Ochsner has stepped up its commitment to community partnership since Katrina, taking health services to the people it serves. A colorful, eye-catching van takes physical education classes to area schools. The Mobile Fitness Unit targets childhood obesity with a range of fitness equipment and weight-loss programs for children.

Tackling childhood obesity has been a particular target for Ochsner. The Centers for Disease Control and Prevention (CDC) ranks Louisiana as the eighth most obese state in the U.S., with almost 30 percent of the state's residents classified as medically obese. The state has the seventh highest rate of overweight youth.

During the summer of 2009, Ochsner partnered with Rouses, a popular local grocery chain, to help local residents make healthier food choices by implementing "healthy shopping guidelines." At a press conference announcing the partnership, Patrick Quinlan explained that "people traditionally get wellness information at the doctor's office, but a local grocery store is a natural setting to talk about nutrition and meal planning. Rouses has given Ochsner a great opportunity to reach people before they make their food choices."[9] He called it "an innovative and unique approach to educating residents on wellness."[10]

REACHING OUT

The partnership with local institutions such as Rouses is by no means the only community outreach program Ochsner supports in the twenty-first century. One popular national program adopted by Ochsner in recent years is Reach Out and Read. Operated in coordination with Supriya Jindal, Louisiana's First Lady, Reach Out and Read enabled medical staff at Ochsner's Department of Pediatrics to promote early literacy and encourage young children to read.[11]

A second major community outreach initiative in local schools launched in 2009 was Change the Kids, Change the Future. Designed to reduce chronic disease by changing the health habits of schoolchildren, Change the Kids, Change the Future encourages exercise, better nutrition and preventative health education.[12]

Ochsner also increased its commitment to local community education in 2008 when it unveiled its new STAR (Science, Technology, Academics, Research) Program, which aimed to encourage and cultivate future generations of physicians and healthcare professionals among local high school students. Ochsner's Library Services Program and the MyOchsner patient portal provide patients with web-based access to healthcare information, as well as access to their electronic medical records.[13]

Increasingly, Ochsner is leveraging its sports medicine affiliations with the New Orleans Saints and New Orleans Hornets to educate the city's children about the importance of integrating fitness and a healthy diet into their daily lives.[14] Ochsner Eat Fit menu options at the Louisiana Superdome and New Orleans Arena are the result of a collaboration between the venues' executive chefs and staff and Ochsner's Elmwood Fitness Center's sports dietitians. Other programs sponsored by Ochsner, including the school-based Health Center at Bonnabel High School, Golden Opportunity and the American Cancer Society Patrick F. Taylor Hope Lodge, all reaffirm the System's goal of making New Orleans a better place for the community's residents.

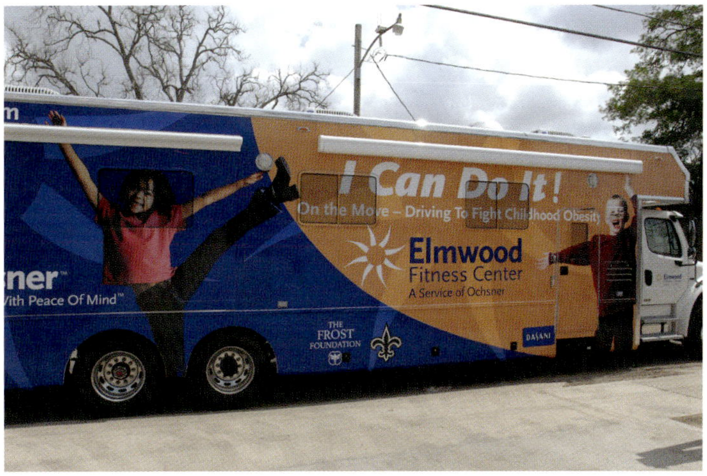

Ochsner brings the value of preventive medicine and fitness to communities and neighborhoods across southeast Louisiana with Elmwood Fitness Center's mobile fitness unit.

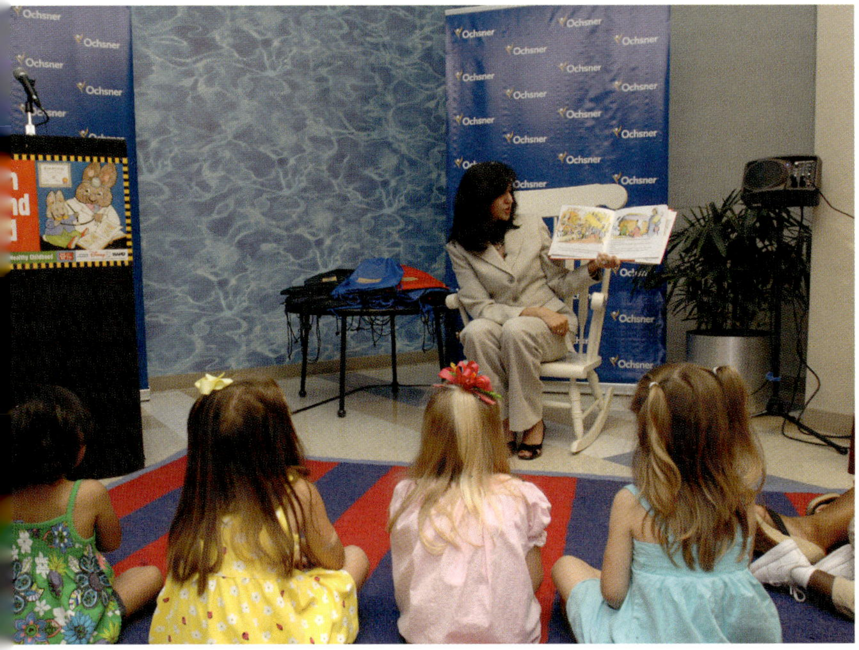

Louisiana First Lady Supriya Jindal reads to a group of attentive children to help them sharpen their reading skills through the Reach Out and Read program. Ochsner partnered with the First Lady in the innovative program that promotes early literacy and encourages young children to read.

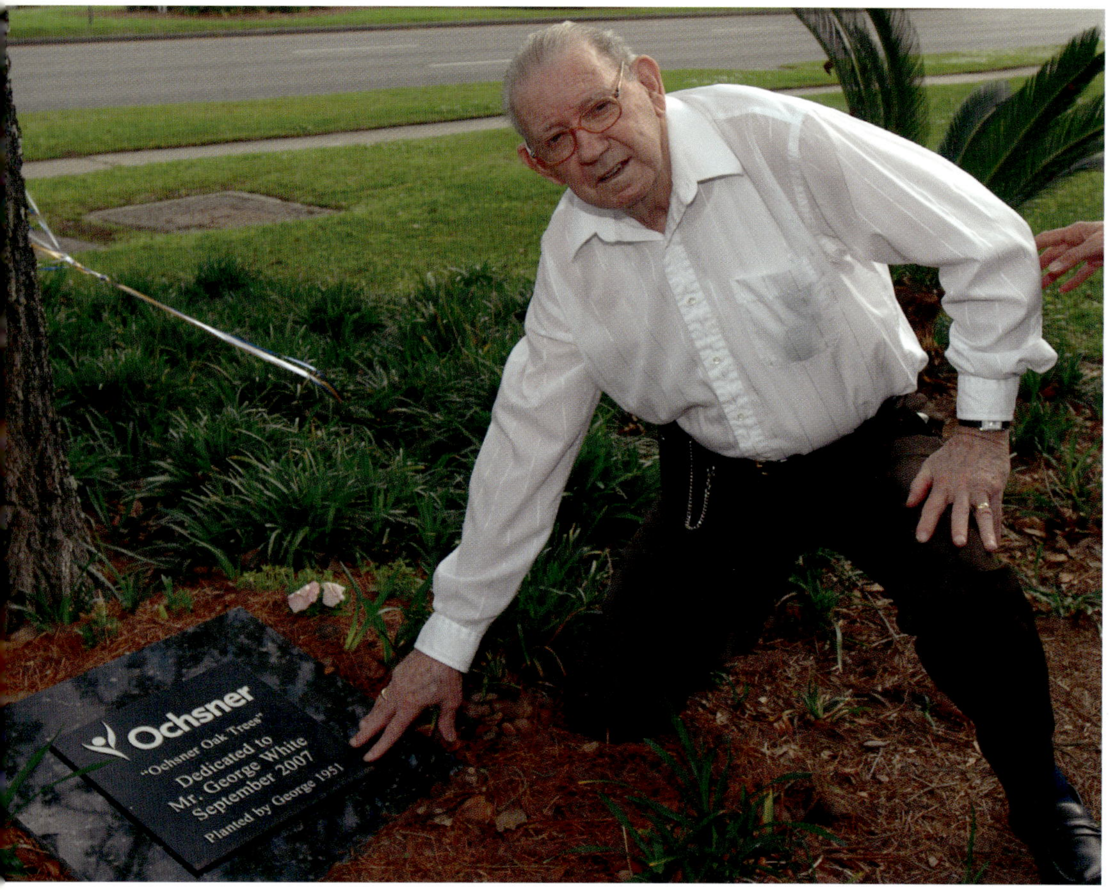

A plaque on the grounds of the Jefferson Highway campus honors longtime employee George White, who planted six-foot oak trees on the site in 1951 for Alton Ochsner. Sixty years later, George White's mammoth oaks shade the grounds of Ochsner's Jefferson Highway campus.

GIVING BACK

With more than 12,500 employees in New Orleans and surrounding parishes, Ochsner has a payroll of more than $750 million each year. That money flows through the community for food, housing, consumer purchases, school tuition and a thousand other activities. As a not-for-profit organization, Ochsner reinvests 100 percent of its annual income back into the healthcare system and community services. In 2010, Ochsner spent nearly $1.78 billion to provide quality care to more than 58,000 patients.[15]

Ochsner has long relied upon strong philanthropic support to maintain quality patient care, as well as research and education efforts. Since 2004, Ochsner has raised more than $26 million to help support its mission. In 2010, that philanthropic care included the continuing renovation of Ochsner Baptist Medical Center and the opening of the Gayle and Tom Benson Cancer Center. Donor money helped to develop the Nurse Family Partnership Program at Ochsner Medical Center – West Bank Campus for an innovative program that serves first-time mothers and their babies.[16] Philanthropy and charitable giving remain pillars of the Ochsner System 70 years after the founders first opened Ochsner's doors.

HEALTHCARE WITH PEACE OF MIND™

One change Alton Ochsner and the founders would definitely approve of is Ochsner's extension into the parishes surrounding New Orleans. With eight hospitals and dozens of neighborhood health centers, Ochsner Health System is bringing quality healthcare to the community in unprecedented fashion. "We've learned that anything is possible," said Patrick Quinlan. "The addition of community hospitals to our system allows us to improve the quality of care experienced by patients throughout the area. Armed with success, we will continue."[17]

At Ochsner Medical Center – Baton Rouge, it must have seemed like *déjà vu* when Hurricane Gustav lashed the area with torrential rains and gale-force winds in the summer of 2008. Ochsner Medical Center – Baton Rouge was the only healthcare provider in Louisiana's capital city to remain open during the storm, caring for hundreds of patients and providing shelter for hundreds of residents. The hospital provided 17,000 free hot meals and more than 15,000 gallons of gasoline for those seeking a safe haven from the storm.[18]

For Ochsner employees, small miracles are an everyday occurrence.

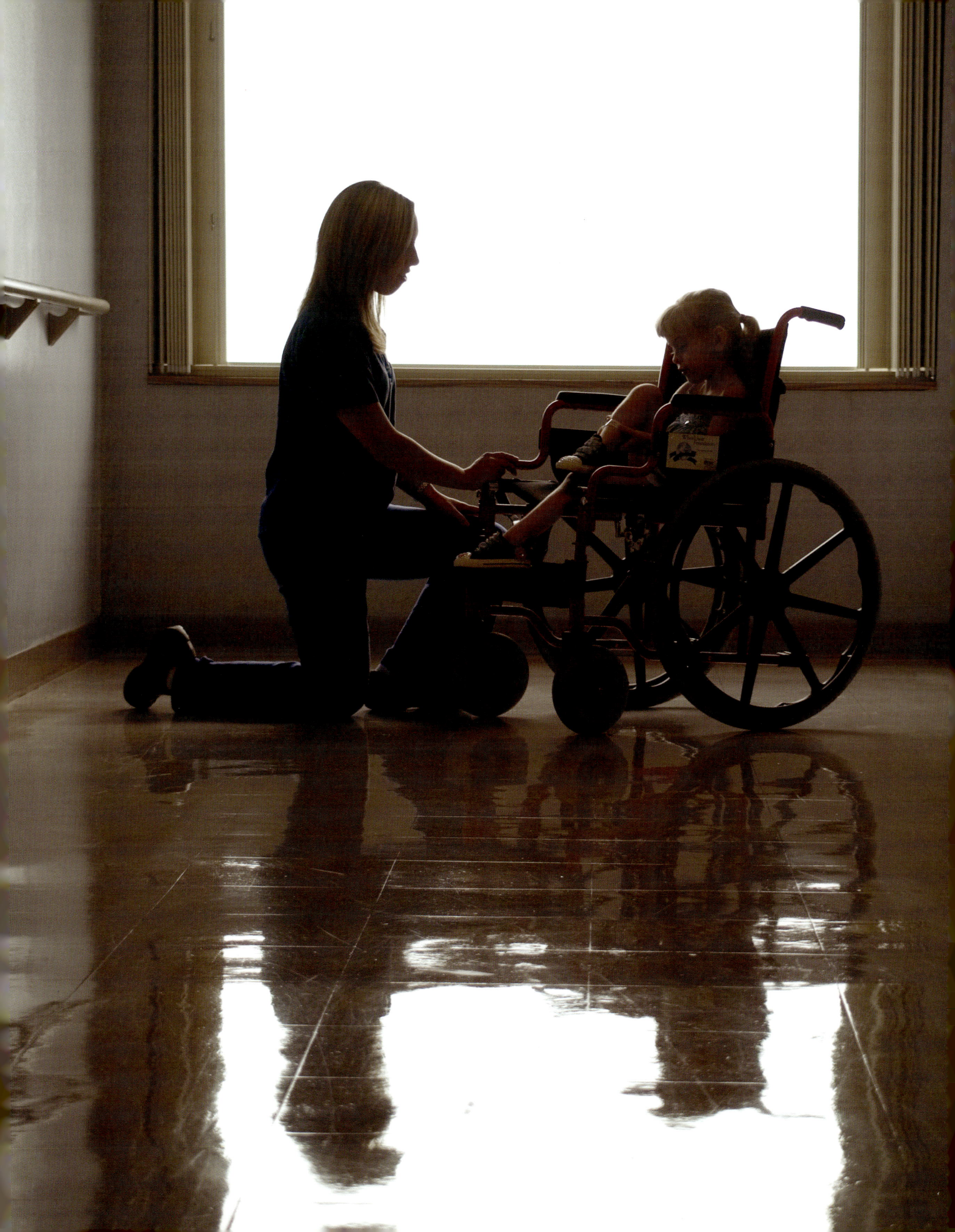

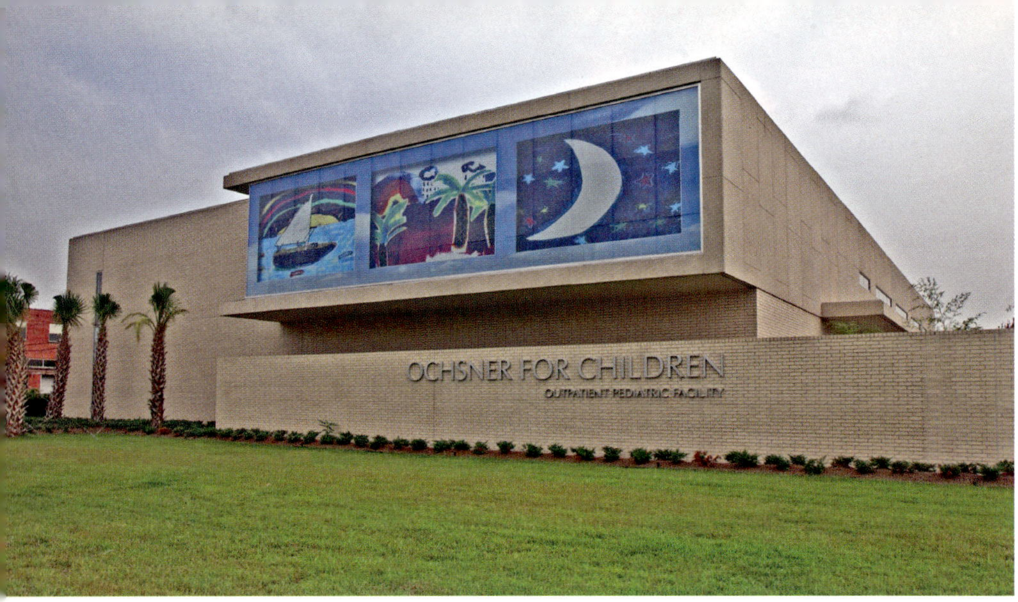

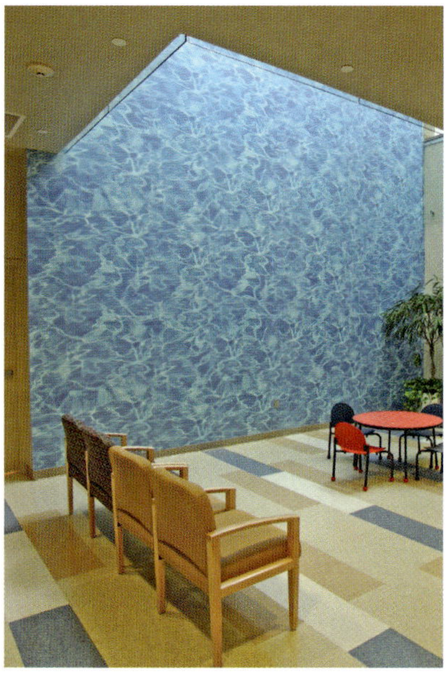

Ochsner's Pediatric Clinic is designed to allay the fears of children and their parents and provide a comfortable healing environment.

'OCHSNER IS ABOUT HOPE'

Joan Rooney was part of the team at Ochsner Medical Center – West Bank Campus that hired 94 full-time staff nurses in 2008. The infusion of nursing staff helped them significantly reduce the need for agency nurses and contributed to strong improvement in patient care. The new nurses joined more than 400 physicians on a dedicated multi-disciplinary team that won prestigious Press Ganey Compass Awards for excellence in Inpatient Services and the Emergency Department.[19]

Rooney, Assistant Vice President of Nursing Services, became a part of Ochsner in 2006 when the predecessor Tenet hospital joined the Ochsner family. At the time, the 22-year veteran of the West Bank recalled being nervous about her future.

As it turned out, she had nothing to worry about. "Immediately, we were welcomed by Ochsner," Rooney said. "Dr. Quinlan and Warner Thomas came over to our campus. They were passionate about welcoming us to Ochsner."[20]

Rooney has seen substantial improvement in the years since Ochsner Medical Center – West Bank Campus joined Ochsner. "Ochsner is about hope, about giving back to the community," Rooney said. "Ochsner is about excellence. We're always striving to be better."[21]

Ochsner St. Anne General Hospital serves a growing population in the bayous surrounding Raceland, Louisiana. In 2008 and 2009, St. Anne increased its staff by nearly a quarter when it reopened its Cath Lab and Cardiology Clinic and opened a new Infusion Center.

Ann Savoie, an outpatient infusion nurse at St. Anne, explained that the new Infusion Center has been a real boon to patients. Savoie said most of her patients are undergoing chemotherapy, and they "used to have to go to the Jefferson Highway campus for infusion. The fact that they don't have to travel as much made a big difference."[22]

Patients come to the St. Anne Infusion Center from as far away as Morgan City, Louisiana, because they like the one-on-one attention. "Ochsner means being able to provide service to the community close to home," Savoie said, "but having the resources if you need them."[23]

Bringing quality healthcare to the community involves partnering with others to broaden Ochsner's reach. In 2009, Ochsner joined with LHC Group Inc., one of the largest providers of home nursing services in the United States and operators of seven long-term acute care hospitals (LTACH) throughout Louisiana, to purchase 25 percent of an LTACH in Kenner. Earlier in 2009, Ochsner joined with LHC Group to provide home health services in southeast Louisiana.[24]

"Caring for our communities is Ochsner's first concern," explained Warner Thomas. "By expanding our joint venture with LHC Group, we're able to broaden services for patients who are most in need and require long-term acute care."[25]

During the spring of 2010, Ochsner welcomed its eighth medical center to the Ochsner System in southeast Louisiana when it purchased Northshore Regional Medical Center, a 165-bed acute care, full-service hospital in Slidell with an ambulatory surgery center and related properties, and incorporated it into the System as Ochsner Medical Center – North Shore. The new facility brings 100 physicians, more than 700 employees and the region's only Pediatric Intensive Care Unit (PICU) into the growing Ochsner family.[26] Ochsner noted its large clinical presence on the North Shore and its strong patient support with more than 250,000 annual visits helped provide a strong base for expansion of medical services at North Shore Regional Medical Center. The addition allows Ochsner to complete its care model in Slidell and to provide an integrated clinical model to patients on the North Shore.

Ochsner worked closely with Scott Boudreaux, Vice President and Chief Executive Officer – North Shore Region, Dr. Edward Martin, Regional Medical Director, and other members of the North Shore team to ensure a smooth transition.

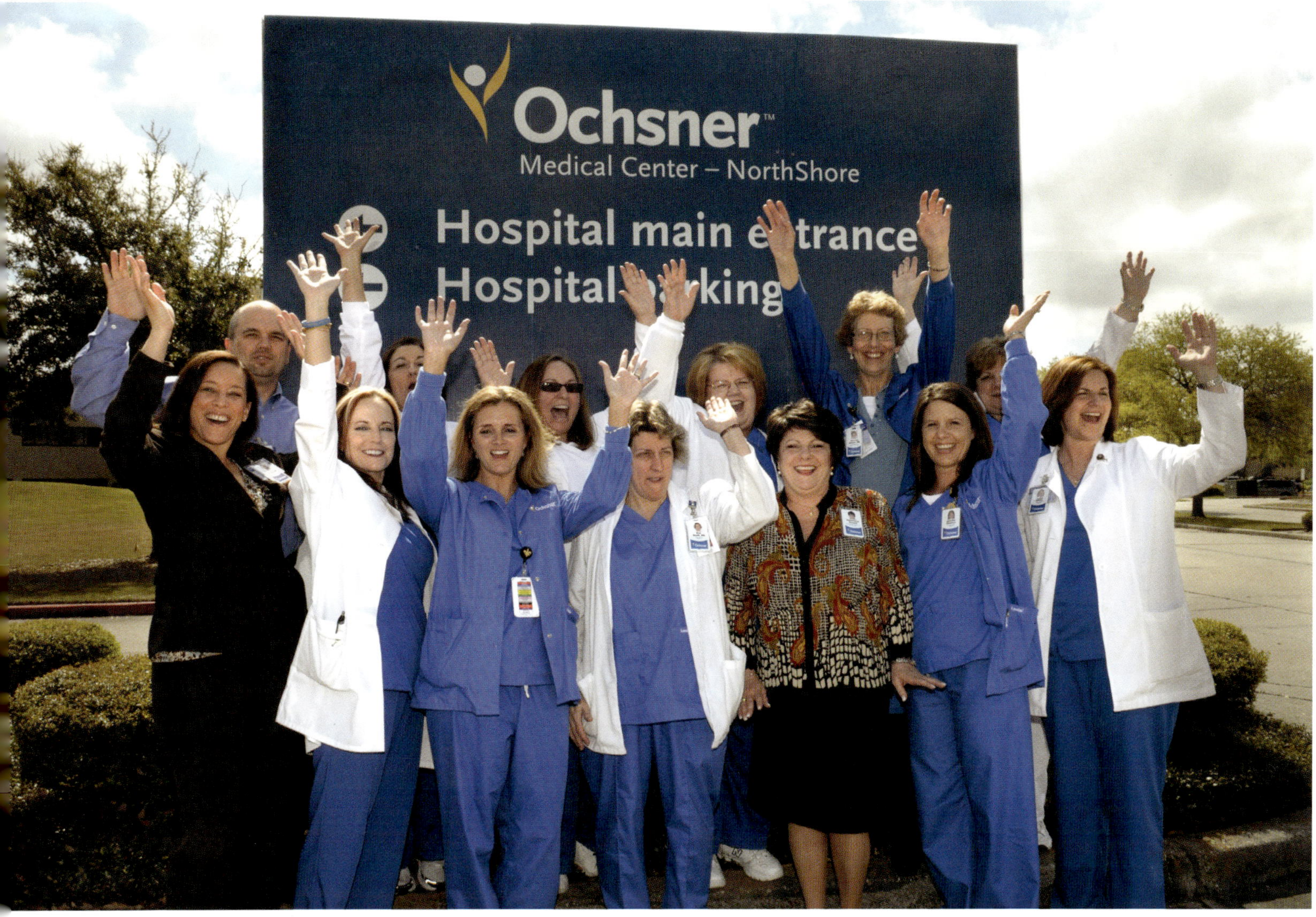

Expanding patient care in the populous St.Tammany-Mississippi Gulf Coast region, Ochsner bought Northshore Regional Medical Center in April 2010. The 165-bed, acute care, full-service hospital located in Slidell, Louisiana, is now Ochsner Medical Center – North Shore.

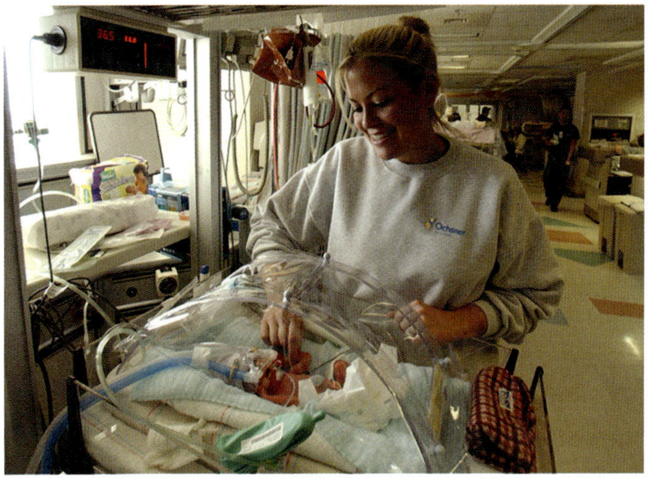

Ochsner's Neonatal Intensive Care Unit prides itself on the care it provides to the youngest and most helpless patients.

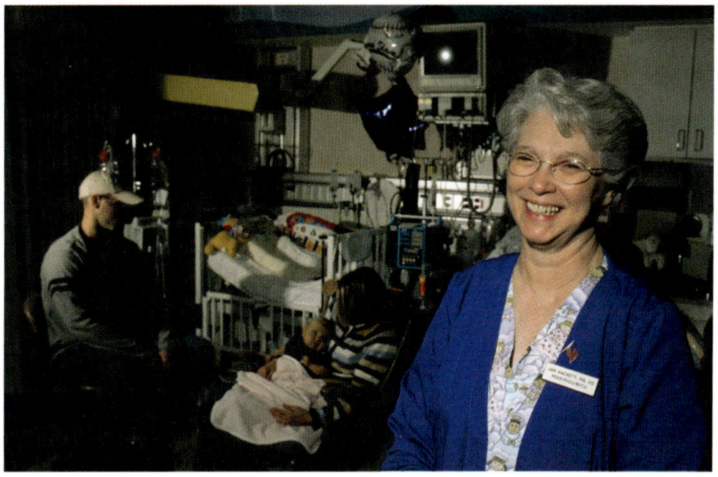

Jan Hackett, R.N., was a Unit Director and nurse at Ochsner's Neonatal Intensive Care Unit, where compassion and technology intersect.

TAKING A STAND

Dr. Alton Ochsner's name is forever associated with the link between cigarette smoking and lung cancer. His path-breaking research during the 1930s led inexorably to the Surgeon General's warnings about cigarette smoking decades later.

So it was fitting during the spring of 2011 when Ochsner Health System prohibited the use of tobacco products at any and all of its properties by physicians, employees, patients and visitors. After April 1, 2011, Ochsner campuses system-wide would no longer provide designated smoking areas or ashtrays.

"As a leader in healthcare, it's important we set the standard for meaningful care and healthy living," said Dr. Patrick Quinlan. "We cannot compromise on this policy because we cannot compromise the health of our patients, our community or our employees."[27]

According to the Centers for Disease Control, cigarette smoking is the single leading cause of preventable death in the U.S., leading to more than 400,000 deaths annually. In fact, more deaths are caused each year by tobacco use than by all deaths from alcohol use, illegal drug use, HIV, motor vehicle injuries, suicides and murders combined.

"These are facts we cannot and will not ignore, and we are doing something about it," said Quinlan, reiterating Ochsner Health System's determination to remain steadfast in its aim to be tobacco-free.[28] He added that Ochsner encourages other companies in Louisiana to join them in becoming completely tobacco-free.

Louisiana residents pay a high price for their addiction to cigarette smoking. "This year alone, 6,500 Louisianians will die from their own smoking," said Dr. Joseph Bisordi, Chief Medical Officer, Ochsner Health System. "Almost 1,000 more nonsmokers will die from exposure to secondhand smoke. Twenty times that many will die from smoking-related diseases. And still, smoking remains the leading cause of preventable deaths in the United States."[29]

To assist the community, Ochsner provides smoking cessation resources, the latest in protocols and information about tobacco-free living, recent news and opportunities to interact with and support others who are also in the process of quitting.[30]

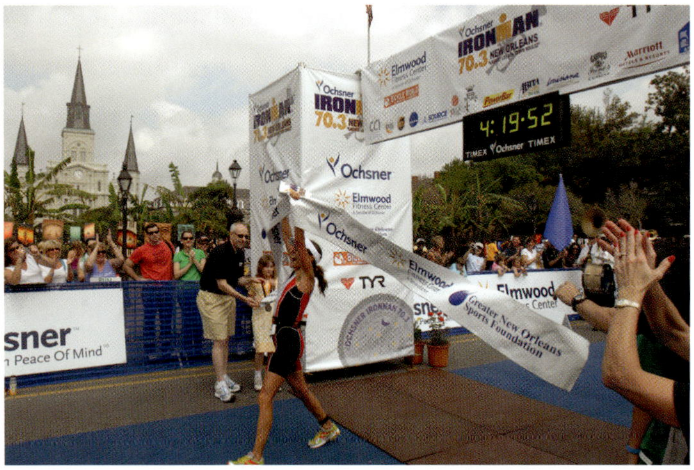

In April 2009 the Ochsner Ironman 70.3 attracted 2,323 athletes to compete in this first-ever New Orleans triathlon and the only event of its kind in the region. A course of 70.3 miles, consisting of a 1.2-mile swim, a 56-mile bike sprint and a 13.1-mile run, took athletes on a scenic tour through the historic city of New Orleans and illustrated Ochsner's commitment to improving and encouraging the health and wellness of the communities it serves.

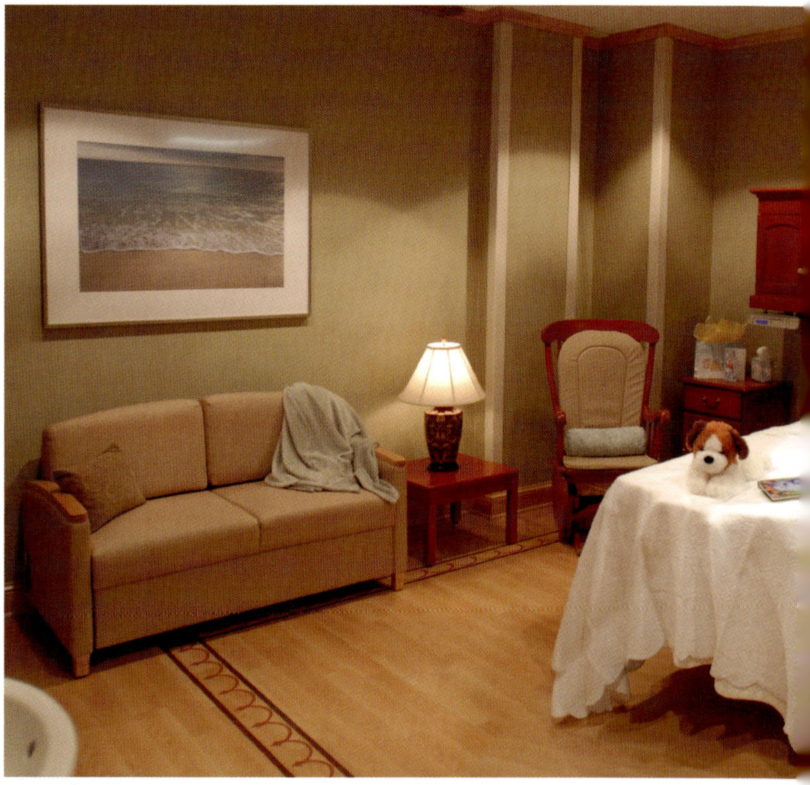

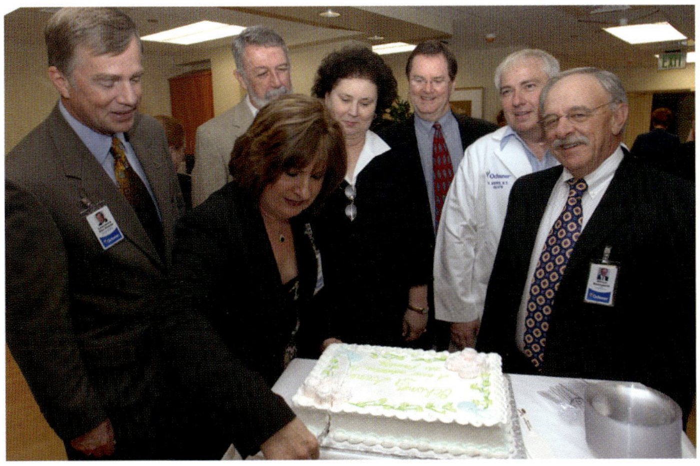

Celebrating the grand opening of Ochsner St. Anne General Hospital's renovated Labor and Delivery suites, pictured below, are (left to right): Lawrence Van Hoose, Senior Vice President – External Relations; Lucia Champagne, R.N.; OB/GYN Physician Charles Faucheux, M.D.; Marsha Arabie, R.N., Vice President – Nursing and Support Services; OB/GYN Physicians J. Frederick Cardwell, M.D. and Gregory Morris, M.D. and Milton Bourgeois Jr., CEO – Ochsner St. Anne General Hospital.

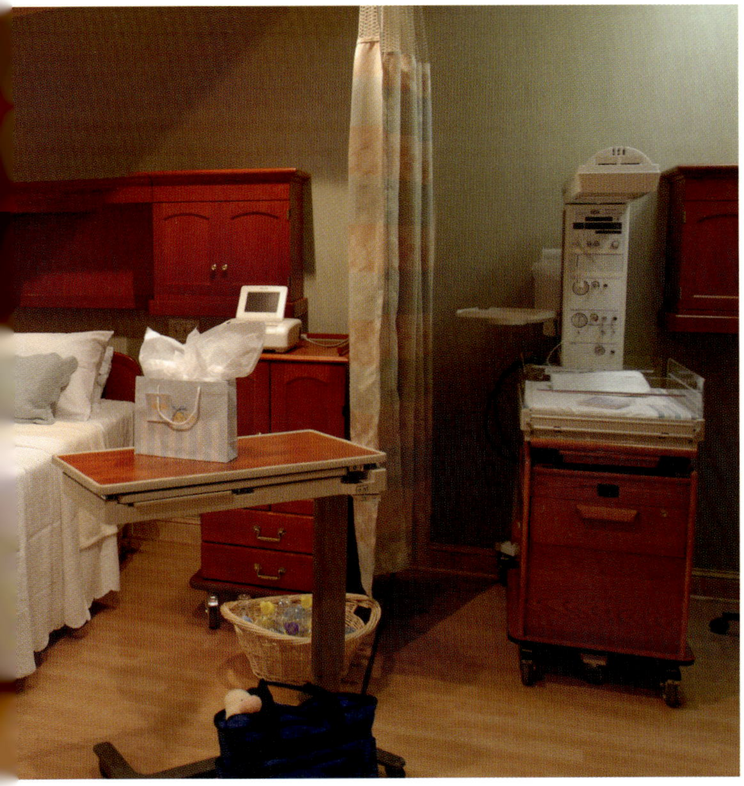

OCHSNER COMMUNITY OUTREACH

Dr. Patrick Quinlan likes to cite an old quote in the medical profession: "Good health doesn't begin at the doctor's office—it starts where we live, work, learn and play."[31]

Quinlan is a passionate champion of community outreach. He believes a successful Ochsner is vital to the community and the proper execution of the Ochsner Mission makes the city of New Orleans, the surrounding region and the state of Louisiana a better place to live.

While the $1 billion in economic impact derived from Ochsner's patient care, research and education is evident, community service and its benefits are more subject to interpretation. Quinlan points out that because of its size and capabilities, Ochsner has the ability to affect the future of the entire region.

Accordingly, Ochsner devised principles to guide its community outreach decision. Ochsner definitely wants to lead or participate in those areas in which its presence matters. It wants to concentrate on those aspects that play to Ochsner's strength. It wants to focus on solving the root causes of problems rather than throw money at the symptoms of the problems. And Ochsner wants, wherever possible, to partner with others in initiatives that will benefit the community.[32]

The Community Outreach Program focuses on many areas and programs including Change the Kids, Change the Future™, Childhood Health and Education, Community Education, Health Partnerships, Workplace Wellness, the Mobile Fitness Unit, Reach Out and Read, the STAR Program, Hello Health Seminars, Rouses Choose Healthy Initiative and the Ochsner Eat Fit menu.

Ochsner reaches out to the community in dozens of ways that might otherwise escape notice. Besides STAR, Ochsner's Academic Community Outreach Department develops and coordinates programs that bring Ochsner into the classroom, including the iLab Student Outreach Lab and School Exploration Educational Visits.[33]

Ochsner physicians host weekly seminars at area restaurants to provide direct access to health topics for residents. Issues covered during the Hello Health seminars have included women's health and heart disease risk factors.

To serve the growing Hispanic population in New Orleans, Ochsner operates a bilingual organization with an international office and offers Spanish language courses for employees so they can better discuss treatments and medical terminology with patients.

"Our diverse clinics and hospitals reflect our belief that healthcare should be close to home," Quinlan said. "We should be where people live in their neighborhood and communities. Our focus on employees and their families involves them in their health at work. Our many partnerships with schools focus on learning, and we target where our neighbors and patients play."[34]

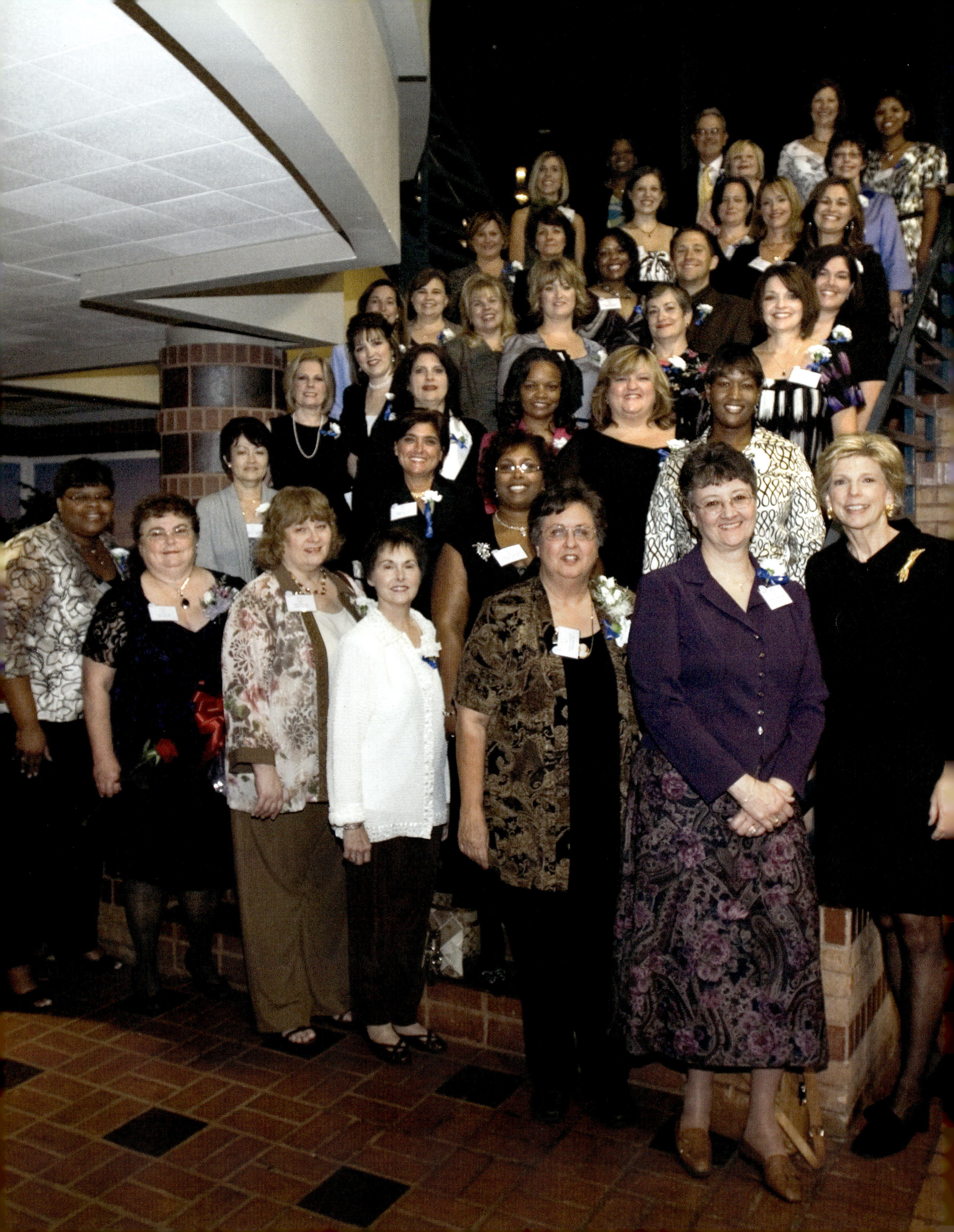

• WHAT OCHSNER MEANS TO ME •

"There's a special TRUST that grows with patients over a period of many years that doesn't happen with just one visit. I have formed lasting relationships with patients and now treat several generations of the same families – grandparents, parents, children and grandchildren."

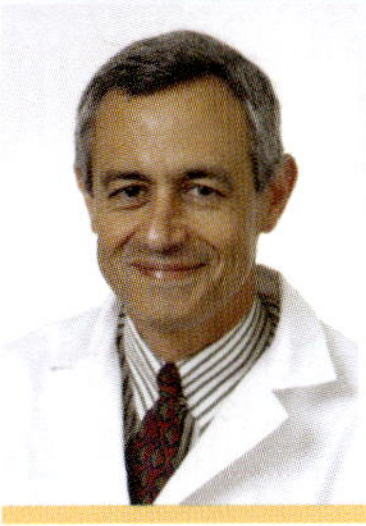

Dr. Leandro Area, Family Physician, Assistant Chairman of Department of Family Medicine, Head Physician, Ochsner Health Center – Lakeview

To watch the full interview with Dr. Leandro Area, visit **ochsner.org/history**.

The Ochsner Leadership Institute develops leadership qualities like knowledge, intelligence and vision, symbolized by the flame logo. The program trains Ochsner managers, physicians and nurses to lead by example, guide, energize and inspire excellence in others.

A NATIONWIDE LEADER

Ochsner's leadership role in establishing a tobacco-free system is manifested in many ways every day. In 2009, Ochsner and GE Healthcare established a Strategic Enterprise Relationship to affect healthcare delivery, operations, management, education and training. GE helped Ochsner expand its Ochsner Leadership Institute (OLI) that trains managers to lead by example and to inspire excellence in those they lead. The OLI program, which is based on a rigorous training model, helps managers, physicians and nurses develop leadership qualities such as knowledge, vision and intelligence.[35] GE Chief Executive Officer Jeff Immelt joined Ochsner executives in 2010 at an Ochsner-sponsored forum that offered more than 900 Gulf Coast business leaders insights into forming successful recovery strategies.[36]

Ochsner deepened its partnership with GE in 2010, particularly in the areas of leadership development and implementation of innovative technologies. Using AgileTrac, a GE technology, Ochsner enhanced its infrastructure and allowed the health system to deliver healthcare more safely and efficiently. Pursuing real-time location technologies frees Ochsner staff to concentrate on patient care.[37]

The System's nurses perhaps best exhibit frontline leadership at Ochsner, and Ochsner is blessed to have some of the best in the business. In 2009–2010, Ochsner nurses made up more than one-third of the 100 Great Nurses in Louisiana. Each year, the foundation sponsoring the coveted award recognizes 100 registered nurses as "great—one who stands out among peers through their natural leadership and mentoring qualities, and one who gives back to the profession and community in their daily lives."[38] More than 50 Ochsner nurses each year receive the national DAISY award for extraordinary and compassionate patient care.

Increasingly, that patient care is represented through Ochsner's Relationship-Based Care practice model. Relationship-Based Care emphasizes the creation of a healing relationship that is the basis of both patient satisfaction and positive patient outcomes.[39]

Nancy Davis, Senior Vice President, Patient Care and System Chief Nursing Officer, far right, heads a nursing team at Ochsner that placed 39 of the top 100 nurses in Louisiana's "Great 100 Nurses Celebration" in 2008.

THE MORE THINGS CHANGE

Quality of care and patient safety have been an Ochsner standard ever since Dr. Alton Ochsner and four colleagues from Tulane opened Ochsner Clinic at the corner of Aline and Prytania Streets in Uptown New Orleans the day after New Year's in 1942. Through the decades since, generations of Ochsner physicians, nurses and employees have kept sacred Alton Ochsner's instruction to treat the patient and not just the disease.

The legacy left by Alton Ochsner and the founders has been one of excellence. Each generation of the Ochsner family has faced challenges and opportunities. Ochsner and his colleagues built the practice of the Clinic in the face of a sometimes-hostile New Orleans medical community. They expanded the Clinic's reach by establishing a not-for-profit Foundation, which in turn opened the first Ochsner Foundation Hospital at Camp Plauché. That first generation then went on to build the second, permanent Ochsner Foundation Hospital on Jefferson Highway.

The next generation made Ochsner synonymous with clinical excellence during the 1960s and 1970s. Ochsner cardiovascular surgeons, under the leadership of Dr. John Ochsner, performed the region's first heart valve replacement, coronary artery bypass, pacemaker implant, heart transplant and lung transplant. Other Ochsner surgical teams performed the first successful adult and pediatric kidney transplants in the region. Meanwhile, Dr. Albert Segaloff advanced Ochsner's research initiatives with 34 years of groundbreaking breast cancer research.

The third generation presided over outreach initiatives that took the Ochsner legacy well beyond the geographical confines of the Jefferson Highway campus. They opened the first of what would become a network of over 38 neighborhood health centers located across the length and breadth of southeast Louisiana. They confronted the challenge of sweeping change in how society consumed and paid for healthcare and involved Ochsner in the brave new world of managed care. Along the way, they succeeded in achieving an accomplishment eluding the two generations preceding them: a unification of the Clinic and Foundation that made the growth of a true Ochsner Health System possible.

Today's generation faces challenges no less difficult than those confronted earlier by Alton Ochsner and the other founders, and later by Drs. Merrill Hines, Frank Riddick, George Porter and Patrick Quinlan. No one could ever have foreseen the devastation that Hurricane Katrina would leave in its wake, and Ochsner's steadfastness in the face of chaos endeared it to a community that felt abandoned. Ochsner and its over 12,500 employees have stepped up in the years following Katrina and given a community hope when it invested in hospitals that had been all but destroyed by the hurricane.

The healthcare institution Alton Ochsner and the founders helped establish at the corner of Aline and Prytania Streets in Uptown New Orleans nearly 70 years ago has become a model of healthcare in the twenty-first century. Ochsner continues to expand on the vision of the founders—serving, healing, leading, educating and innovating for the people of New Orleans and southeast Louisiana. Alton Ochsner's legacy is a guidepost to the future of American healthcare, and Ochsner Health System is helping to foster that legacy for future generations. Follow our story as it continues to unfold at ochsner.org/history.

Warner Thomas put it best when he emphatically told employees: "We're here to do great things for the community."[40]

Great Things. Community. They define what it means to be part of Ochsner.

Alton Ochsner would be proud.

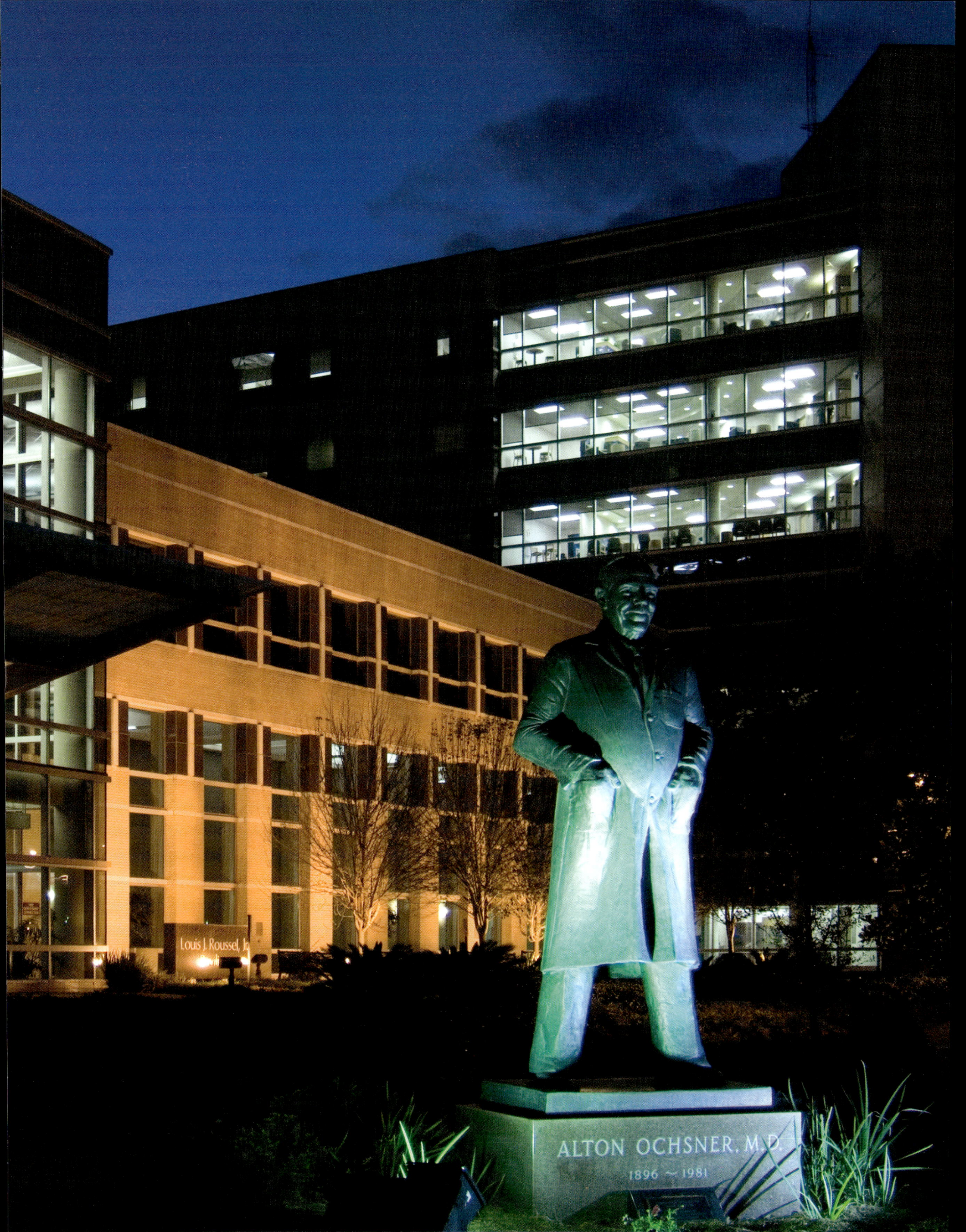

ALTON OCHSNER, M.D.
1896 ~ 1981

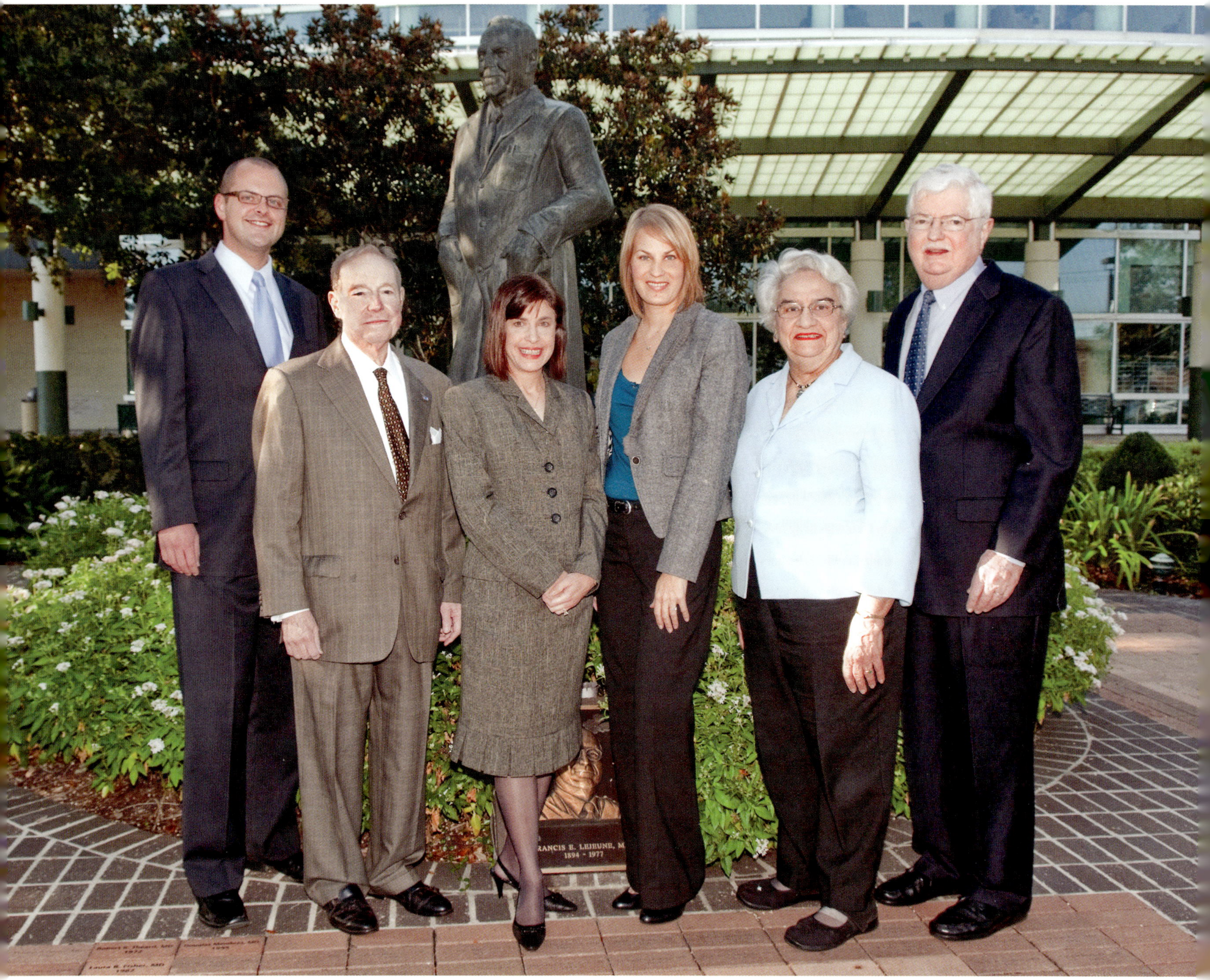

Members of the Ochsner History Book Team included (pictured from left to right) Cade Farmer, Frank A. Riddick, M.D., Ethel Madden, Lynne Bischof, Marion Stafford and Michael A. Sullivan, M.D.

THANK YOU

Ochsner would like to thank these individuals for sharing their time and their memories, without which this book would not have been possible.

PERSONAL INTERVIEWS:

Bobby Brannon
Mary Brown
Nancy Davis
Rudolph Ehrensing, M.D.
Bernard Ferrari, M.D.
Richard Freeman Jr.
Edward D. Frolich, M.D.
Harley Ginsberg, M.D.
Richard Guthrie, M.D.
Charlie Heim
Charles Kantrow Jr., M.D.
Carl Kardinal, M.D.
Francis "Duke" LeJeune Jr., M.D.
Evelyn LeTard
J. Thomas Lewis
George Loss, M.D.
John Ochsner, M.D.
John Lockwood Ochsner, M.D.
William Pinsky, M.D.
George Porter, M.D.
Scott Posecai
Patrick Quinlan, M.D.
Richard Ré, M.D.
Frank A. Riddick, M.D.
Terry Shilling
Michael Sullivan, M.D.
Warner Thomas
Michael Tooke, M.D.
Catherine Tremaine
Hector Ventura, M.D.
Grant Walker

OCHSNER HISTORY BOOK TEAM:

Frank A. Riddick, M.D.
Michael A. Sullivan, M.D.
Stanton E. Shuler, M.D.
Lynne Bischof
Jessica Delgado
Jackson Ellisor
Cade Farmer
Siobhan Flahive
Stephen Legendre
Ethel Madden
Lori Monteleone
Tammy Nocito
Nital Sheridan
Marion Stafford
Shelley Sullivan
Lawrence Van Hoose

The H Agency Team including writer Bill Beck

ENDNOTES

CHAPTER 1

1. "Surgeon's Speech," *TIME Magazine,* November 15, 1926
2. "Rudolph Matas, 1860-1957," www.knowsouthernhistory.net
3. Ibid.
4. Hector O. Ventura, M.D., "Alton Ochsner, M.D.: Physician," *The Ochsner Journal,* v.4, no.1, Winter 2002, pp.48–52
5. Digitally Recorded Oral History Interview with John Lockwood Ochsner, New Orleans, Louisiana, January 20, 2009
6. Ventura, "Alton Ochsner, M.D.: Physician," pp.48–52
7. Guy Alvin Caldwell, *curriculum vitae,* p.1
8. "Guy Alvin Caldwell, M.D.," *The Journal of Bone and Joint Surgery,* v.64, 1982, p.472
9. Hector O. Ventura, M.D., "Guy Alvin Caldwell, M.D.: Physician and Administrator," *The Ochsner Journal,* v.4, no.2, Spring 2002, p.113
10. "Guy Alvin Caldwell, M.D.," *The Journal of Bone and Joint Surgery,* p.473
11. Ibid.
12. Hector O. Ventura, M.D., "Guy Alvin Caldwell, M.D.: Physician and Administrator," p.114
13. Ventura, "Alton Ochsner, M.D.: Physician," pp.48–52
14. Ibid.
15. Ibid.
16. Ibid.
17. "Alton Ochsner's Memoirs"
18. Eddy Randrup, M.D., and Hector O. Ventura, M.D., "Edgar Burns," *The Ochsner Journal,* v.4, no.3, Summer 2002, p.182
19. Ibid.
20. Ochsner Archives Interview with Catherine Burns Tremaine, New Orleans, Louisiana, 2000
21. Randrup and Ventura, "Edgar Burns," p.182
22. "Alton Ochsner's Memoirs"
23. Ibid.
24. Ibid.
25. Ibid.
26. Ibid.
27. Digitally Recorded Oral History Interview with Dr. Francis "Duke" LeJeune Jr., New Orleans, Louisiana, January 21, 2009
28. Hector O. Ventura, M.D. and Eddy Randrup, M.D., "Francis Ernest ("Duke") LeJeune Sr. MD," *The Ochsner Journal*, v.5, no.1, Winter 2003, p.47
29. Duke LeJeune Jr. Interview
30. Francis E. LeJeune Sr., *Curriculum Vitae*
31. Ventura and Randrup, "Francis Ernest ("Duke") LeJeune Sr. MD," p.47
32. Duke LeJeune Jr. Interview
33. Ventura and Randrup, "Francis Ernest ("Duke") LeJeune Sr. MD," p.48
34. "Francis E. LeJeune Sr., MD, 1894-1977," Tulane-Otolaryngology, www.mcl.tulane.edu
35. "New Orleans Imbroglio," *TIME Magazine,* October 6, 1930
36. Ibid.
37. T. Harry Williams, *Huey Long* (New York: Alfred A. Knopf, 1969), pp.542–545
38. "Death of a Dictator," *TIME Magazine,* September 16, 1935
39. Ochsner, A., DeBakey, M., "Primary Pulmonary Malignancy. Treatment by total pneumonectomy: analysis of 79 collected cases and presentation of 7 personal cases," *Surgery, Gynecology and Obstetrics,* v.68, February 15, 1939, pp.435–451
40. Curtis Hartman Tyrone, *curriculum vitae*
41. Hector O. Ventura, M.D. and Eddy Randrup, M.D., "Curtis Tyrone, MD," *The Ochsner Journal,* v.4, no.4, Autumn 2002, p.245
42. Ibid.
43. "News From The Ochsner Medical Institutions," July 14, 1982, p.1
44. Ventura and Randrup, "Curtis Tyrone, MD," p.246
45. Ibid.

CHAPTER 2

1. "Rochester, Minn.," *TIME Magazine,* May 19, 1923
2. "Alton Ochsner Memoirs"
3. Ibid.
4. Ibid.
5. Ibid.
6. Guy A. Caldwell, M.D., *Early History of the Ochsner Medical Center: The First Twenty-Two Years* (Springfield, Illinois: Charles C. Thomas Publisher, 1965), p.6
7. Ibid., p.7
8. Catherine Burns Tremaine Interview, p.4
9. John Wilds, *Ochsner's: An Informal History of the South's Largest Private Medical Center* (Baton Rouge: Louisiana State University Press, 1985), p.30
10. Duke LeJeune Jr. Interview, p.4
11. Ibid.
12. Ibid.
13. Ibid.
14. "Physicians ponder 'Little Mayo Clinic' for New Orleans," *New Orleans States-Item,* December 4, 1940
15. Henry E. Chambers, *A History of Louisiana* (Chicago and New York: American Historical Society, Inc: 1925), pp.380–381
16. Western Union Telegram, Francis LeJeune Sr. to Alton Ochsner, March 27, 1941; Copy located in Ochsner Archives
17. Caldwell, *Early History of the Ochsner Medical Center,* p.13
18. Ibid.
19. Ibid.
20. "Alton Ochsner Memoirs"
21. Ibid.

22. Ibid.

23. Mildred Little, "Alton Ochsner Medical Foundation Formed Here," *New Orleans States,* January 25, 1944

24. Caldwell, *Early History of the Ochsner Medical Center,* p.13

25. Ibid., pp.22–24

26. Ibid., p.27

27. Evelyn LeTard, "History of Ochsner Medical Center, 1940-1983;" Manuscript copy located in Ochsner Archives

28. Digitally Recorded Oral History Interview with Evelyn LeTard, New Orleans, Louisiana, January 19, 2009

29. LeTard, "History of Ochsner Medical Center, 1940-1983," p.4

30. Evelyn LeTard Interview

CHAPTER 3

1. "NOAA/NHC Deadliest Hurricanes," http://www.nhc.noaa.gov/pastdeadly.shtml; See also, Caldwell, *Early History of The Ochsner Medical Center,* p.40

2. Caldwell, Early History of The Ochsner Medical Center, p.41

3. Ibid., p.49

4. "Alton Ochsner Memoirs"

5. Larry Schwartz, "Remarkable Hogan wins '50 U.S. Open," www.espn.go.com/classic/s/addhoganben.html

6. Quoted in Caldwell, *Early History of The Ochsner Medical Center,* pp.54–55

7. Wilds, Ochsner's, p.18

8. "The Hooded Falcon," *Time,* August 4, 1958

9. John Ochsner Interview

10. Ibid.

11. "Alton Ochsner Memoirs"

12. Ibid.

13. Caldwell, *Early History of The Ochsner Medical Center,* p.58

14. Paul Starr, *The Social Transformation of American Medicine* (New York: Basic Books, 1982)

15. Caldwell, *Early History of The Ochsner Medical Center,* p.64

16. Ibid., pp.64–65

17. Ibid., p.65

18. Ibid., p.64

19. "The Texas Tornado," Time, May 28, 1965

20. Ibid.

21. John Lockwood Ochsner Interview

22. Ibid.

23. "In Memoriam: Idys Mims Gage, M.D.," *newsletter: Report of the Alton Ochsner Medical Foundation,* v.VI, September 1958, p.1

24. "Libby Dufour Residence Nearing Completion," *newsletter: Report of the Alton Ochsner Medical Foundation,* v.II, April 1954

25. "New Research Building of Alton Ochsner Medical Foundation," op.cit., v.III, October 1955

26. Caldwell, *Early History of The Ochsner Medical Center,* p.84

27. Caldwell, *Early History of the Ochsner Medical Center,* p.76

28. Memo, Marine Board of Investigation, United States Coast Guard, to Commandant, 8th Coast Guard District, New Orleans, 4 December 1958

29. Caldwell, *Early History of the Ochsner Medical Center,* p.76

CHAPTER 4

1. Wilds, *Ochsner's,* p.178

2. Ibid.

3. Alan Sheldon, *Managing Change and Collaboration in the Health System,* p.10

4. Wilds, *Ochsner's,* p.179

5. Ibid., p.152

6. Caldwell, *Early History of the Ochsner Medical Center,* p.101; See also, "Cornerstone Ceremony Set for New Ochsner Clinic," *newsletter,* v.IX, July 1962

7. "In Memoriam: J. Blanc Monroe, 1880-1960," *newsletter,* June 1960

8. "In Memoriam: Mercer G. Lynch, M.D., Edward H. Leveroos, M.D.," *newsletter,* June 1960

9. "In Memoriam: Edmund Ernest Richardson," *newsletter,* July 1962

10. Wilds, *Ochsner's,* pp.174–176

11. Ibid., pp.143–146

12. John Lockwood Ochsner Interview

13. Ibid.

14. Tape Recorded Oral History Interview with Frank Riddick, M.D., New Orleans, Louisiana, September 20, 2001

15. Digitally Recorded Oral History Interview with Frank Riddick, M.D., New Orleans, Louisiana, January 21, 2009

16. Frank Riddick September 20, 2001 Interview

17. Wilds, *Ochsner's,* pp.147–148

18. Ibid., p.148

19. "Construction Begun on $1,500,000 Rawley M. Penick Memorial building," *newsletter,* v.XII, February 1966

20. Ibid.

21. R.F. Robison, "The Race for Megavoltage," *Acta Oncologica,* v.34, no.8, 1995, pp.1055–1074

22. "In Memoriam: Rawley M. Penick, Jr., M.D.," *newsletter: Alton Ochsner Medical Foundation,* v.X, August 1963

23. Wilds, *Ochsner's,* p.182

CHAPTER 5

1. "AOMF Development Campaign Fund Approaching 90%," *The Newsletter,* November 1971

2. Ibid.

3. W. E. Kittredge, M.D., "Dr. Edgar Burns, In Memoriam," *The Newsletter,* November–December 1973

4. Ibid.

5. Frank Riddick January 21, 2009 Interview

6. Ibid.

7. "Chairman, Board of AOMF Trustees," *The Newsletter*, June 1975

8. "Ochsner Clinic Medical Director," *The Newsletter*, June 1975

9. "Annual Report Ochsner '74"

10. Digitally Recorded Oral History Interview with Bobby Brannon, New Orleans, Louisiana, January 20, 2009

11. "Construction Costs & Financing," *The Newsletter*, June 1975

12. Ibid.

13. Digitally Recorded Oral History Interview with Edward Frohlich, New Orleans, Louisiana, February 18, 2009

14. Ibid.

15. Ibid.

16. Digitally Recorded Oral History Interview with Richard Re, New Orleans, Louisiana, January 22, 2009

17. Hector O. Ventura, M.D., "Research at Ochsner Clinic: Highlights in its History," *The Ochsner Journal*, v.7, no.2, Summer 2007

18. Wilds, *Ochsner's*, p.228

19. Ventura, "Research at Ochsner Clinic"

20. "Dr. Albert Segaloff, 68, Dies; A Breast Cancer Researcher," *New York Times*, February 28, 1985

CHAPTER 6

1. "Dr. Alton Ochsner Dies At 85; Co-Founder of Health Center," *New York Times*, September 25, 1981

2. "Entertainment, Medical Sessions Highlight Dr. Ochsner's Eightieth Birthday," *Ochsner Report*, v.1, no.1, Spring 1976, p.1

3. "Alton Ochsner Memoirs"

4. Ibid.

5. "Entertainment, Medical Sessions Highlight Dr. Ochsner's Eightieth Birthday"

6. "New X-Ray System Is Better, Cheaper," *Ochsner Report*, v.10, no.2, Spring 1985

7. Digitally Recorded Oral History Interview with Michael Sullivan, New Orleans, Louisiana, January 20, 2009

8. Ibid.

9. "An Evaluation of Past, Present, and Future Relationships Between Ochsner Clinic And Alton Ochsner Medical Foundation," 1985, p.3; Unpublished manuscript, Ochsner Archives

10. Ibid., p.4

11. Digitally Recorded Oral History Interview with George Porter, New Orleans, Louisiana, January 21, 2009

12. "An Evaluation of Past, Present, and Future Relationships Between Ochsner Clinic And Alton Ochsner Medical Foundation," 1985, p.13

13. George Porter Interview

14. "Ochsner Bronze Portrait Placed At Campus Entrance," Inside Ochsner, v.10, no.1, January 1986, p.5; See Also, *Ochsner Medical Institutions, Annual Report, 1986*, p.1

15. "Ochsner Bronze Portrait Placed At Campus Entrance"

16. *Ochsner Medical Institutions, Annual Report, 1987,* p.24

17. "Division of Planning," *Ochsner Medical Institutions, Annual Report, 1986,* p.22

18. Ibid.

CHAPTER 7

1. "The Ochsner Health Plan," *Ochsner Medical Institutions, Annual Report 1987*, p.23

2. George Porter Interview

3. Bobby Brannon Interview

4. "The Ochsner Health Plan"

5. "Governance of the Ochsner Medical Institutions," 1991, p.9; Copy located in Ochsner Archives

6. "The Ochsner Health Plan," *Ochsner Medical Institutions, Annual Report 1994*, p.14

7. "Neighborhood Clinics Expand To Meet Growing Needs," *Inside Ochsner*, v.14, no.1, January 1990, p.1

8. Ibid.

9. "The Growing Ochsner Network," *Inside Ochsner*, v.18, no.2, April 1994, pp.1–2

10. "Ochsner Purchases Elmwood Fitness Center," *Inside Ochsner*, v.15, no.4, August 1991, p.1

11. "Governance of the Ochsner Medical Institutions," p.2

12. Ibid., p.6

13. Digitally Recorded Oral History Interview with Richard Guthrie, New Orleans, Louisiana, January 19, 2009

14. "Governance of the Ochsner Medical Institutions," p.8

15. Richard Guthrie Interview

16. "Governance of the Ochsner Medical Institutions," p.9

17. Ibid., p.9

18. Frank Riddick September 20, 2001 Interview, Part 2

19. "Tooke: Service To Play Larger Role At Ochsner," *Inside Ochsner*, v.17, no.1, February 1993

20. Digitally Recorded Telephone Oral History Interview with Michael Tooke, Easton, Maryland, February 18, 2009

21. "Research," *Ochsner Medical Institutions, 1993 Annual Report*, p.20

22. "Ochsner and Tulane End Affiliations Talks," *Inside Ochsner*, v.18, no.2, April 1994

23. Michael Tooke Interview

24. "Ochsner, SCH Plan Louisiana's First Statewide Health Network," *Inside Ochsner*, v.18, no.2, April 1994

25. Frank Riddick January 21, 2009 Interview

CHAPTER 8

1. "Ochsner Foundation Hospital One of the Nation's 'Best' in Heart, Gynecology, Rheumatology and Urology," for OnlYou, v.1, no.8, August 2000

2. "Medical Milestone – Surgeons Perform 500th Heart Transplant," *for OnlYou*, v.1, no.3, February 2000

3. Ibid.

4. Ibid.

5. Ibid.

6. "Critical Care Tower 2000," *for OnlYou*, v.1, no.5, April 2000

7. Digitally Recorded Oral History Interview with Charles Heim, New Orleans, Louisiana, January 19, 2009

8. Ibid.

9. Richard Guthrie Interview

10. Frank Riddick January 21, 2009 Interview

11. "Former Ochsner Leader Leaves Behind a Remarkable Legacy," *for OnlYou*, v.1, no.3, February 2000

12. Digitally Recorded Oral History Interview with Mary Brown, New Orleans, Louisiana, January 21, 2009

13. John Lockwood Ochsner Interview

14. Ibid.

15. Ibid.

16. Ibid.

17. Ibid.

CHAPTER 9

1. Digitally Recorded Oral History Interview with Patrick Quinlan, New Orleans, Louisiana, January 20, 2009

2. Frank A. Riddick Jr., M.D., "Message From Senior Management," *for OnlYou*, v.1, no. 2, December 9, 1999, p.1

3. Patrick Quinlan Interview

4. Ibid.

5. Ibid.

6. Digitally Recorded Oral History Interview with Richard Freeman, New Orleans, Louisiana, January 21, 2009

7. Ibid.

8. Patrick Quinlan Interview

9. Richard Freeman Interview

10. Patrick Quinlan Interview

11. Ibid.

12. Digitally Recorded Oral History Interview with Warner Thomas, New Orleans, Louisiana, February 19, 2009

13. Patrick Quinlan, "The Ochsner New Year," *For OnlYou,*" v.2, no.1, February 2001

14. Richard Freeman Interview

15. "chief concerns," *in the know @ Ochsner*, Winter 2001, p.2

16. Memorandum, Frank A. Riddick Jr. to AOMF Division Directors, AOMF Department Managers, August 10, 2001

17. Chris Bonura, "Power of One," New Orleans City Business, August 20, 2001, p.1

18. Ronette King, "Ochsner operations are merging," *The Times-Picayune*, September 6, 2001

19. Patrick Quinlan Interview

20. Frank A. Riddick Jr., "Remarks at Press Conference," September 6, 2001, p.3; Typescript copy located in Ochsner Archives

21. Ibid.

22. Patrick Quinlan Interview

23. Ibid.

24. Ibid.

25. Patrick Quinlan Interview

26. "chief concerns," *in the know @ Ochsner*, Winter 2001, p.2

27. Patrick Quinlan Interview

28. Ibid.

CHAPTER 10

1. Digitally Recorded Telephone Oral History Interview with Patrick Quinlan, New Orleans, Louisiana, October 23, 2009

2. Ibid.

3. Ibid.

4. Digitally Recorded Oral History Interview with Grant Walker, New Orleans, Louisiana, January 20, 2009

5. Ibid.

6. Ibid.

7. Ibid.

8. Grant Walker, "Hurricane Katrina Journal," p.2

9. Ibid.

10. Ibid.

11. Ibid.

12. Betty M. Wells Video Interview, ftp://mediaservices.ochsner.org/history_book/

13. Ibid.

14. Ibid.

15. Warner Thomas Interview

16. Grant Walker, "Hurricane Katrina Journal," August 27, 2005, p.1

17. Ibid.

18. Ibid.

19. Digitally Recorded Oral History Interview with Scott Posecai, New Orleans, Louisiana, March 18, 2009

20. Ibid.

21. Grant Walker Interview

22. Ibid.

23. Patrick Quinlan October 23, 2009 Interview

24. Richard Guthrie Interview

25. Ibid.

26. Grant Walker Interview

27. Grant Walker, "Hurricane Katrina Journal," p.3

28. Ibid.

29. Patrick Quinlan October 23, 2009 Interview

CHAPTER 11

1. *Ochsner Outreach*, September 5, 2005

2. Warner Thomas, Weekly Phone Call with Employees, Transcript, October 24, 2005, p.2

3. Patrick Quinlan October 23, 2009 Interview

4. Grant Walker, "Hurricane Katrina Journal," p.6

5. Ibid.

6. Ibid.

7. Ibid., p.7

8. Ibid.

9. Ibid.

10. Ibid., p.8

11. Patrick Quinlan October 23, 2009 Interview

12. Ibid.

13. Grant Walker, "Hurricane Katrina Journal," p.9

14. Grant Walker Interview

15. Ibid.

16. Ibid.

17. Charles Heim Interview

18. Betty M. Wells Video Interview

19. Grant Walker, "Hurricane Katrina Journal," p.15

20. Ibid., p.17

21. Patrick Quinlan October 23, 2009 Interview

22. John Lockwood Ochsner Interview

23. Ibid.

CHAPTER 12

1. Ochsner 2005–2006 Annual Report

2. "New Orleans hospitals struggle since Katrina," *USA Today*, April 26, 2006

3. Ochsner 2005–2006 Annual Report

4. News item, *Lake Charles American Press*, April 24, 2006

5. Ochsner 2005–2006 Annual Report

6. "St. Anne," www.louisianamedicalnews.com/hospital-spotlight-ochsner-health-system-cms-1048

7. "New Orleans hospitals struggle since Katrina"

8. Ibid.

9. Ibid.

10. "Ochsner buying 3 hospitals," *New Orleans Times-Picayune*, July 19, 2006

11. Ibid.

12. Sheri Fink, "Strained by Katrina, A Hospital Faced Deadly Choices," *The New York Times*, August 25, 2009

13. Ibid.

14. Bobby Brannon Interview

15. Digitally Recorded Oral History Interview with Terry Shilling, New Orleans, Louisiana, March 18, 2009

16. Ibid.

17. Scott Posecai Interview

18. "Baptist is back," *New Orleans Times-Picayune,* October 8, 2006

19. "Ochsner Baptist Medical Center adds beds, services," *New Orleans City-Business*, September 10, 2007

20. "Turning a corner," *New Orleans CityBusiness*, April 27, 2009

21. Ochsner 2005–2006 Annual Report

22. Warner Thomas Remarks, Baptist Imaging Center Ribbon Cutting, November 14, 2007

23. Ibid.

24. Patrick Quinlan Remarks, Baptist Imaging Center Ribbon Cutting, November 14, 2007

25. Curtis Dosch Remarks, Baptist Imaging Center Ribbon Cutting, November 14, 2007

26. Ibid.

27. Arnie Fielkow Remarks, Baptist Imaging Center Ribbon Cutting, November 14, 2007

28. Ochsner Archives Video Interview with Joanne Cardaro, New Orleans, Fall 2009

29. Ibid.

30. Ibid.

31. James Maurin Remarks, Baptist ER and Clara Wing Ribbon Cutting, January 12, 2009

32. Rob Wolterman Remarks, Baptist ER and Clara Wing Ribbon Cutting, January 12, 2009

33. Patrick Quinlan Remarks, Baptist ER and Clara Wing Ribbon Cutting, January 12, 2009

34. Joanne Cardaro Video Interview

35. Patrick Quinlan Remarks, Baptist ER and Clara Wing Ribbon Cutting, January 12, 2009

CHAPTER 13

1. "Make Life Happen," Transplant Press Conference, Brent House Conference Center, New Orleans, Louisiana, January 22, 2008

2. Patrick Quinlan Remarks, op.cit.

3. Ibid.

4. Hector Ventura Remarks, op.cit.

5. Ibid.

6. Warner Thomas November 13, 2009 Interview

7. "America's Best Hospitals," *U.S. News & World Report*, July 15, 2009

8. Patrick Quinlan Remarks, Brent House Conference Center, New Orleans, Louisiana, August 4, 2009

9. Ochsner Press Release, "Ochsner Medical Center Only Louisiana Hospital Ranked Top 5% in Nation," January 26, 2010

10. Ibid.

11. Ibid.

12. Ibid.

13. Warner Thomas November 13, 2009 Interview

14. Ibid.

15. Ochsner Clinic Foundation Library and Archives, "Medical Library Recovery for Southeastern Louisiana," 2006 Project Summary & Highlights, p.1

16. Digitally Recorded Oral History Interview with Dr. William Pinsky, New Orleans, Louisiana, January 23, 2009

17. Patrick Quinlan October 23, 2009 Interview

18. Ibid.

19. Ibid.

20. Undated William Pinsky Remarks, Ochsner Communications Department

21. Ibid.

22. Ibid.

23. Ibid.

24. Ibid.

25. "Fitness & Performance," www.elmwoodfitness.com/Club/

26. "Mind & Body," www.elmwoodfitness.com/Club/

27. "Personal Training/Weight Loss," www.elmwoodfitness.com/Club/

28. "Kids Corner," www.elmwoodfitness.com/Club/

29. Ibid.

30. Ochsner Health System Press Release, "Elmwood Fitness Center Links Video Games with Exercise to Fight Childhood Obesity," August 3, 2010

31. Patrick Quinlan October 23, 2009 Interview

32. Ibid.

33. Warner Thomas November 13, 2009 Interview

34. Ibid

35. Ibid.

36. Patrick Quinlan October 23, 2009 Interview

37. Ibid.

38. Ibid

CHAPTER 14

1. Ochsner Health System, 2010 Annual Report

2. Ibid.

3. Ochsner Health System, 2009 Annual Report

4. Ochsner Health System, 2009 Annual Report

5. Ibid.

6. Ochsner Health System, 2010 Annual Report

7. Ochsner Health System, 2009 Annual Report

8. Patrick Quinlan October 23, 2009 Interview

9. Ibid.

10. Ibid.

11. Prepared Remarks, Dr. Danny Bronfin, Ochsner Communications Department, n.d.

12. Ochsner Health System, 2009 Annual Report

13. Ochsner Health System, 2008 Annual Report

14. Ibid.

15. Ochsner Health System, 2010 Annual Report

16. Ibid.

17. Ochsner Health System, 2008 Annual Report

18. Ibid.

19. Ibid.

20. Ochsner Archives Video Interview with Joan Rooney, www.ochsner.org

21. Ibid.

22. Ochsner Archives Video Interview with Ann Savoie, www.ochsner.org

23. Ibid.

24. "LHC Group And Ochsner Health System Announce LTACH Joint Venture," May 4, 2009

25. Ibid.

26. Ochsner Health System, 2010 Annual Report

27. Ochsner Press Release, "Ochsner Takes Stand Against Preventable Deaths," March 15, 2011

28. Ibid.

29. Ibid.

30. Ibid.

31. "Community Outreach," http://www.ochsner.org/community/

32. Ibid.

33. Ochsner Health System, 2007 Annual Report

34. Ibid.

35. Ochsner Health System, 2009 Annual Report

36. Ochsner Health System, 2010 Annual Report

37. Ibid.

38. Ochsner Health System, 2009 Annual Report

39. Ibid.

40. Ochsner Health System, 2005–2006 Annual Report

ABOUT THE AUTHOR

Writer and historian Bill Beck has established a reputation as one of the nation's most accomplished healthcare historians. Beck has more than 80 published books to his credit. Recent books include illustrated anniversary histories for Presbyterian Hospital in Albuquerque, New Mexico; St. Vincent Hospital in Indianapolis, Indiana; and the American Society for Therapeutic Radiation Oncology in northern Virginia. His book celebrating the 150th anniversary history of the American Dental Association in Chicago, Illinois, was published in 2009.

Beck is a 1971 graduate of Marian College, Indianapolis, and did graduate work in American History at the University of North Dakota. Beck started Lakeside Writers' Group more than twenty years ago following ten years as a reporter for newspapers in Minnesota and North Carolina and seven years as the senior writer in the public affairs department at Minnesota Power & Light Company in Duluth, Minnesota.

Ochsner Campus, 2011

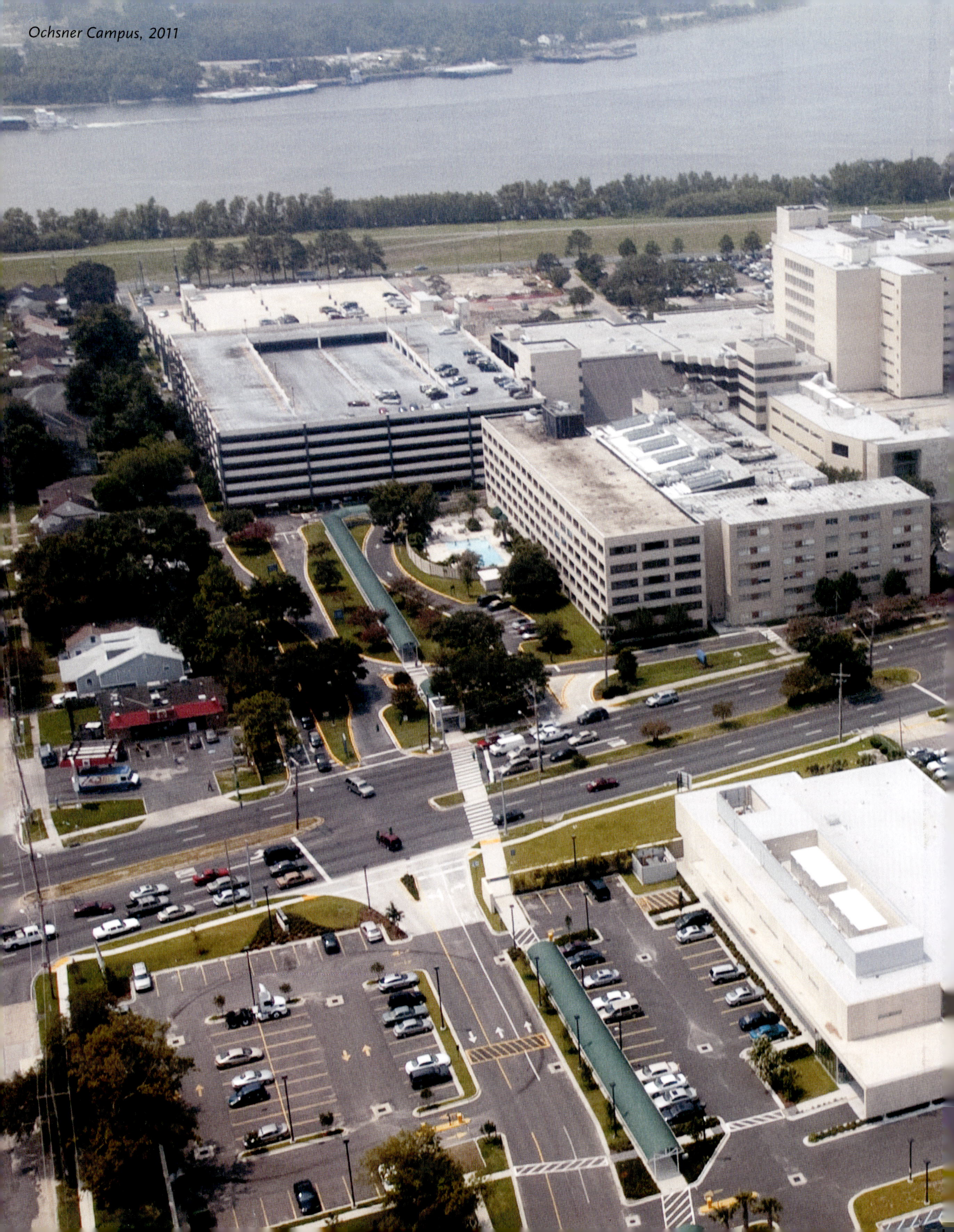